Diseases of the Esophagus

Volume I

Malignant Diseases

Editors:

Mark K. Ferguson, M.D.
Chief, Section of Thoracic Surgery
The University of Chicago
Chicago, Illinois

Alex G. Little, M.D.
Chairman, Department of Surgery
University of Nevada School of Medicine
Las Vegas, Nevada

David B. Skinner, M.D.
President, New York Hospital
Cornell Medical Center
New York, New York

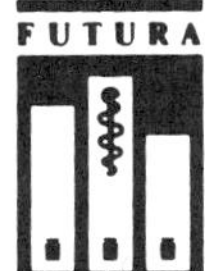

Futura Publishing Company, Inc.
Mount Kisco, NY
1990

Library of Congress Cataloging-in-Publication Data

Diseases of the esophagus / editors, Mark K. Ferguson, Alex G. Little, David B. Skinner.
p. cm.
Based on the Fourth World Congress of the International Society for Diseases of the Esophagus, held Sept. 6–8, 1989 in Chicago, Ill.
Includes bibliographical references.
Contents: Vol. 1 Malignant diseases—v. 2. Benign diseases / editors, Alex G. Little, Mark K. Ferguson, David B. Skinner.
ISBN 0-87993-367-4 (v. 1).—ISBN 0-87993-368-2 (v. 2)
1. Esophagus—Diseases—Congresses. 2. Esophagus—Cancer—Congresses. I. Ferguson, Mark K. II. Little, Alex G. III. Skinner, David B., 1935– . IV. International Society for Diseases of the Esophagus. Congress (4th : 1989 : Chicago, Ill.)
[DNLM: 1. Esophageal Diseases—congresses. WI 250 D61105 1989]
RC815.7.D574 1990
616.3′2—dc20
DNLM/DLC
for Library of Congress 90-2918
CIP

Published by:
Futura Publishing Company, Inc.
2 Bedford Ridge Road, P.O. Box 330
Mount Kisco, New York 10549

LC #: 90-2918
ISBN #: 0-87993-367-4

Printed in the United States of America.

To Phyllis,
for her patient support and understanding.

Mark K. Ferguson

To Louise, Ashley, and Jody,
without whose support this book
would not have been possible.

Alex G. Little

To the many Residents and Fellows
who have contributed so much to our work
on esophageal diseases over the past 20 years.

David B. Skinner

Contributors

Osahiko Abe, M.D.
Professor, Department of Surgery, School of Medicine, Keio University, Tokyo, Japan

Takashi Akaishi, M.D.
2nd Department of Surgery, Tohoku University, School of Medicine, Sendai, Japan

Hiroshi Akiyama, M.D.
Chairman, Department of Surgery, Toranomon Hospital, Tokyo, Japan

Tetsu Akiyama, M.D.
Department of Oncology, Institute of Medical Science, Tokyo University, Tokyo, Japan

Nasser K. Altorki, M.D.
Assistant Professor of Surgery, The New York Hospital-Cornell Medical Center, New York, New York 10021

Nobutoshi Ando, M.D.
Assistant Professor, Department of Surgery, School of Medicine, Keio University, Tokyo, Japan

Marco Baessato, M.D.
1st Department of Surgery, University of Padua, Padua, Italy

Romeo Bardini, M.D.
1st Department of Surgery, University of Padua, Padua, Italy

Holger Bartels, M.D.
Department of Surgery, Technical University of Munich, Munich, West Germany

Jacques Belghiti, M.D.
Professor, Department of Digestive Surgery, Beaujon Hospital, Paris, France

Luigi Bonavina, M.D.
1st Department of Surgery, University of Padua, Padua, Italy

P. Borelli, M.D.
1st Department of Surgery, University of Padua, Padua, Italy

J. L. Buard, M.D.
Center de Chirurgie Digestive et Unit de Transplantation; Centre Hospitalier and Universitaire de Rennes, Rennes, France

E. Bücheler, M.D.
Department of Radiology, University Hospital, Hamburg, West Germany

N. Campioni, M.D.
Department of Surgery, Istituto dei Rumori Regina Elena, Rome, Italy

C.U. Casciani, M.D.
Department of Surgery, University of Rome-Tor Vergata, Rome, Italy

Carlo Castoro, M.D.
1st Department of Surgery, University of Padua, Padua, Italy

Franco Cavazzini, M.D.
1st Department of Surgery, University of Padua, Padua, Italy

Vincent Chasseray, M.D.
Centre Hopitalier and Universitaire de Rennes, Rennes, France

André Chatelain, Ph.D
Professor, Institute of Experimental Physics, Swiss Federal Institute of Technology, Lausanne, Switzerland

John Kevin Collins, M.D.
Senior Lecturer, Virology/Immunology, Department of Microbiology, University College-Cork, Cork, Ireland

Aine Corbett, M.D.
Department of Microbiology, University College-Cork, Mercy Hospital, Cork, Ireland

M.H. Cullen, M.D.
Consultant Oncologist, Queen Elizabeth Hospital, Edgbaston, Birmingham, United Kingdom

Antonino Cusumano, M.D.
1st Department of Surgery, University of Padua, Padua, Italy

Pietro DeBesi, M.D.
Department of Oncology, University of Padua, Padua, Italy

A.-K. Eckstein, M.D.
University of Kiel, Department of General Surgery, Kiel, West Germany

C. Edwards, M.D.
Consultant Pathologist, Department of Histopathology, East Birmingham Hospital, Birmingham, United Kingdom

Mitsuo Endo, M.D.
Professor, Tokyo Medical and Dental University, Tokyo, Japan

François Fékété, M.D.
Professor, Department of Digestive Surgery, Beaujon Hospital, Paris, France

Mark K. Ferguson, M.D.
Associate Professor of Surgery, Chief, Section of Thoracic Surgery, The University of Chicago, Chicago, Illinois

Charlotte Fontolliet, M.D.
Associate Pathologist, Institut Universitaire de Pathologie, Lausanne, Switzerland

P. Franz, M.D.
Department of Radiology, University Hospital, Hamburg, West Germany

S. Freys, M.D.
University of Kiel, Department of General Surgery, Kiel, West Germany

G.B. Friehs, M.D.
Professor, Department of Thoracic and Hyperbaric Surgery, University Medical School of Graz, Graz, Austria

K.-H. Fuchs, M.D.
University of Kiel, Department of General Surgery, Kiel, West Germany

Masao Fujimaki, M.D.
Professor and Chairman, 2nd Department of Surgery, Toyama Medical and Pharmaceutical University, Toyama, Japan

Hiromasa Fujita, M.D.
1st Department of Surgery, Kurume University School of Medicine, Kurume, Japan

Brice Gayet, M.D.
Professor, Department of Digestive Surgery, Beaujon Hospital, Paris, France

P. Ginevri, M.D.
Department of Surgery, University of Rome-Tor Vergata, Rome, Italy

Yuji Goukon, M.D.
2nd Department of Surgery, Tohoku University, School of Medicine, Sendai, Japan

Horst Grimm, M.D.
Surgical Endoscopy Unit, University Hospital, Hamburg, West Germany

Xian Zhi Gu, M.D.
Cancer Hospital and Research Institute, Chinese Academy of Medical Sciences, Beijing, China

A. Hackl, M.D.
Professor, Department of Radiology, Radiotherapeutical Division, University Medical School, Graz, Austria

Chariya Hahnvajanawong, M.D.
Department of Microbiology, University College-Cork, Cork, Ireland

K. Hamper, M.D.
Department of Pathology, University Hospital, Hamburg, West Germany

Masao Hanaoka, M.D.
Professor, Department of Pathology, Institute for Virus Research, Kyoto University, Kyoto, Japan

Tateo Hanaoka, M.D.
Associate Professor, 2nd Department of Surgery, Kyorin University School of Medicine, Tokyo, Japan

Fujio Hanyu, M.D.
Professor and Chairman, Department of Surgery, Institute of Gastroenterology, Tokyo Women's Medical College, Tokyo, Japan

Hisao Hayakawa, M.D.
Staff Member, Foundation of Detection of Early Gastric Carcinoma, Tokyo, Japan

Hiroto Hayashi, M.D.
2nd Department of Surgery, Yamaguchi University School of Medicine, Ube City, Yamaguchi, Japan

Katsu Hirayama, M.D.
2nd Department of Surgery, Tohoku University School of Medicine, Sendai, Japan

Arnulf H. Holscher, M.D.
Department of Surgery, Technical University of Munich, Munich, West Germany

Kiichi Honma, M.D.
2nd Department of Surgery, Yamaguchi University School of Medicine, Ube City, Yamaguchi, Japan

Guo Jun Huang, M.D.
Professor of Thoracic Surgery, Cancer Hospital and Research Institute, Chinese Academy of Medical Sciences, Beijing, China

C. Iascone, M.D.
Department of Surgery, University of Rome-La Sapienza, Rome, Italy

Hiroko Ide, M.D.
Assistant Professor, Department of Surgery, Institute of Gastroenterology, Tokyo Women's Medical College, Tokyo, Japan

Yukihiko Ikehata, M.D.
Department of Surgery, School of Medicine, Keio University, Tokyo, Japan

Masayuki Imamura, M.D.
1st Department of Surgery, Faculty of Medicine, Kyoto University, Kyoto, Japan

Nakao Ishida, M.D.
President, Tohoku University, Sendai, Japan

Koichi Ishigami, M.D.
Emeritus Professor, 2nd Department of Surgery, Yamaguchi University School of Medicine, Ube City, Yamaguchi, Japan

Kaichi Isono, M.D.
Professor, Department of Surgery, School of Medicine, Chiba University, Chiba, Japan

Kunihiko Itoh, M.D.
Department of Pharmaceutical Sciences, Tohoku University Hospital, Sendai, Japan

F.M. Juettner, M.D.
Associate Professor, Department of Thoracic and Hyperbaric Surgery, University Medical School of Graz, Graz, Austria

Teruo Kakegawa, M.D.
Professor, Department of Surgery, Kurume University School of Medicine, Kurume, Japan

Chouo Kaku, M.D.
2nd Department of Surgery, Kyorin University School of Medicine, Tokyo, Japan

Hoichi Kato, M.D.
Department of Surgery, National Cancer Center Hospital, Tokyo, Japan

Hiroshi Katoh, M.D.
2nd Department of Surgery, Toyama Medical and Pharmaceutical University, Toyama, Japan

Osamu Kimura, M.D.
2nd Department of Surgery, Kyorin University School of Medicine, Tokyo, Japan

G. K. Kiroff, M.D.
Centre de Chirurgie Digestive et Unit de Transplantation; Centre Hospitalier and Universitaire de Rennes, Rennes, France.

Michihiko Kitamura, M.D.
2nd Department of Surgery, Tohoku University, School of Medicine, Sendai, Japan

Ataru Kobayashi, M.D.
Chief Resident of Gastroenterological Surgery, Tokyo Women's Medical College, Tokyo, Japan

Kenji Kobayashi, M.D.
2nd Department of Surgery, Osaka University Medical School, Osaka, Japan

Seiichiro Kobayashi, M.D.
Professor and Director of Gastroenterological Surgery, Tokyo Women's Medical College, Tokyo, Japan

P.H. Kohek, M.D.
Department of Thoracic and Hyperbaric Surgery, University Medical School of Graz, Graz, Austria

Hiroyuki Kuwano, M.D.
Department of Surgery II, Faculty of Medicine, Kyushu University, Fukuoka, Japan

Jochen Lange, M.D.
Department of Surgery, Technical University of Munich, Munich, West Germany

R. Pasquali Lasagni, M.D.
Department of Surgery, Istituto dei Tumori Regina Elena, Rome, Italy

Bernard Launois, M.D.
Centre Hospitalier and Universitaire de Rennes, Rennes, France

Stefano Lazzaro, M.D.
1st Department of Surgery, University of Padua, Padua, Italy

Alex G. Little, M.D.
Professor and Chairman, Department of Surgery, University of Nevada School of Medicine, Las Vegas, Nevada

Fu Sheng Liu, M.D.
Cancer Hospital and Research Institute, Chinese Academy of Medical Sciences, Beijing, China

R. Maas, M.D.
Department of Radiology, University Hospital, Hamburg, West Germany

Yasushi Masaki, M.D.
2nd Department of Surgery, Yamaguchi University School of Medicine, Ube City, Yamaguchi, Japan

Masayuki Masuda, M.D.
2nd Department of Surgery, Tohoku University School of Medicine, Sendai, Japan

Hiroyuki Matsuda, M.D.
Department of Surgery II, Faculty of Medicine, Kyushu University, Fukuoka, Japan

Norio Matsumoto, M.D.
2nd Department of Surgery, Yamaguchi University School of Medicine, Ube City, Yamaguchi, Japan

Hugoe R. Matthews, M.D.
Consultant Thoracic Surgeon, East Birmingham Hospital, Birmingham, United Kingdom

Yves Menu, M.D.
Radiology Department, Beaujon Hospital, Paris, France

E. Meyer-Pannwitt, M.D.
Department of Surgery, University Hospital, Hamburg, West Germany

Taizo Minami, M.D.
Department of Surgery, Kurume University School of Medicine, Kurume, Japan

Michinao Mizugaki, Ph.D.
Professor, Department of Pharmaceutical Sciences, Tohoku University Hospital, Sendai, Japan

G. Molas, M.D.
Department of Anatomy and Pathologic Cytology, Beaujon Hospital, Paris, France

Philippe Monnier, M.D.
Chief Resident, Ear, Nose, and Throat Department, University Canton Hospital, Lausanne, Switzerland

A. Moraldi, M.D.
Department of Surgery, University of Rome-Tor Vergata, Rome, Italy

Masaki Mori, M.D.
Department of Surgery II, Faculty of Medicine, Kyushu University, Fukuoka, Japan

Shozo Mori, M.D.
Professor, 2nd Department of Surgery, Tohoku University School of Medicine, Sendai, Japan

Takesada Mori, M.D.
2nd Department of Surgery, Osaka University Medical School, Osaka, Japan

Takuo Murakami, M.D.
Associate Professor, 2nd Department of Surgery, Yamaguchi University School of Medicine, Ube City, Yamaguchi, Japan

Yoko Murata, M.D.
Department of Surgery, Tokyo Metropolitan Komagome Hospital, Tokyo, Japan

Kin-ichi Nabeya, M.D.
Professor, 2nd Department of Surgery, Kyorin University School of Medicine, Tokyo, Japan

Masaaki Nagamatsu, M.D.
Department of Surgery II, Faculty of Medicine, Kyushu University, Fukuoka, Japan

Yujiro Nanba, M.D.
Associate Professor, Department of Pathology, Institute for Virus Research, Kyoto University, Kyoto, Japan

Kyooo Nanaumi, M.D.
Department of Diagnostic Radiology, Toranomon Hospital, Tokyo, Japan

Surendra Narne, M.D.
1st Department of Surgery, University of Padua, Padua, Italy

V. Nicolas, M.D.
Department of Radiology, University Hospital, Hamburg, West Germany

Tetsuro Nishihira, M.D.
2nd Department of Surgery, Tohoku University, School of Medicine, Sendai, Japan

Kinji Nishiyama, M.D.
Department of Radiology, Osaka University Medical School, Osaka, Japan

Mamoru Nishizawa, M.D.
Tokyo Metropolitan Cancer Detection Center, Tokyo, Japan

Hiroshi Nogami, M.D.
2nd Department of Surgery, Kyorin University School of Medicine, Tokyo, Japan

Lorenzo Norberto, M.D.
1st Department of Surgery, University of Padua, Padua, Italy

Tetsuya Nyumura, M.D.
Instructor, 2nd Department of Surgery, Kyorin University School of Medicine, Tokyo, Japan

Fiona O'Brien, M.D.
Department of Microbiology, University College-Cork, Mercy Hospital, Cork, Ireland

Takenori Ochiai, M.D.
Assistant Professor, Department of Surgery, School of Medicine, Chiba University, Chiba, Japan

Maurice O'Donoghue, M.D.
Department of Microbiology, University College-Cork, Mercy Hospital, Cork, Ireland

Tai Ohmori, M.D.
Department of Surgery, School of Medicine, Keio University, Tokyo, Japan

Shinji Ohno, M.D.
Department of Surgery II, Faculty of Medicine, Kyushu University; Fukuoka, Japan

Noriaki Ohuchi, M.D.
2nd Department of Surgery, Tohoku University School of Medicine, Sendai, Japan

Akihiko Okayama, M.D.
2nd Department of Surgery, Tohoku University, School of Medicine, Sendai, Japan

Masaaki Oka, M.D.
Assistant Professor, 2nd Department of Surgery, Yamaguchi University School of Medicine, Ube City, Yamaguchi, Japan

Toshikuni Okada
Tokyo Metropolitan Cancer Detection Center, Tokyo, Japan

Satoshi Okura, M.D.
Assistant Professor, 2nd Department of Surgery, Kyorin University School of Medicine, Tokyo, Japan

Kazuaki Okuyama, M.D.
Instructor, Department of Surgery, School of Medicine, Chiba University, Chiba, Japan

Alison O'Mahony, M.D.
Department of Microbiology, University College-Cork, Mercy Hospital, Cork, Ireland

Yoshimasa Ono, M.D.
Department of Surgery, Toranomon Hospital, Tokyo, Japan

Kimio Onozawa, M.D.
Assistant Professor, 2nd Department of Surgery, Kyorin University School of Medicine, Tokyo, Japan

Gerald C. O'Sullivan, M.D.
Consultant Surgeon and Lecturer in Surgery, Department of Surgery, University College-Cork, Cork, Ireland

B. Pakisch, M.D.
Department of Radiology, Radiotherapeutical Division, University Medical School of Graz, Graz, Austria

Laurent Palazzo, M.D.
Department of Gastroenterology, Beaujon Hospital, Paris, France

J.A. Paolaggi, M.D.
Professor, Department of Gastroenterology, Beaujon Hospital, Paris, France

Alberto Peracchia, M.D.
1st Department of Surgery, University of Padua, Padua, Italy

E. Poier, Ph.D.
Department of Radiology, Radiotherapeutical Division, University Medical School of Graz, Graz, Austria

Shigen Ri, M.D.
Instructor, 2nd Department of Surgery, Kyorin University School of Medicine, Tokyo, Japan

Jürgen D. Roder, M.D.
Department of Surgery, Technical University of Munich, Munich, West Germany

Antonella Ruffatto, M.D.
1st Department of Surgery, University of Padua, Padua, Italy

Alberto Ruol, M.D.
1st Department of Surgery, University of Padua, Padua, Italy

Kazuyoshi Sakamoto, M.D.
1st Department of Surgery, Kurume University School of Medicine, Kurume, Japan

Takashi Sakamoto, M.D.
2nd Department of Surgery, Toyama Medical and Pharmaceutical University, Toyama, Japan

Yoshiharu Sato, M.D.
2nd Department of Surgery, Tohoku University School of Medicine, Sendai, Japan

Marcel Savary, M.D.
Professor and Chairman, Department of Otolaryngology-Head and Neck Surgery, University of Lausanne School of Medicine, Lausanne, Switzerland

H. Schaube, M.D.
University of Kiel, Department of General Surgery, Kiel, West Germany

Andrea Segalin, M.D.
1st Department of Surgery, University of Padua, Padua, Italy

Yutaka Shimada, M.D.
1st Department of Surgery, Faculty of Medicine, Kyoto University, Kyoto, Japan

Ryuzaburo Shineha, M.D.
2nd Department of Surgery, Tohoku University, School of Medicine, Sendai, Japan

Yohtaroh Shinozawa, M.D.
Instructor, Department of Surgery, School of Medicine, Keio University, Tokyo, Japan

Hitoshi Shiozaki, M.D.
2nd Department of Surgery, Osaka University Medical School, Osaka, Japan

Hikoo Shirakabe, M.D.
Chairman, Foundation for Detection of Early Gastric Carcinoma, Tokyo, Japan

Genzan Shirozu, M.D.
1st Department of Surgery, Kurume University School of Medicine, Kurume, Japan

Jörg Rüdiger Siewert, M.D.
Professor of Surgery, Department of Surgery, Technical University of Munich, Munich, West Germany

David B. Skinner, M.D.
President and CEO, The New York Hospital, Professor of Surgery, Cornell Medical College, New York, New York

N. Soehendra, M.D.
Surgical Endoscopy Unit, University Hospital, Hamburg, West Germany

Paolo Sorrentino, M.D.
1st Department of Surgery, University of Padua, Padua, Italy

A. Steel, M.D.
Senior Medical Registrar, Regional Department of Thoracic Surgery, East Birmingham Hospital, Birmingham, United Kingdom

Janet K. Stephens, M.D., Ph.D.
Department of Pathology, University of Colorado Health Sciences, Denver, Colorado

S. Stipa, M.D.
Department of Surgery, University of Rome-La Sapienza, Rome, Italy

G. Stuecklschweiger, Ph.D.
Department of Radiology, Radiotherapeutical Division, University Medical School of Graz, Graz, Austria

Keizo Sugimachi, M.D.
Professor and Chairman, Department of Surgery II, Faculty of Medicine, Kyushu University, Fukuoka, Japan

Ke Lin Sun, M.D.
Department of Thoracic Surgery, Cancer Hospital and Research Institute, Chinese Academy of Medical Sciences, Beijing, China

Masatoshi Suzuki, M.D.
Department of Surgery, Toranomon Hospital, Tokyo, Japan

Shigeru Suzuki, M.D.
Professor, Department of Gastroenterology, Tokyo Women's Medical College, Tokyo, Japan

Hiroshi Tachimori, M.D.
Department of Surgery, National Cancer Center Hospital, Tokyo, Japan

Hideaki Tahara, M.D.
2nd Department of Surgery, Osaka University Medical School, Osaka, Japan

Ryo Takano, M.D.
2nd Department of Surgery, Tohoku University School of Medicine, Sendai, Japan

Toru Takiguchi, M.D.
Assistant Professor, Tokyo Medical and Dental University, Tokyo, Japan

Shigeyuki Tamura, M.D.
2nd Department of Surgery, Osaka University Medical School, Osaka, Japan

Kenji Tazawa, M.D.
Associate Professor, 2nd Department of Surgery, Toyama Medical and Pharmaceutical University, Toyama, Japan

Takayoshi Tobe, M.D.
1st Department of Surgery, Faculty of Medicine, Kyoto University, Kyoto, Japan

Silvia Toso, M.D.
Oncology Department, Padua Hospital, Padua, Italy

Carlo Tremolada, M.D.
1st Department of Surgery, University of Padua, Padua, Italy

Masahiko Tsurumaru, M.D.
Chief of Surgery, Department of Surgery, Toranomon Hospital, Tokyo, Japan

Shin-ichi Tsutsui, M.D.
Department of Surgery II, Faculty of Medicine, Kyushu University, Fukuoka, Japan

Harushi Udagawa, M.D.
Department of Surgery, Toranomon Hospital, Tokyo, Japan

Hubert Van den Bergh, Ph.D.
Laboratory of Chemical Technology, Swiss Federal Institute of Technology, Lausanne, Switzerland

Valerie Vilgrain, M.D.
Radiology Department, Beaujon Hospital, Paris, France

Corinne Vons, M.D.
Chief of Clinic, Department of Digestive Surgery, Beaujon Hospital, Paris, France

Georges Wagnières
Research Assistant, Institute of Experimental Physics, Swiss Federal Institute of Technology, Lausanne, Switzerland

Steven J. Walker, M.D.
Esophageal Cancer Fellow, Regional Department of Thoracic Surgery, East Birmingham Hospital, Birmingham, United Kingdom

Liang Jun Wang, M.D.
Cancer Hospital and Research Institute, Chinese Academy of Medical Sciences, Beijing, China

Mei Wang, M.D.
Cancer Hospital and Research Institute, Chinese Academy of Medical Sciences, Beijing, China

Zhen Yan Wang, M.D.
Cancer Hospital and Research Institute, Chinese Academy of Medical Sciences, Beijing, China

Goro Watanabe, M.D.
Department of Surgery, Toranomon Hospital, Tokyo, Japan

Hiroshi Watanabe, M.D.
Head, Department of Surgical Oncology, National Cancer Center Hospital, Tokyo, Japan

Yasuaki Watanabe, M.D.
2nd Department of Surgery, Tohoku University, School of Medicine, Sendai, Japan

Akira Yamada, M.D.
2nd Department of Surgery, Toyama Medical and Pharmaceutical University, Toyama, Japan

Akiyoshi Yamada, M.D.
Professor, Department of Gastroenterology, Tokyo Women's Medical College, Tokyo, Japan

Goro Yamaki, M.D.
Department of Diagnostic Radiology, Toranomon Hospital, Tokyo, Japan

Isamu Yamamoto, M.D.
Department of Radiology, Teikyoo University, Ichihara, Japan

Hideaki Yamana, M.D.
1st Department of Surgery, Kurume University School of Medicine, Kurume, Japan

Iwao Yamashita, M.D.
2nd Department of Surgery, Toyama Medical and Pharmaceutical University, Toyama, Japan

Sigeru Yamazaki, M.D.
Assistant Professor, Tokyo Medical and Dental University, Tokyo, Japan

Hiroshi Yano, M.D.
2nd Department of Surgery, Osaka University Medical School, Osaka, Japan

Tokiharu Yano, M.D.
2nd Department of Surgery, Osaka University Medical School, Osaka, Japan

Wei Bo Yin, M.D.
Cancer Hospital and Research Institute, Chinese Academy of Medical Sciences, Beijing, China

Mitchel Mitsuo Yokoyama, M.D.
Professor, Department of Immunology, Kurume University School of Medicine, Kurume, Japan

Misao Yoshida, M.D.
Chief Surgeon, Department of Surgery, Tokyo Metropolitan Komagome Hospital, Tokyo, Japan

Kunihide Yoshino, M.D.
Assistant Professor, Tokyo Medical and Dental University, Tokyo, Japan

M. Zerilli, M.D.
Department of Surgery, University of Rome-La Sapienza, Rome, Italy

Da Wei Zhang, M.D.
Cancer Hospital and Research Institute, Chinese Academy of Medical Sciences, Beijing, China

Ru Gang Zhang, M.D.
Cancer Hospital and Research Institute, Chinese Academy of Medical Sciences, Beijing, China

Foreword

The fourth triennial congress of the International Society for Diseases of the Esophagus (ISDE) was successfully held in Chicago, Illinois, under the presidency of David B. Skinner, M.D. It included unforgettable events that particularly featured a well-organized and high-quality scientific program from which contributions were solicited for a publication representing the state-of-the-art of our understanding of esophageal physiology and pathology. I hope that the publication will make these efforts available to wider scientific readership in this field. I am also pleased that the ISDE is now firmly established and I am sure that we can look forward to even more development with the fifth congress.

Finally, I would like to express my heartfelt appreciation to Professor Skinner and his staff for their great contribution toward the huge success of the congress.

Kiyoshi Inokuchi, M.D.
The Immediate-past President of
International Society for
Diseases of the Esophagus

Preface

Recent years have witnessed the publication of numerous authoritative books devoted to diseases of the esophagus. This is not surprising, given the advances in diagnostic and therapeutic techniques that occurred during the previous 15 years. For example, as of 1970, the following were not in routine clinical use: flexible esophagoscopy, transhiatal esophagectomy, radical en bloc esophageal resection, extended pH monitoring, computed tomography, therapeutic lasers, and chemotherapy for esophageal cancer. During the decade between 1970 and 1980, all of these modalities became commonplace in the treatment of either benign or malignant diseases of the esophagus, representing major technological advances in the management of such problems. The many books published on esophageal diseases represent the fruition of these scientific and clinical efforts.

Why, then, another work devoted to the esophagus? Our aim has not been to provide an encyclopedic rendering of available knowledge of the organ, but to highlight new areas of investigation and to address issues of both evaluation and therapy that are controversial. To this end, we requested chapters based on presentations at the Fourth World Congress of the International Society for Diseases of the Esophagus held in Chicago, Illinois. The selection process ensured origin of the chapters from among the many disciplines involved with diseases of the esophagus and resulted in a distinct international flavor. The authors represent the highest level of clinical and scientific accomplishment from around the world.

Publication of this book would not have been possible without efforts of a number of important individuals. The Scientific Committee for the Fourth World Congress of the ISDE, listed below, selected over 350 papers for presentation at the meeting, from which these chapters have been chosen. The leadership of the ISDE organized the Fourth World Congress, permitting a unique level of interaction among physicians of varying specialties and nationalities, a process that is important in sharing and advancing our knowledge. Ms. Darlene Buczak had the responsibility for initial collection and collation of the material. Finally, Ms. Linda Shaw, our editor, provided unerring guidance in producing the final text from a jumble of unintelligible scribbles.

This book is intended for those who already have a working knowledge of esophageal diseases and who wish an update on issues that are at the frontiers of current practice. The chapters are divided into sections, for which the editors have written overviews to provide a contextual setting for the material. The book may be used in many ways. Most readers will find certain sections particularly pertinent, using the remaining sections as a source of up-to-date reference material. Those who manage esophageal diseases as a full-time occupation will, no doubt, benefit from a close scrutiny of the entire text. Considering the multiple uses to which this book can be put, and given the topic, the following seems appropriate:

Some books are to be tasted,
others to be swallowed,
and some few are to be chewed and digested.
–Bacon

Mark K. Ferguson, M.D.
Alex G. Little, M.D.
David B. Skinner, M.D.

Members of the Scientific Program Committee Fourth World Congress of the International Society for Diseases of the Esophagus

President: David B. Skinner, New York, New York

Steering:

Hiroshi Akiyama
Tokyo, Japan
Tom R. DeMeester
Omaha, Nebraska
Andre Duranceau
Montreal, Quebec, Canada
Mark K. Ferguson
Chicago, Illinois
E. Moreno Gonzalez
Madrid, Spain
Glyn G. Jamieson
Adelaide, Australia
Bernard Launois
Rennes, Cedex, France
Toni Lerut
Leuven, Belgium
Alex G. Little
Las Vegas, Nevada
Hugoe R. Matthews
Birmingham, England
Alberto Peracchia
Padua, Italy
Charles S. Winans
Chicago, Illinois
John Wong
Hong Kong
Bruno Zilberstein
Sao Paulo, Brazil

Advisory:

C. Thomas Bombeck
Chicago, Illinois
Attila Csendes
Santiago, Chile
Henry F. Ellis
Boston, Massachusetts
François Fékété
Paris, France
Robert Giuli
Paris, France
Vincente Guarner
Mexico City, Mexico
Min-Hsiung Huang
Taipei, Taiwan, R.O.C.
Jean-Min Sheh
Taipei, Taiwan, R.O.C.
Mark B. Orringer
Ann Arbor, Michigan
Henrique Walter Pinotti
Sao Paulo, Brazil
Sergio Stipa
Rome, Italy
Anthony Watson
Lancaster, England

Ex-Officio:

G. Castrini
Rome, Italy
M. Endo
Tokyo, Japan
J. Rudiger Siewert
Munich, West Germany
K. Inokuchi
Saga-shi, Japan
K. Nabeya
Tokyo, Japan

Contents

I.

Tumor Biology: Editors' Overview

The variable response of esophageal cancer patients to therapeutic intervention has been a continual source of concern. Poorly defined characteristics of tumor growth have always been better determinants of prognosis than any physician-prescribed remedy. Taking the iconoclastic view, Mr. Ronald Belsey has said that in the treatment of esophageal cancer, "cure must be regarded as a fortunate and unpredictable accident . . ." As evidenced in the eight chapters on tumor biology, however, considerable technological progress has enabled the characterization of tumor development and growth to a far greater extent than was previously possible. One recent research development is the use of explant/cell-culture systems for the investigation of cell lines derived from human esophageal cancer. In Chapter 1, Collins and his coauthors lay the groundwork for studies using these cell lines by describing cell surface receptors, ultrastructural characteristics, tumorigenicity, and production of immunosuppressive products. Efforts at further characterization of specific components of esophageal cancer tissues are described in this section as well. In Chapter 2, monoclonal antibodies are used to evaluate the production and urinary excretion of nucleosides derived from transfer RNA in esophageal cancer cells. These techniques offer the potential for early noninvasive diagnosis of these cancers. In Chapter 3, Nogami and associates explore the use of immunohistochemical assays to evaluate alterations in cell surface glycoprotein moieties during transformation of dysplastic columnar esophageal epithelium to malignant tissue. These techniques also permit differentiation between Barrett's adenocarcinoma and gastric cancer. The two studies illustrate how immunohistochemical methods can assist in the diagnosis of human esophageal cancers and in understanding their biology.

Growth of esophageal cancer and other cancers is undoubtedly dependent in part on circulating factors. In Chapters 4 and 5, the relationships between epidermal growth factor (EGF) receptors and both cancer cell proliferation and prognosis are described. Using an immunohistochemical staining technique on human cancer tissue, the number of EGF receptors is shown to be inversely correlated with prognosis. Employing more sophisticated techniques of assaying cultured human esophageal cancer cell lines for EGF-stimulated proliferation, Shimada et al. report this effect is cell-line-dependent as well as culture-medium-dependent. While it seems clear that considerable work remains before the mechanisms governing growth of esophageal cancer cells are completely elucidated, the dependence of at least some esophageal cancers on EGF is clear. Chapters 4 and 6 investigate the relationship between lymphocyte infiltration and prognosis in esophageal cancer. While the degree of lymphocytic infiltration is directly correlated with prognosis in the work by Yano and others, O'Sullivan and his coauthors show that some esophageal cancers release a soluble mediator that actually suppresses the activity of local lymphocytes. This mediator is effective against both B cell and T cell lymphocytes, and may facilitate the spread of malignant cells to regional lymph nodes.

In Chapter 7, Minami and others characterize DNA content in human esophageal cancer using flow cytometry. This technique has been used to assess DNA content in a variety of human cancers, but has been used only rarely for esophageal cancers. Of interest, they report that half of the esophageal cancers are aneuploid, a finding that is more common in moderately and well-differentiated cancers than in those that are poorly differentiated. This is in distinct contrast to squamous cell carcinomas of other organs. DNA content is inversely correlated with prognosis, a finding that has been reported in other solid tumors. Clearly, with improved technology, DNA flow cytometry may prove clinically useful in assessing prognosis and, perhaps, in selecting therapy for certain patients.

Okura and his coauthors report studies on the growing time of esophageal cancer in Chapter 8. Their interesting findings indicate that the growth rate of esophageal cancer is significantly faster than that of gastric and colon cancers, and correlates well with the developing time of depth of esophageal wall invasion. Because it takes an average of 16 months for invasive cancer to develop, they suggest that further efforts should be expended toward developing mass cancer screening programs.

1

Characterization of Cell Lines Derived from Human Squamous Carcinomas of the Esophagus

John K. Collins, Gerald O'Sullivan, Maurice O'Donoghue, Fiona O'Brien, Alison O'Mahony, Aine Corbett, Chariya Hahnvajanawong

Introduction

Squamous carcinoma of the esophagus is an infrequent but particularly lethal tumor, which is refractory to current chemotherapy, radiotherapy, surgery, and in the few cases where tried, biological therapy. It has traditionally been argued that the site of the tumor with consequent dysphagia and nutritional deprivation, along with the generally advanced age of the patients, contributes to the lethal nature of this tumor. At present, most patients have apparent metastases or occult metastases which present following esophagectomy. Treatment therefore must not only be aimed at the primary tumor but also at metastases. While the primary causative agents would appear to be dietary or environmental carcinogens, little is known about the subsequent development and molecular biology of

Ferguson MK, Little AG, Skinner DB: Diseases of the Esophagus, Vol. I: Malignant Diseases. Futura Publishing Company, Inc., Mount Kisco, NY, © 1990.

these tumors. The factors contributing to the particular virulence of esophageal carcinoma are not well understood and, as with most human tumors, are not amenable to study in vivo.

The establishment of continuously growing tumor-derived cell lines provides an accessible and convenient model to study human tumors at a cellular and molecular level. Worldwide, feeder-independent tumorigenic continuous cell lines from human squamous carcinomas of the esophagus have not generally been available for such studies.[1,2] We have in our laboratory established two such cell lines and report their properties. These cell lines may facilitate the identification, isolation, and characterization of biological agents such as tumor-derived growth factors and immune suppressor factors which may be specific to this tumor. In addition, the study of sensitivity patterns to cytotoxic agents and radiation therapy is useful prior to the clinical application of new therapeutic modalities.

Techniques

The first esophageal cell line designated OC1 was established from malignant ascites in a 40-year-old male Caucasian known to suffer from esophageal carcinoma. Cytological analysis confirmed the ascitic fluid to be packed with squamous carcinoma cells. The second cell line OC2 was established from a metastatic lymph node of a 65-year-old female Caucasian diagnosed as suffering from squamous carcinoma of the esophagus. Both cell lines are carried in Dulbecco's modified Eagle's medium supplemented with 10% fetal bovine serum.

Morphology and Intermediate Filament Expression

OC1 cells in tissue culture exhibit a typical squamous polygonal epithelial morphology with a tendency to organize into multilayered colonies ultimately forming a clumpy monolayer. OC2 cells seem more dedifferentiated, almost fibroblastic in type with less ability to form clumps and a greater propensity to form confluent monolayers. The morphological and cultural characteristics have remained stable through 2 years of continuous cell culture when compared with cells cryopreserved immediately after their establishment in cell culture.

Table I
Cytokeratin Profiles of Cell Lines Derived from Squamous Carcinoma of the Esophagus (OC1 and OC2), Normal Esophageal Tissue and Primary Squamous Carcinoma of the Esophagus

Cytokeratin	MW (kd)	54	48	68	58	56	54	52	56.5	56	45	40
	* Number	13	16									19
Cell Line	OC1		+ +					+ +				+ + + +
	OC2		+					+				+ + +
Normal Esophagus			ND					+				+ +
Squamous Carcinoma of Esophagus			ND					+				+ + + +

* Based on the numerical classification of Moll et al.[3]
ND = Not determined.

Both cell lines were confirmed to be epithelial in origin by staining positive for both acidic and basic cytokeratins using monoclonal antibodies (Table I).[3] Cytokeratin 19 (40 kd) is the subtype most abundant in tumors and was predominantly expressed by both cell lines. Higher molecular weight cytokeratins could be induced on retinoid (vitamin A) treatment, indicating the capability to re-establish a more normal differentiated phenotype.

Of particular interest was the finding that vimentin, another intermediate filament normally found only in mesenchymal cells, was coexpressed in both cell lines. This expression may be a consequence of tissue culture establishment and growth. The alteration of cytokeratin expression and coexpression of vimentin may alter a configurational constraint on epithelial cells. Vimentin expression has been particularly associated with metastatic lesions.[4]

Under both scanning and transmission electron microscopy, OC1 cells demonstrate features typical of squamous carcinoma.[5] Surface morphology displays large cells with a centrally placed rounded nucleus with numerous villiform projections, surrounded by a thin layer of cytoplasm, attached to the substratum by several adhesion plaques. Desmosomes are apparent at cell junctions. A notable feature is the densely packed cytoplasm with numerous secretory type structures and large arrays of ribosome-bound endoplasmic reticulum. The OC2 cell line appears to have a more fibroblast-like morphology and lacks evidence of desmosomes or tonofilaments. The cells contain large nuclei often with pseudoinclusions and prominent marginated nucleoli. The cytoplasm is exceedingly rich in secretory vesicles, ribosome-bound endoplasmic reticulum, and dense mitochondria.

Tumorigenicity Studies

The ultimate demonstration that tumor-derived cell lines are really transformed or malignant is the induction of xenograft tumors in immunocompromised experimental animals. Both OC1 and OC2 cells induce tumors in athymic nude mice, OC2 cells being the most efficient, giving 100% tumor induction with 10^7 cells and also exhibiting faster growth.

Consistent with their ability to induce tumors in nude mice, both cell lines demonstrate anchorage-independent growth in soft agar—a valuable in vitro measurement of the transformed or malignant phenotype. Growth in reduced serum, e.g., 1% fetal calf serum versus 10% for normal cells, is another indicator of transformation. This reflects the autocrine or paracrine nature of tumor cells reducing their dependence on exogenous scarce growth factors in vivo. Both OC1 and OC2 cells exhibited clonogenic growth in serum-free medium and in media supplemented with 0.1%, 0.5%, 1%, and 10% serum. The growth of tumor cells in serum-free medium is quite unusual and demonstrates a remarkable independence from exogenous growth factor requirements.

Yet another trait of tumorigenicity is invasiveness. This property was assessed using the embryonic chick heart invasion assay of Mareel et al.[6] Both cell lines demonstrated an aggressive ability to engulf and invade the normal embryonic chick heart tissue.

Transforming Growth Factor Production

Cancers are masses of transformed or malignant cells with normal stromal elements such as fibroblasts, vascular endothelial cells, etc. Some tumor cells produce transforming growth factors which are capable of inducing normal stromal cells such as fibroblasts to have phenotypically abnormal, for example, anchorage-independent growth. Both the OC1 and OC2 cell lines produce a transforming growth factor which drives normal rat kidney fibroblasts to grow in soft agar, therefore exhibiting a transformed phenotype.

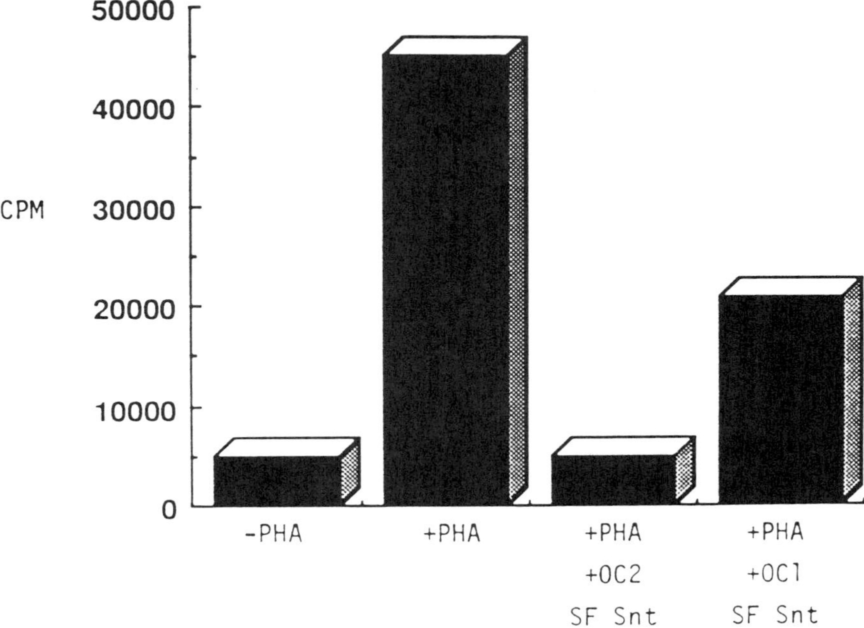

Figure 1: Suppression of donor peripheral blood lymphocyte (PBL) mitogenic responses by OC1 and OC2 squamous carcinoma cell lines. Proliferation was measured using ^{3}H-thymidine incorporation.[7] PBLs were stimulated with phytohemagglutinin (PHA) at a concentration of 3 μg/mL. Serum-free supernatant (SF Snt) was medium conditioned by OC1 or OC2 cells for 48 hours. CPM = counts per minute.

Immune Suppressor Production

Fundamental to survival and growth of a tumor in vivo is the evasion/suppression of an activated antitumor immune response. Most human tumors are immunogenic yet survive and proliferate in immunocompetent hosts. They do this through a number of mechanisms including the local production by the tumor of a molecule which is capable of paralyzing antitumor immune mechanisms. As shown in Figures 1 and 2, both OC1 and OC2 cells produce a potent immune suppressor molecule which inhibits proliferation of cells of lymphoid origin. (See also O'Sullivan et al., Chapter 7 of this volume.)

Another escape mechanism is the suppression of HLA (MHC class I) antigen expression, thus evading cytotoxic T-cell corecognition

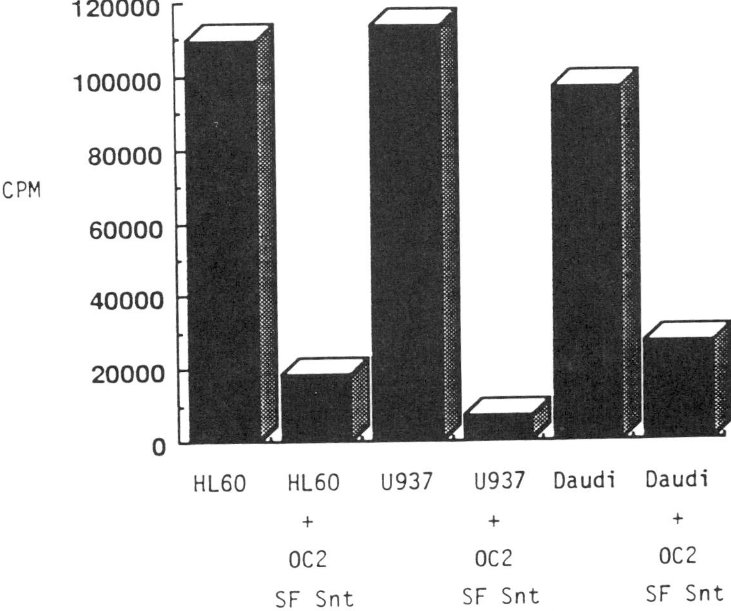

Figure 2: Suppression of proliferation of human malignant lymphoid cell lines with OC2-derived esophageal carcinoma suppressor (conditioned 48 hour serum-free medium). Proliferation was measured using ^{3}H-thymidine incorporation.[7] HL6O = progranulocyte, U937 = promonocyte, Daudi = B cell lymphoma, CPM = counts per minute, SF Snt = serum-free supernatant.

and killing. Using anti-MHC class I (MHC-I) monoclonal antibodies, both OC1 and OC2 cells were found to lack appreciable MHC-I antigen expression. On treatment with α2 interferon (intron A), both cells demonstrated a marked expression of MHC-I antigen. Interferon may have a role as a component of a biological therapy schedule.

Preliminary analyses for oncogene amplification in these cells highlight genetic rearrangement differences. We have found amplification of L-myc[8] in both and in a number of primary esophageal tumors. We have, however, not found amplification of N-ras oncogene in the cell lines or in esphageal tumors. Interestingly, gross amplification of C-sis, which codes for a platelet-derived growth factor-like molecule, could be demonstrated in OC1 cells. Thus the two cell lines differ not only at the morphological level but also at the level of oncogene expression.

Table II
Chemosensitivity of Esophageal Carcinoma Cell Lines Using the MTT Assay as Described[9] [ID_{50} Concentration (μg/mL)]

Cell Line	*Cis-platin*	*5-Fluoro-uracil*	*Metho-trexate*	*Pharmo-rubiciin*	*Doxo-rubicin*	*Vin-blastine*	*Vin-cristine*
OC1	18.0	1.7	0.09	0.09	0.09	ND	ND
OC2	7.1	0.09	0.07	0.15	0.03	0.65	0.34

Chemosensitivity Profiles of Esophageal Cell Lines

Since squamous carcinomas of the esphagus are generally refractory to chemotherapy, it was of interest to look at the drug resistance/sensitivity of these esophageal cell lines. Using the MTT assay of Denizot,[9] we found significant differences between both cell lines (Table II). With the exception of cisplatinum, both cell lines were sensitive to concentrations of anticancer drugs achieved in clinical practice.

Radiation sensitivity studies were also done using ^{60}Co irradiation and survival was measured by clonogenic growth. An LD_{50} response between 100 and 200 rads was recorded for both cell lines, a response indicative of a radiosensitive nature.

Conclusions

Two continuous cell lines have been established from esophageal squamous cell carcinomas. These show the highly developed characteristics of tumorigenicity, invasiveness, and exogenous growth factor independence. These properties, coupled with an ability to produce a potent immunosuppressing agent, provide at least a partial explanation for the poor prognosis associated with this tumor. Oncogene analyses show genomic rearrangement in these cells which are possibly initiated by the precipitating carcinogenic insult. Surprisingly, the cell lines showed no intrinsic drug resistance.

Future therapeutic prospects will involve biological response modifiers and biological therapy programs. Reversal of immune suppression, activation of an effective immune response, and neutralization of tumor-derived growth factors are prospective areas for development in the treatment of esophageal cancer.

The findings presented give a basis for the poor prognosis and a platform on which to construct more effective and less toxic chemo/immuno/biotherapy treatments for esophageal carcinoma.

ACKNOWLEDGMENTS: This work was supported by grants from the Irish Health Research Board, The Mercy Hospital Cancer Research fund, and from PARC Hospital Management. Intron A was a gift from Schering Plough (Avondale Brinny Chemical Company Ltd., Ireland) and r-interleukin-2 was a gift from Eurocetus Amsterdam, The Netherlands. We would also like to acknowledge the assistance of Mr. Robert Bond of the Biological Services Unit, University College, Cork, Ireland.

References

1. Yang CS: Research on esophageal cancer in China: A review. Cancer Res 40:2633, 1980.
2. Banks-Schegel SP, Quintero J: Growth and differentiation of human esophageal carcinoma cell lines. Cancer Res 46:250, 1986.
3. Moll R, Franke WW, Schiller DL, et al: The catalog of human cytokeratins: Patterns of expression in normal epithelia, tumors and cultured cells. Cell 31:11, 1982.
4. Ben-Zeev A: Cell configuration-related control of vimentin biosynthesis and phosphorylation in cultured mammalian cells. J Cell Biol 97:858, 1983.
5. Rafferty D, O'Donoghue M, O'Sullivan G, Collins JK: Ultrastructural characterisation of two cell lines derived from human oesophageal squamous carcinoma. Proc R Mic Soc 23:4, 1988.
6. Mareel M, Kint J, Meyvisch C: Methods of study of the invasion of malignant C3H-mouse fibroblasts into embryonic chick heart in vitro. Virchows Arch B Cell Pathol 30:95, 1979.
7. Hoon DSB, Bowker RJ, Cochran AJ: Suppressor cell activity in melanoma-draining lymph nodes. Cancer Res 47:1529, 1987.
8. Kingston RE, et al: Regulation of heat shock protein 70 gene expression by C-myc. Nature (London) 312:280, 1984.
9. Denizot F, Long R: Rapid colorimetric assay for cell growth and survival: Modifications to the tetrasodium dye procedure giving improved sensitivity and reliability. J Immunol Methods 89:271, 1986.

2

An Immunohistochemical Analysis for Cancer of the Esophagus Using Monoclonal Antibodies Specific for Modified Nucleosides

Masayuki Masuda, Tetsuro Nishihira,
Katsu Hirayama, Noriaki Ohuchi, Ryo Takano,
Yoshiharu Sato, Kunihiko Itoh, Michinao Mizugaki,
Nakao Ishida, Shozo Mori

Introduction

Modified nucleosides such as 1-methyladenosine (m^1Ado) and pseudouridine (ψ) derived predominantly from transfer ribonucleic acids (tRNA) have been shown to be excreted in abundance in the urine of patients with various types of cancer. In this study, we attempted to evaluate the expression of these modified nucleosides in esophageal cancer tissues using monoclonal antibodies (MAbs), termed AMA-2 specific for m^1Ado, and APU-6 specific for ψ, by immunohistochemical assays. Furthermore, urine levels of m^1Ado and ψ in patients with esophageal cancer were examined using these MAbs and enzyme-linked immunosorbent assay (ELISA).

Ferguson MK, Little AG, Skinner DB: Diseases of the Esophagus, Vol. I: Malignant Diseases. Futura Publishing Company, Inc., Mount Kisco, NY, © 1990.

Materials and Methods

For the immunohistochemical study, formalin-fixed, paraffin-embedded tissues of esophageal cancer were collected from surgical specimens obtained at Tohoku University Hospital from 1985 to 1987. Urine samples were collected from patients with esophageal cancer for the study of m^1Ado or ψ expression by ELISA. Murine IgG2b MAb, termed AMA-2 specific for m^1Ado, and murine IgG1 MAb, termed APU-6 specific for ψ, were prepared and characterized as previously described.[1]

An immunohistochemical assay was performed using the avidin-biotin-peroxidase complex (ABC) method (Vectastain ABC kit, Vector Lab. Inc.). The inhibition ELISA system using these MAbs, AMA-2 or APU-6, was previously established.[1] The concentration of the modified nucleosides (m^1Ado or ψ) in the urine was corrected by the amount of creatinine and expressed as nmol per μmol creatinine.

All reactivity in each section was evaluated by percent cellular reactivity and staining intensity. Percent reactivity was an estimation of the number of epithelial cells (or cancer cells) reactive with MAbs divided by the total number of epithelial cells (or cancer cells) of the same histologic lesion ×100. Intensity was classified in three ranks: negative (-), weak (±), positive (+). The significance of differences was established by using a *t*-test.

Results

Formalin-fixed, paraffin-embedded esophageal cancer tissues were analyzed for expression of m^1Ado or ψ using AMA-2 and APU-6 and the ABC immunohistochemical method (Figs. 1, 2). All of the 31 esophageal cancer lesions generally reacted strongly (+) with AMA-2 in the cytoplasm but rarely in the nuclei. Twenty-eight out of the 31 (90%) also reacted strongly (+) with APU-6 in the cytoplasm but rarely in the nuclei. However, a spinous layer of the dysplastic epithelium reacted weakly (±) or strongly (+) with AMA-2 or APU-6 in the cytoplasm. Normal epithelium of the esophagus did not react with either MAbs except for very weak staining in the basal layer. Other cancerous tissue also reacted strongly (+) with both MAbs. Among the benign tumors examined, two fibroadenomas of the mammary gland and three follicular adenomas of the thyroid gland were reactive with AMA-2 or APU-6, but the staining intensity was very

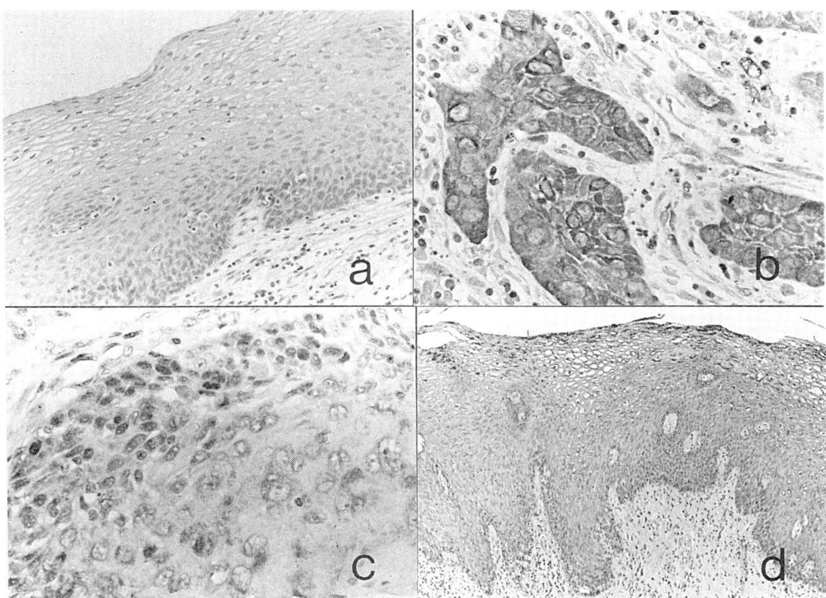

Figure 1: (a) Normal esophageal tissue stained with MAb AMA-2 using ABC immunohistochemical method. Epithelial cells in the basal layer are weakly reactive. Counterstained with hematoxylin. Similar results were seen with MAb APU-6. (b) Moderately differentiated squamous cell carcinoma reactive with MAb AMA-2. Note the strong cytoplasmic staining of carcinoma cells. Similar results were seen with MAb APU-6. (c) Moderately differentiated squamous cell carcinoma showing immunoreactivity of the nucleus as well as the cytoplasm to MAb AMA-2. The nuclear staining was frequently observed before carcinoma invasion. Similar results were seen with MAbs APU-6. (d) Dysplastic lesion of the esophagus stained with MAbs AMA-2. Note the heterogenous reactivity of MAb AMA-2 with the dysplastic epithelial cells.

weak (±). Epithelial cells in cases of appendicitis were not reactive with either MAbs.

Two staining patterns were observed: one was a cytoplasm dominant type and the other was a nuclear dominant type. The cytoplasmic staining was seen frequently, and the nuclear staining was rarely seen in the border of the tumor. No significant relationship between the percent reactivity of the cancer tissues and prognostic factors such as stage, lymph node metastasis, and histological differentiation of the tumor was observed.

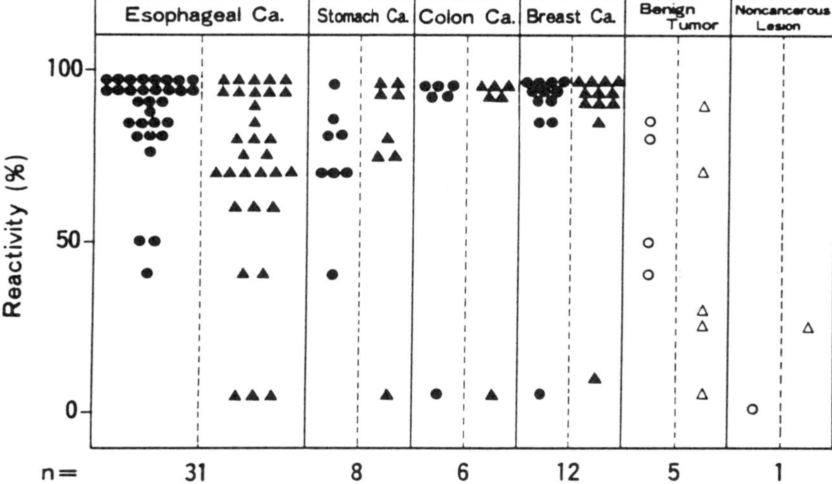

Figure 2: Immunohistochemical reactivity of AMA-2 or APU-6 for various cancers and benign lesions. Benign tumors: two fibroadenomas of the mammary gland, three follicular adenomas of the thyroid gland. Noncancerous lesions: epithelium in cases of appendicitis. Closed circle = percent reactivity to AMA-2 stained with positive (+) intensity. Closed triangle = percent reactivity to APU-6 with positive (+) intensity. Open circle = percent reactivity to AMA-2 with weak (±) intensity. Open triangle = percent reactivity to APU-6 with weak (±) intensity.

Fifty-one urine samples were collected from patients with esophageal cancer (including five patients with early stage cancer). The excretion of the m^1Ado or ψ in the urine before operation was examined using AMA-2 or APU-6 and inhibition ELISA assay (Fig. 3). Significantly higher levels of m^1Ado and ψ were found in the urine of the patients with esophageal cancer as compared with those of healthy donors. Nine of the 51 patients (17.6%) showed elevated levels of m^1Ado above the cut-off level (3.23 nmol/μmol creatinine; mean +2SD from healthy donors), and 28 of the 51 patients (54.9%) showed high urinary excretion level of ψ above the cut-off level (51.04 nmol/μmol creatine; mean +2SD).

Discussion

At present, more than 50 different modified nucleosides have been characterized. These modified nucleosides are found predom-

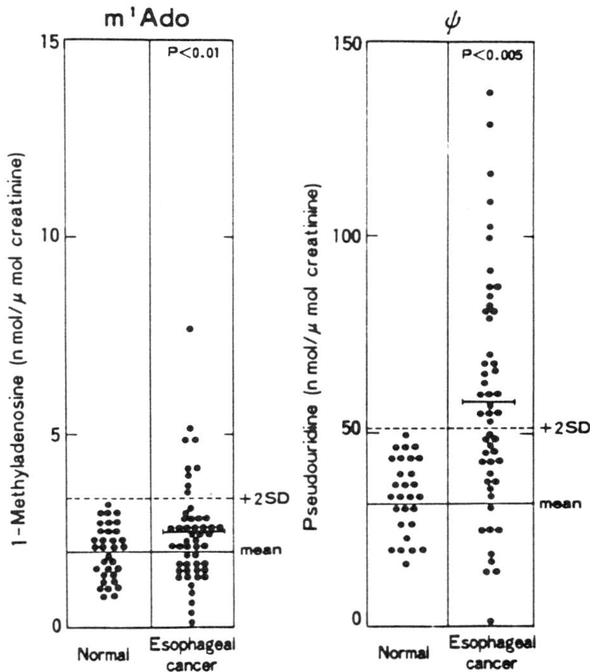

Figure 3: Urine levels of m^{1}Ado or ψ in patients with esophageal cancer before operation.

inantly in tRNA as a trace component and are considered to play an important role in the fine tuning of tRNA.[2] The synthesis of most modified nucleosides is known to occur at the polynucleotide level after the transcription of the tRNA genes. Many studies have shown that the levels of certain modified nucleosides in the urine are elevated in a wide variety of cancer patients.[3–5] The elevation of modified nucleosides in the urine of cancer patients has been suggested to be caused by the higher turnover of tRNA in the tumor tissue rather than by the destruction of the tissue.[6]

One of the these modified nucleosides, 1-methyladenosine (m^{1}Ado), has been shown to have a potent immunosuppressive effect,[7,8] impairing the resistance to *Listeria* infection in mice. This implies that m^{1}Ado may contribute to the creation of an immunosuppressive environment of cancerous lesions.

In this study, we analyzed the expression of two modified nucleosides, m^1Ado and ψ, in cancer of the esophagus. This immunohistochemical study has demonstrated enhanced expression of these modified nucleosides in the cancer tissues compared with that in normal epithelium, though there was no relationship between the percent reactivity and standard prognostic factors.

We also investigated the urinary excretion of these modified nucleosides. The levels of m^1Ado or ψ were significantly higher in the patients with esophageal cancer than those in healthy donors. Detection of these modified nucleosides by MAbs in the urine of patients with esophageal cancer may be useful for monitoring the effectiveness of therapy or the recurrence of the tumor.

References

1. Itoh K, Mizugaki M, Ishida N: Preparation of a monoclonal antibody specific for 1–methyladenosine and its application for the detection of elevated levels of 1-methyladenosine in urines from cancer patients. Jpn J Cancer Res 79:1130, 1988.
2. Björk GR, Ericson JU, Gustafsson CED, et al: Transfer RNA modification. Ann Rev Biochem 56:263, 1987.
3. Waalkes TP, Dinsmore SR, Mrochek JE: Urinary excretion by cancer patients of the nucleosides N^2,N^2-dimethylguanosine, 1-methylinosine, and pseudouridine. J Natl Cancer Inst 51:271, 1973.
4. Waalkes TP, Gehrke CW, Zumwalt RW: The urinary excretion of nucleosides of ribonucleic acid by patients with advanced cancer. Cancer 36:390, 1975.
5. Gehrke CW, Kuo KC, Waalkes TP: Patterns of urinary excretion of modified nucleosides. Cancer Res 39:1150, 1979.
6. Borek E, Baliga BS, Gehrke CW: High turnover rate of transfer RNA in tumor tissue. Cancer Res 37:3362, 1977.
7. Ishida N: Isolation of factors responsible for the immunosuppression found in tumor-bearing animals. Yakugaku Zasshi 105:91, 1985.
8. Itoh K, Majima T, Edo K: Suppressive effect of 1-methyl- adenosine on the generation of chemiluminescence by mouse peritoneal macrophages stimulated with opsonized zymosan. Tohoku J Exp Med 157:205, 1989.

3

Glycoprotein Alterations in Barrett's Esophagus, Adenocarcinoma Arising in Barrett's Epithelium and Adenocarcinoma of the Gastroesophageal Junction

Hiroshi Nogami, Janet K. Stephens, Mark K. Ferguson, Kin-ichi Nabeya

Introduction

Patients with Barrett's esophagus have an increased risk for the development of adenocarcinoma.[1,2] Epithelial dysplasia is thought to be both the earliest morphologic evidence of malignancy in the esophagus as well as its direct precursor. Given the consequences to a patient when a diagnosis of severe dysplasia is rendered, it is disturbing that the classification of dysplasia remains complicated and difficult to apply.[3] In some organs, the distribution and expression of mucosal glycoproteins in glandular epithelium may change with the development of neoplasia. The glycoprotein profile may therefore be a reliable marker of dysplastic change in columnar type epithelium.[4] In addition, the distribution of these compounds may help in distin-

Ferguson MK, Little AG, Skinner DB: Diseases of the Esophagus, Vol. I: Malignant Diseases. Futura Publishing Company, Inc., Mount Kisco, NY, © 1990.

guishing those carcinomas that are of gastroesophageal junction origin from adenocarcinomas arising in Barrett's epithelium where this is not possible clinically.

Assessment of mucosal glycoprotein distribution may be accomplished by cytochemical methods using lectins.[4–13] Lectins are glycoproteins which are able to bind to specific carbohydrate residues. Over a hundred lectins have been purified but the number of these which are applicable to probe intestinal glycoproteins is small. These include gorse seed lectin (*Ulex europaeus*, UEA-1) with specificity for alpha-1 fructose; horse gram lectin (*Dolichos biflorus*, DBA) with specificity for N-acetylgalactosamine-alpha 1,3N-acetylgalactosamine; peanut lectin (*Arachis hypogaea*, PNA) with specificity for the disaccharide D-galactose-beta 1,3N-acetylgalactosamine, and soybean agglutinin (*Glycine max*, SBA) with specificity for alpha-D-galactosamine-N-acetylgalactosamine. Using these four compounds, we examined a group of patients with Barrett's esophagus, some of whom had adenocarcinomas of the distal esophagus which arose in Barrett's type epithelium and some with associated dysplastic changes only, and compared them to patients with adenocarcinomas which arose in the region of the cardia or gastroesophageal junction.

Materials and Methods

We examined tissue from 32 patients which included a series of 13 cases of Barrett's (benign) esophagus, 13 adenocarcinomas arising in Barrett's lesions with associated mucosal dysplasia (four cases), and six cases of adenocarinoma arising at the gastroesophageal junction (GEJ). Tissues from these various specimens were fixed in phosphate-buffered formalin (3.7%), embedded in paraffin, and sectioned at 4 microns. Sections were stained with hematoxylin and eosin and the following features were noted: type of Barrett's epithelium, degree of dysplasia present,[3] histologic type of adenocarcinoma, and degree of differentiation. Parallel slides were stained with a battery of lectins. The staining procedure consisted of deparaffinizing sections which had been placed on albumin-coated slides and rehydrated through graded alcohols.[14] Sections were then stained with biotinylated lectins (Vector Laboratories, Burlingame, CA) in phosphate-buffered saline and visualized using the avidin-biotin horseradish peroxidase system (ABC, Vector Laboratories) after incubation in diaminobenzidine-hydrogen peroxidase. The distribution of cellular

Table I
Distribution of Lectin Binding Sites of Barrett's Esophagus, Barrett's Adenocarcinoma, and GEJ Carcinoma

Lectins Used/ Sugar Specificity	*Ulex Europaeus Agglutinin-1 (UEA-1) /L-Fuc*	*Peanut Agglutinin (PNA) /Gal Gal-NAC*	*Soybean Agglutinin (SBA) /Gal Gal-NAC*	*Dolichos Biflorus Agglutinin (DBA) /Gal-NAC*
Barrett's				
Fundic	A, G	A, G	A, G	—
Gastric	A, G, C	—	A, G, C	A, G, C
Specialized	A, G, C	—	—	—
Barrett's Dysplasia	A, C	—	A, C	—
Barrett's Adenocarcinoma	A, G, C	—	—	—
GEJ Adenocarcinoma	C	C	C	C

L-Fuc = L-fucose, Gal = galactose, GalNac = N-acetylgalactosamine, A = Apex, G = Glycocalyx, C = Cytoplasm

staining (glycocalyceal, apical, intracytoplasmic) was then determined.

Results

The pattern of reaction of neoplastic and non-neoplastic epithelial cells labeled with the various lectins is summarized in Table I. Gastric (junctional) type Barrett's (four cases) bound the lectins UEA, SBA, and DBA to the apex and glycocalyx of the cell, as well as intracytoplasmically (Fig. 1a). Fundic Barrett's (two cases) bound UEA, PNA, and SBA but only to the apex and glycocalyx (Fig. 1b). Seven cases of Barrett's with specialized (intestinal) epithelium bound only the lectin UEA to the apex and glycocalyx of the cell with focal intracytoplasmic staining (Fig. 1c). Dysplastic foci of Barrett's (four cases) which arose in specialized (intestinal) epithelium adjacent to the carcinomas, bound UEA as well as SBA to the apex of the cells and focally within the cytoplasm. Adenocarcinomas arising in Barrett's epithelium all bound the lectin UEA, usually in a cytoplasmic distribution (Fig. 1d). While the other lectins were detected, their presence was only focal and of weak intensity, especially in more poorly differentiated tumors. In contrast, six carcinomas of the gastroesophageal

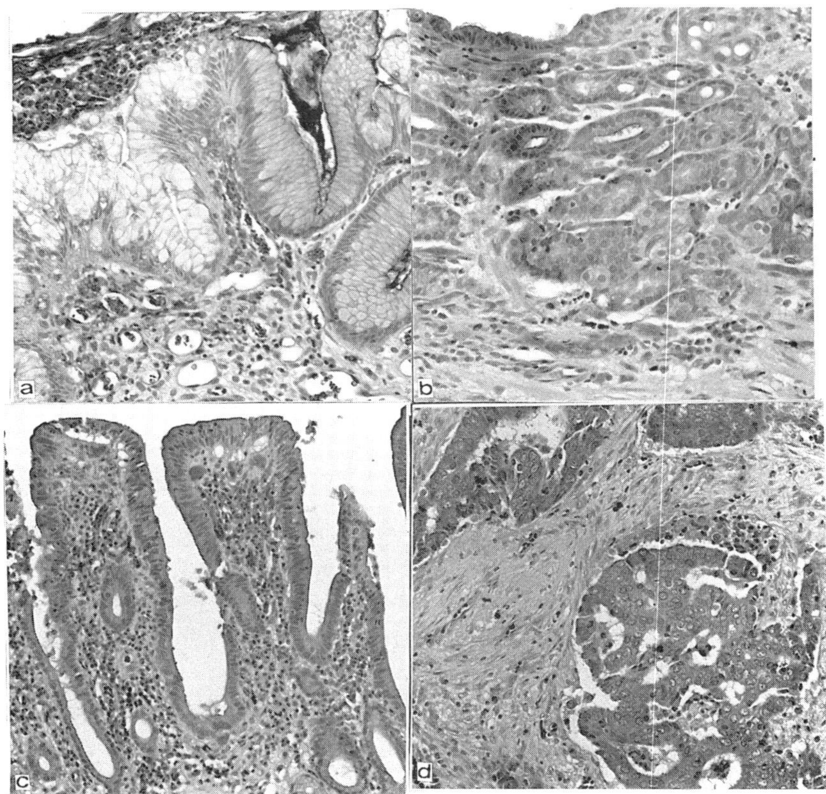

Figure 1: Light micrographs of Barrett's esophagus and Barrett's adenocarcinoma stained with horseradish-peroxidase labeled lectins. (a) Barrett's esophagus, gastric (junctional) type epithelium stained with PNA. Reaction product is identified predominately in the apex and glycocalyx (200×). (b) Barrett's esophagus, fundic type epithelium stained with SBA. Reaction product is identified within the apex and glycocalyx and focally within the cytoplasm (200×). (c) Barrett's esophagus, intestinal (specialized columnar) epithelium stained with UEA-1. Reaction product is identified within the apex, glycocalyx and cytoplasm (150×). (d) Barrett's adenocarcinoma reacted with UEA-1. Reaction product is present predominantly within the cytoplasm but is also identified within the apex and glycocalyx (150×).

junction bound nearly all lectins in a predominantly cytoplasmic distribution similar to that of the adjacent normal gastric epithelium. The intensity of the staining reaction was similar in all positive cases.

Discussion

It is known that intestinal epithelium undergoes an alteration in carbohydrate structure during cellular differentiation and malignant transformation.[4] These changes can be detected by several means including the selective binding of lectins, specific proteins capable of binding to the carbohydrate portion of a glycoconjugate. Because of the risk of malignant transformation in Barrett's lesions of the esophagus and the present difficulties in accurately determining the presence and degree of dysplasia in endoscopic biopsies, it is of considerable importance to identify a reliable, objective means to do this. In addition, there is often clinical disagreement as to the origin of certain distal esophageal neoplasms, that is whether these arise from the proximal stomach or the distal esophagus when Barrett's epithelium is not clearly identified either clinially or histologically.

To accomplish these objectives, we examined the differential lectin reactivity of distal esophageal adenocarcinomas, junctional carcinomas, and different histologic types of Barrett's epithelium. Fundic and gastric type Barrett's exhibited binding of UEA, PNA, and SBA to apex, glycocalyx, and/or cytoplasm, with gastric type epithelium also binding DBA. Intestinal type Barrett's epithelium bound only UEA. With the development of dysplasia in the intestinal epithelium, some reaction with SBA was also noted. The profile of the invasive adenocarcinomas was very similar to that of intestinal type Barrett's. Of interest was the fact that the GEJ adenocarcinomas bound all four lectins in a predominantly cytoplasmic distribution. These findings are similar to those previously reported in Barrett's esophagus[18] and gastric lesions.[11] These results suggest that the pattern of glycoprotein distribution and expression changes with neoplastic transformation of Barrett's esophagus and is in turn different from those of normal gastric mucosa and adenocarcinomas arising in the GEJ. This suggests a possible role for the use of lectin cytochemistry in endoscopic surveillance biopsies to improve the sensitivity of detection of premalignant change. It may also prove valuable when combined with other techniques such as flow cytometry or image analysis.

References

1. Berenson LJ, Riddell RH, Skinner DB, Preston JW: Malignant transformation of esophageal columnar epithelium. Cancer 41:554, 1978.
2. Cameron AJ, Ott BJ, Payne WS: The incidence of adenocarcinoma in columnar-lined (Barrett's) esophagus. N Engl J Med 313:857, 1985.
3. Reid BJ, Haggitt RC, Rubin CE, et al: Observer variation in the diagnosis of dysplasia in Barrett's esophagus. Hum Pathol 19:166, 1988.
4. Boland CR, Montgomerry CK, Kim YS: Alterations in human colonic mucin occurring with cellular differentiation and malignant transformation. Proc Natl Acad Sci USA 79:2051, 1982.
5. Boland CR, Montgomery CK, Kim YS: A cancer-associated mucin alteration in benign colonic polyps. Gastroenterology 82:664, 1982.
6. Cooper HS: Peanut lectin-binding sites in large bowel carcinoma. Lab Invest 47:383, 1982.
7. Yonezawa S, Nakamura T, Tanaka S, et al: Binding of *Ulex europaeus* agglutinin-1 in polyposis CO11: Comparative study with solitary adenoma in the sigmoid colon and rectum. JNCI 71:19, 1983.
8. Yonezawa S, Nakamura T, Tanaka S, Sato E: Glycoconjugate with *Ulex europaeus* agglutinin-1 binding sites in normal mucosa, adenoma and carcinoma of the human large bowel. JNCI 69:777, 1982.
9. Fischer J, Klein PJ, Vierbuchen M, et al: Characterization of glycoconjugates of human gastrointestinal mucosa by lectins. I. Histochemical distribution of lectin binding sites in normal alimentary tract as well as in benign and malignant gastric neoplasms. J Histochem Cytochem 32:681, 1984.
10. Fischer J, Klein RJ, Vierbuchen M, et al: Characterization of glycoconjugates of human gastrointestinal mucosa by lectins. II. Lectin binding to the isolated glycoproteins of normal and malignant gastric mucosa. J Histochem Cytochem 32:690, 1984.
11. Bur M, Franklin WA: Lectin binding to human gastric adenocarcinomas and adjacent tissues. Am J Pathol 119:279, 1985.
12. Ito M, Takata K, Saito S, et al: Lectin-binding pattern in normal human gastric mucosa. Histochemistry 83:189, 1985.
13. Compton CC: Premalignancy in chronic ulcerative colitis: Lectin binding as a diagnostic adjuvant. Hum Pathol 20:407, 1989.
14. Nogami H, Nabeya K, Ho M, et al: Changes in lectin binding pattern of human esophagus in association with malignancy. In: Diseases of the Esophagus, Siewert JR, Holscher AH (eds), Berlin, Springer-Verlag, 1986, p 55.
15. Kalish RJ, Clancy PE, Orringer MB, Appelman HD: Clinical, epidemiologic and morphologic comparison between adenocarcinomas arising in Barrett's esophageal mucosa and in the gastric cardia. Gastroenterology 86:461, 1984.
16. Wang HH, Antoniolli DA, Goldman H: Comparative features of esophageal and gastric adenocarcinomas: Recent changes in type and frequency. Hum Pathol 17:482, 1986.

17. MacDonald WC, MacDonald JB: Adenocarcinoma of the esophagus and/or gastric cardia. Cancer 60:1094, 1987.
18. Haggitt RC, Reid BJ, Rubin CE, Rabinovitch PS: Barrett's esophagus: Mucin histochemistry correlated with histologic diagnosis and flow cytometric data. Gastroenterology 92:1421, 1987.

4

The Relationship Between Tumor-Infiltrating Lymphocytes and Epidermal Growth Factor Receptor Expression in Esophageal Cancer

Hiroshi Yano, Hitoshi Shiozaki, Kenji Kobayashi, Tokiharu Yano, Hideaki Tahara, Shigeyuki Tamura, Takesada Mori

Introduction

In esophageal cancer, patients with many tumor-infiltrating lymphocytes (TILs) in their lesions generally have a better prognosis than those with few TILs. In squamous cell carcinoma, the epidermal growth factor receptor (EGF-R) plays an important role in the initial mediation of tumor proliferation. In this study, the relationship between the presence of TILs and EGF-R expression was examined by immunohistological staining of esophageal cancer specimens.

Materials and Methods

Esophageal squamous cell carcinoma tissue specimens were obtained from 24 patients who had never received irradiation or anti-

Ferguson MK, Little AG, Skinner DB: Diseases of the Esophagus, Vol. I: Malignant Diseases. Futura Publishing Company, Inc., Mount Kisco, NY, © 1990.

cancer chemotherapy. The specimens were frozen by dry ice acetone immediately after surgical removal. Frozen tissues were cut into 4 μm thick sections with a cryostat and were fixed with cold acetone for 10 minutes. The avidin-biotin-peroxidase complex (ABC) method was used for immunostaining in this study.[1] To detect EGF-R, anti-EGF-R monoclonal antibody (Oncor, Inc.) was used. To detect the subpopulations of lymphocytes, anti-Leu 1 (pan T cell), anti-Leu 7 (NK/K cell), and anti-Leu 12 (pan B cell) monoclonal antibodies (Becton Dickinson Monoclonal Center, Inc.) were employed.

TILs were counted using a light microscope (×400) in the five areas surrounding the most invasive cancer nest, and all specimens were classified into one of four groups (Fig. 1): Group (±): scanty TILs (less than 10 lymphocytes per visual field); Group (+): mild TIL infiltrate (10–100 lymphocytes); Group (+ +): moderate TIL infiltrate (100–200 lymphocytes); Group (+ + +): marked TIL infiltrate (more than 200 lymphocytes). According to the intensity of EGF-R staining, all the specimens were divided into three groups (Fig. 3): Group (+): faint staining with anti-EGF-R; Group (+ +): moderate staining with anti-EGF-R; Group (+ + +): strong staining with anti-EGF-R. The pathological classification was based on the Guidelines for Clinical and Pathologic Studies on Carcinoma of the Esophagus established by the Japanese Society for Esophageal Diseases.[2]

Results

EGF-R was expressed faintly in the basal and parabasal layers of normal esophageal epithelia, and strongly in all areas of dysplastic epithelia (Fig. 2). In the invading cancer nests, EGF-R was located on the cancer cell membranes which were stained either strongly or faintly (Fig. 3). There were four cases showing strong staining for EGF-R, and the histologic diagnosis was moderately differentiated squamous cell carcinoma in all four cases. Faint staining for EGF-R was seen in 15 cases, which comprised three well-differentiated, four moderately differentiated, and eight poorly differentiated carcinomas.

The cases with moderate and marked TIL infiltrates numbered 15. In these groups, there were no cases strongly expressing EGF-R (Table I). On the other hand, nine cases had scanty or mild TIL infiltration, and four of them (44%) strongly expressed EGF-R (Table II). Among the seven superficial carcinomas, one patient (No. 18) with

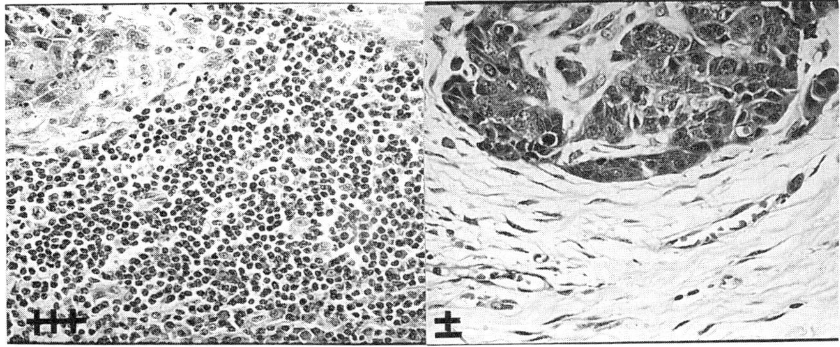

Figure 1: TILs surrounding the most invasive cancer nest. A case of marked TIL infiltrate (+ + +) (left) and a case of scanty TILs (±) (right) are shown (H&E, ×400).

few TILs and strong expression of EGF-R had lymph node metastases, but patients (Nos. 1, 2, 3) with marked TIL infiltrates and weak expression of EGF-R did not. When TILs were stained with anti-Leu antibodies, the lymphocytes in contact with the cancer nests were found to be mostly Leu 1 positive cells (Fig. 4).

Discussion

It has been reported that in various cancers, patients with many TILs have a better prognosis than those with few TILs.[3] The amount of T cell infiltration has also been shown to correlate well with the patient's prognosis.[4] The lymphocytes surrounding cancer nests in our patients were mostly Leu 1 positive cells (pan T cells). Therefore, it appears that T cells play an important role in host resistance to esophageal cancer. Which of the T cell subsets (cytotoxic, suppressor, helper, or inducer cells) was most important in this respect remains unknown.

EGF-R is a glycoprotein with an MW of 170 kilodaltons. Many squamous cell carcinomas show heightened expression of EGF-R, and a positive correlation between EGF-R expression and the prognosis in esophageal cancer has been reported.[5] We found that EGF-R was expressed on the basal and parabasal layers of normal esophageal epithelium. In the cancer cell nests, EGF-R was prominent in moderately differentiated tumors composed of pleomorphic cells with se-

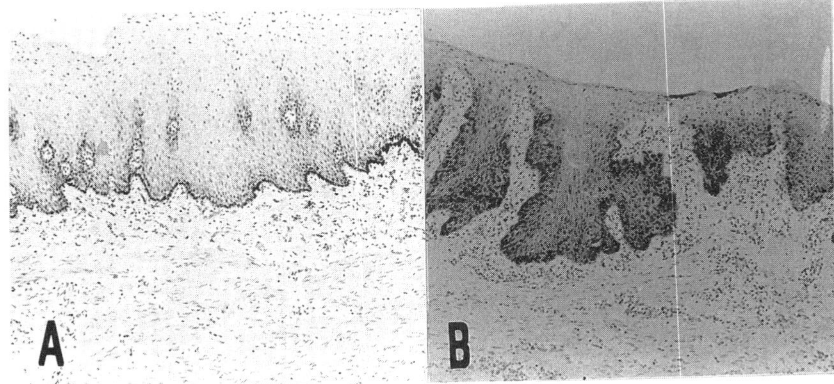

Figure 2: EGF-R is expressed faintly in the basal and parabasal layers of normal esophageal epithelia (A), and strongly in all areas of dysplastic epithelia (B) (ABC method, ×200).

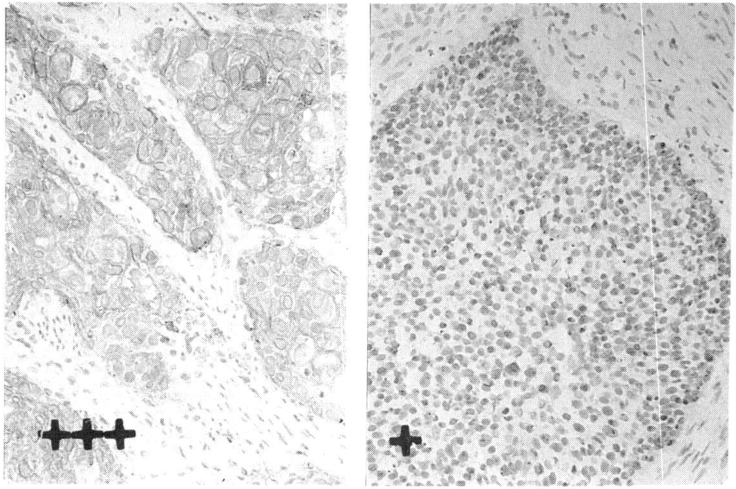

Figure 3: A case of strong staining (+ + +) with anti-EGF-R (left) and a case of faint staining (+) with anti-EGF-R (right) are shown (ABC method, ×400).

Table I
The Clinical Profiles of the Cases with Marked or Moderate TIL Infiltration

Case No.	*Age*	*Sex*	*TILs*	*EGF-R*	*Depth of Invasion**	*Histologic Type***
1	67	♂	+ + +	+	sm	por
2	71	♀	+ + +	+	sm	por
3	58	♂	+ + +	+	sm	mod
4	63	♂	+ + +	+	mp	por
5	53	♂	+ + +	+	mp	por
6	76	♂	+ + +	+	mp	por
7	44	♂	+ + +	+	mp	well
8	49	♀	+ + +	+ +	mm	mod
9	59	♂	+ + +	+ +	sm	por
10	47	♂	+ +	+	sm	mod
11	52	♀	+ +	+	mp	por
12	69	♀	+ +	+	mp	well
13	43	♂	+ +	+	a2	mod
14	73	♂	+ +	+ +	a2	well
15	73	♂	+ +	+ +	a2	por

* mm = to muscularis mucosae, sm = to submucosa, mp = to muscularis propria, a2 = definite invasion to adventitia.
** well = well-differentiated squamous cell carcinoma (SCC), mod = moderately differentiated SCC, por = poorly differentiated SCC.

Table II
The Clinical Profiles of the Cases with Scanty or Mild TIL Infiltration

Case No.	*Age*	*Sex*	*TILs*	*EGF-R*	*Depth of Invasion**	*Histologic Type***
16	67	♂	±	+ + +	a1	mod
17	71	♀	±	+ + +	a2	mod
18	54	♂	±	+ + +	sm	mod
19	67	♂	±	+ + +	a1	mod
20	60	♀	±	+	a1	por
21	56	♂	±	+	a3	mod
22	61	♂	+	+ +	a3	well
23	56	♂	+	+	a2	por
24	74	♂	+	+	a1	well

* sm = to submucosa, a1 = invasion reaching the adventitia, a2 = definite invasion of the adventitia, a3 = invasion into neighboring structures.
** well = well-differentiated squamous cell carcinoma (SCC), mod = moderately differentiated SCC, por = poorly differentiated SCC.

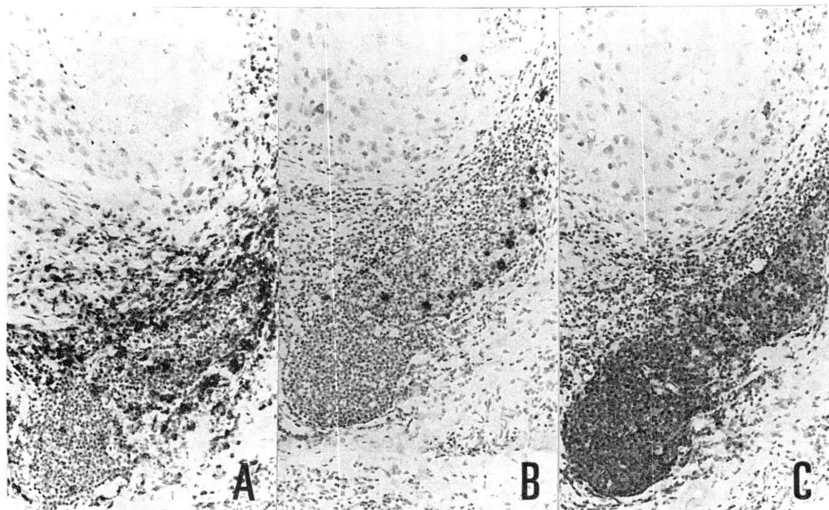

Figure 4: The lymphocytes in contact with the cancer nest are mostly Leu 1 positive cells (A), and few Leu 7 (B) and/or Leu 12 (C) positive cells (ABC method, ×200).

vere nuclear atypia. It was faintly expressed by well-differentiated or poorly differentiated carcinoma cells.

TILs were found in small numbers near cancer cell nests that strongly expressed EGF-R. Therefore, it may be that cancer cells with strong expression of EGF-R produced an immunosuppressive factor. It has been reported that transforming growth factor β (TGFβ) suppressed the growth and differentiation of human B and T lymphocytes,[6] and increased the expression of EGF-R.[7] Thus, the immunosuppressive factor may possibly be TGFβ, but further investigation is necessary on this subject. In superficial carcinomas, cases with strongly expressed EGF-R and few TILs readily developed lymphatic metastasis, and it was thought that they would have a poor prognosis. On the other hand, cases with little expression of EGF-R and many TILs should have a better prognosis. From these results, T cell infiltration and EGF-R expression appear to be important prognostic factors in esophageal cancer.

ACKNOWLEDGMENT: This study was supported in part by a Grant-in-Aid for Cancer Research from the Ministry of Health and Welfare of Japan (63-2).

References

1. Hsu SM, Raine L, Fanger H: Use of avidin-biotin-peroxidase complex (ABC) in immunoperoxidase techniques: A comparison between ABC and unlabeled antibody (PAP) procedures. J Histochem Cytochem 29:577, 1981.
2. Japanese Society for Esophageal Diseases: Guidelines for the Clinical and Pathologic Studies on Carcinoma of the Esophagus, 7th edition, Tokyo, Kanehara & Co. Ltd., 1989.
3. Bennet SH, Futtrell JW, Roth JA, Hoye RC, Ketcham AS: Prognostic significance of histologic host response in cancer of the larynx or hypolarynx. Cancer 28:1255, 1971.
4. Shimokawara I, Imamura M, Yamanaka N, et al: Identification of lymphocyte subpopulations in human breast cancer tissue and its significance: An immunoperoxidase study with anti-human T- and B-cell sera. Cancer 49:1456, 1982.
5. Ozawa S, Ueda M, Ando N, et al: Prognostic significance of epidermal growth factor receptor in esophageal squamous cell carcinomas. Cancer 63:2169, 1989.
6. Kehrl JH, Alvarez-Mon M, Fauci AS: Type β transforming growth factor suppresses the growth and differentiation of human B and T lymphocytes. Clin Res 33:610, 1985.
7. Assoian RK, Frolik CA, Roberts AB, et al: Transforming growth factor-β controls receptor levels for epidermal growth factor in NRK fibroblasts. Cell 36:35, 1984.

5

Effect of Epidermal Growth Factor on the Proliferation of Esophageal Cancer Cell Lines

Yutaka Shimada, Masayuki Imamura, Takayoshi Tobe, Yujiro Nanba, Masao Hanaoka, Tetsu Akiyama

Introduction

Recent studies have shown a relationship between the number of epidermal growth factor (EGF) receptors of various cancer cells and the grade of the malignancy. Regarding the growth of cultured esophageal cancer cells, two conflicting results have been reported. Kamata et al.[1] reported that the growth of squamous carcinoma cell (SCC) lines including esophageal cancer cells is inhibited by EGF and that the degree of inhibition of EGF correlates well with the number of EGF receptors. In contrast, Banks-Schlegel and Quintero[2] reported that esophageal carcinomas have fewer receptors with increased ligand affinity compared to normal esophageal epithelial cells, and that growth is not inhibited by EGF as determined by monolayer assays.

In this study, we used 16 human esophageal cancer cell lines which had been recently established to examine the relationship between the levels of expression of EGF receptors and the effects of EGF on cell proliferation. We observed that EGF-mediated growth

Ferguson MK, Little AG, Skinner DB: Diseases of the Esophagus, Vol. I: Malignant Diseases. Futura Publishing Company, Inc., Mount Kisco, NY, © 1990.

inhibition in a monolayer culture was not a common property of esophageal cancer cells. We also observed that the growth of the cells whose monolayer growth was inhibited by EGF was stimulated by EGF in soft agar.

Effects of EGF on the Proliferation of Esophageal Cancer Cells

We used 16 human esophageal cancer cell lines (KYSE-series), which were established from surgical specimens. The effects of EGF on the proliferation of these cell lines in a monolayer culture was first studied. EGF at concentrations of 25 pM–6.4 nM was added 16 hours after plating 2×10^4 cells in a 24-well culture plate and cell growth was measured on day 4.

As shown in Figure 1, we observed three types of responses to EGF. For four cell lines, KYSE-70, KYSE-140, KYSE-200, and KYSE-360, EGF significantly stimulated cellular proliferation. In contrast, the growth of KYSE-30 cells was markedly inhibited by the addition of EGF. Similarly, EGF inhibited the growth of A431 cells. The growth of three cell lines—KYSE-50, KYSE-111, and KYSE-270—was moderately inhibited, while that of KYSE-390 cells was slightly inhibited by the addition of EGF. There was little effect of EGF on the growth of the other seven cell lines.

Quantification of the EGF Receptor in Esophageal Cancer Cells

In order to determine whether the three different responses of esophageal cancer cell lines to EGF were related to the number of EGF receptors, the number of the EGF receptors on these cells was measured by three methods: ^{125}I-EGF binding assay, immunoprecipitation, and Western blot analysis of the EGF receptors with anti-EGF receptor antibodies.

Table I summarizes the data obtained from Scatchard analysis of the binding of ^{125}I-EGF to esophageal cancer cells at 15°C for 2 hours. Of the 10 cell lines examined, five cell lines were found to possess two classes of binding sites and the other five cell lines were found to possess a single class of binding site. The Kd values of these receptors varied from 0.2 nM to 2.2 nM. The number of receptors in

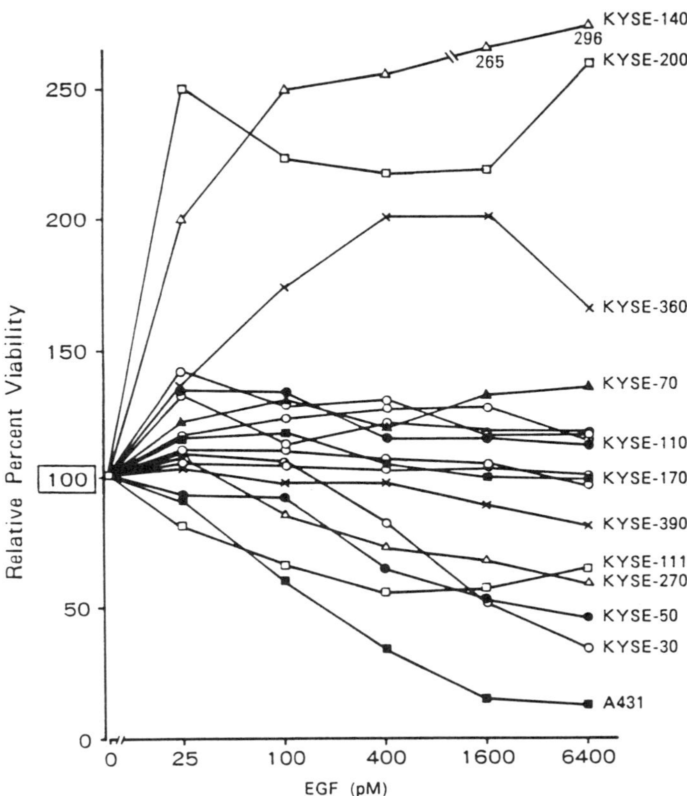

Figure 1: Effects of EGF on anchorage-dependent growth of the KYSE-series. Cells were seeded at 2×10^4 cells/well in 24 well culture plates and cultured for 96 hours in the presence of various concentrations of EGF (25 to 6400 pM). The relative percent viability (RPV) was calculated as follows: RPV = [mean OD (EGF-treated)/mean OD (non-EGF-treated)] $\times$ 100, where the mean absorbance represents the average OD from four wells.

9 of 10 cell lines ranged from 10^4 to 10^5 binding sites/cell. KYSE-30 cells contained 1.2×10^7 binding sites/cell, 6 times that of A431 cells. The numbers of EGF receptors measured by immunoprecipitation and Western blot analysis were similar to those determined by ^{125}I-EGF binding assay. When DNA from each cell line was analyzed by Southern blot analysis, only that of KYSE-30 was found to carry an amplified EGF receptor gene.

Table I
Effects of EGF on the Growth of Esophageal Cancer Cell Lines

Cell Line	No. of EGF Receptors ($\times 10^5$/cell)		kd (nM)		Anchorge-Dependent Growth: Percentage of Relative Viability in the Presence of EGF 6.4 nM (%)
A431	21	1.2		5.2	12.1
KYSE-30	120	0.5		2.0	32.5
KYSE-50	3.0		0.6		45.7
KYSE-111	2.1	0.6		2.2	64.3
KYSE-270	2.1		0.7		58.7
KYSE-390	ND		ND		80.6
KYSE-180	6.0		1.4		116.4
KYSE-170	2.7		1.4		98.8
KYSE-150	2.0	0.4		1.2	105.7
KYSE-220	1.3	0.2		0.9	98.8
KYSE-110	0.9	0.2		0.6	111.5
KYSE-350	ND		ND		115.3
KYSE-410	ND		ND		112.1
KYSE-140	0.6		1.1		296.7
KYSE-200	ND		ND		259.5
KYSE-360	ND		ND		164.5
KYSE-70	ND		ND		134.6

Inhibition and stimulation of anchorage-dependent growth in the presence of EGF at 6.4 nM are expressed as percentages of growth of the control group, which was not administered EGF. The number and affinity of EGF receptors were quantitated by Scatchard analysis of the binding of ^{125}I-EGF.
ND = not done.

Quantification of the EGF Receptor Kinase Activity

Since the tyrosine kinase activity of the EGF receptor is thought to play an important role in cell growth and cell transformation, the EGF receptor kinase activity of all the esophageal cancer cell lines was measured. The immunoprecipitated EGF receptors prepared from detergent lysates of the cell lines were examined for their autophosphorylation activities by incubating them in the presence of γ-^{32}P-ATP. The amount of ^{32}P incorporated into the immunoprecipitated EGF receptors was proportional to the number of EGF receptors in each cell line.

For quantification of the level of tyrosine phosphorylation in vivo, the cells were labeled with ^{32}P-phosphate and then the tyrosine-phosphorylated proteins were immunoprecipitated with antiphosphotyrosine antibodies. As was the case for autophosphorylation of the EGF receptors in vitro, the level of phosphorylation in vivo was also related to the number of EGF receptors contained in each cell.

Relationship Between the Response to EGF and Number of EGF Receptors on Esophageal Cancer Cells

Figure 2 shows the relationship between the response to EGF, taken from Figure 1, and the number of EGF receptors, taken from Table 1. The growth of cells possessing extremely large numbers of EGF receptors (KYSE-30; $>10^7$/cell) was inhibited by EGF as was the case for A431 cells. Conversely, the growth of cell lines containing small numbers of EGF receptors ($<10^5$/cell), such as KYSE-70 and KYSE-140, was stimulated by EGF. The growth of the other eight esophageal cell lines, which possess EGF receptors in the order of 10^5 receptors/cell, were not significantly correlated with the numbers of EGF receptors in these cells.

Effects of EGF on Anchorage-Independent Proliferation of Esophageal Cancer Cells

Since the ability of cells to proliferate under anchorage-independent conditions is considered to be one of the best assays for showing the tumorigenicity of a cell, the effects of EGF on the growth of 15 esophageal cancer cells under anchorage-independent conditions was examined. As shown in Figure 3, the cells whose monolayer growth was inhibited by EGF were on the contrary stimulated by EGF in soft agar in a dose-dependent manner (Fig. 3A). The cells whose monolayer growth was not inhibited by EGF were not stimulated by EGF in soft agar (Fig. 3B).

Discussion

It is well known that the growth of some cultured squamous carcinoma cells is inhibited by EGF. Kamata et al.[1] reported that EGF

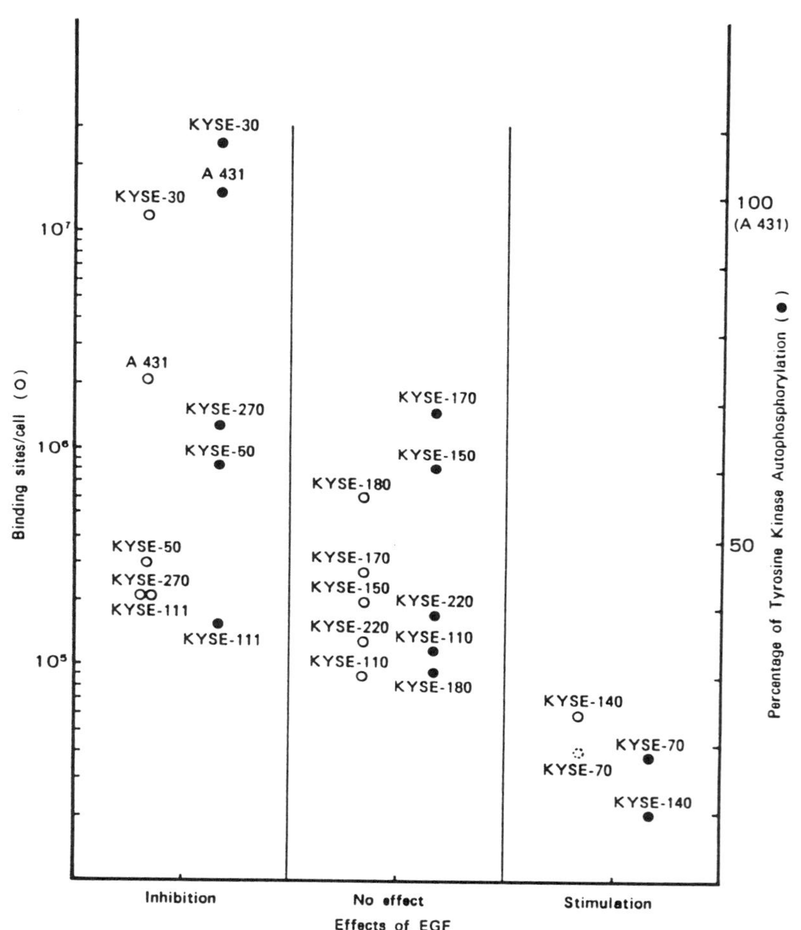

Figure 2: Relationship between the number of EGF receptors and the effects of EGF on anchorage-dependent growth of esophageal cancer cell lines. The cell lines were divided in three groups (inhibition, no effect, stimulation). The number of EGF receptors in KYSE-70 cells and the tyrosine kinase activities of 12 cell lines were calculated from immunoprecipitation experiments.

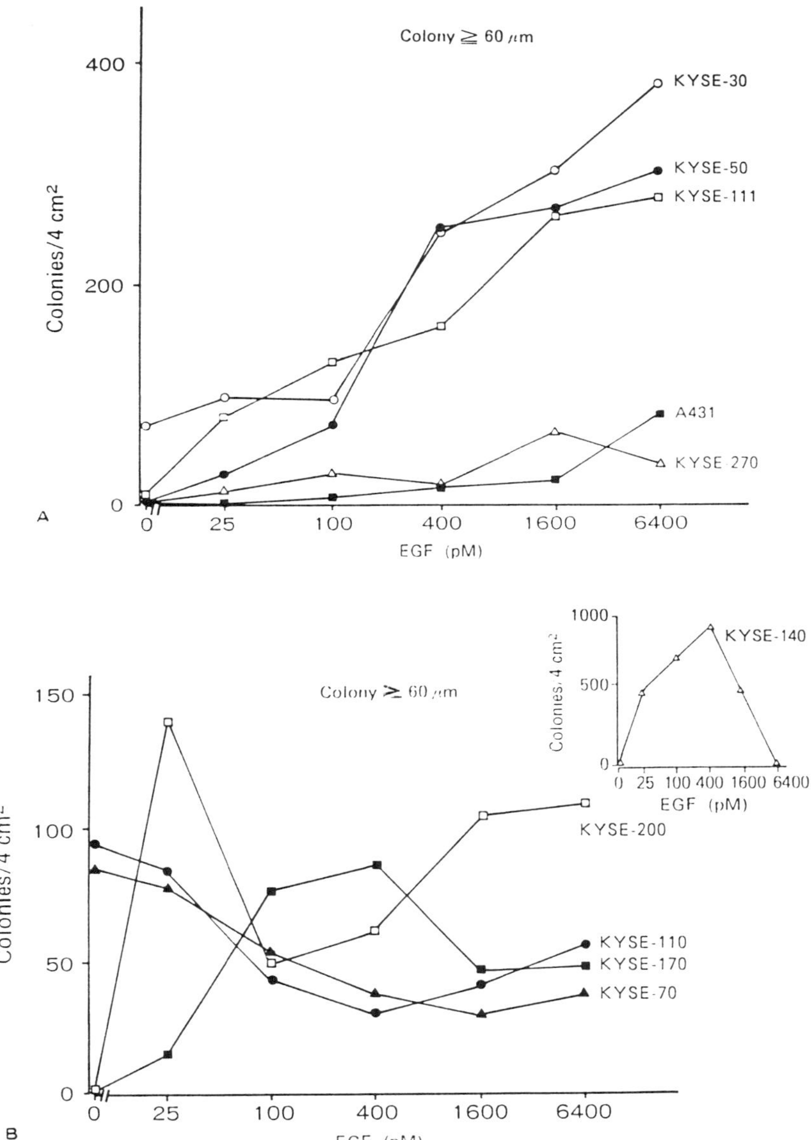

Figure 3 A,B: Effects of EGF on anchorage-independent growth of esophageal cancer cells. Cells were plated in 1 mL of 0.3% agar overlayed on 0.5% agar in 35-mm petri dishes. After 10–14 days, colonies larger than 60 μm were counted.

specifically inhibited the growth of all of the seven esophageal cancer cell lines that they examined as well as that of seven cell lines derived from the skin and oral cavity. On the other hand, Banks-Schlegel and Quintero reported that the growth of esophageal cancer cells was not inhibited by EGF.[2] In this study, we observed three types of responses of esophageal cancer cells to EGF; the growth of five cell lines was inhibited, and that of four cell lines was stimulated, while that of the other seven cell lines was unaffected. Thus, EGF-mediated growth inhibition did not seem to be a common property of all the esophageal cancer cell lines.

From the studies with variant A431 cell lines and other SCC cell lines, it has been suggested that the number of EGF receptors per cell is closely related to the cell's response to EGF.[3–5] However, in our experiments, the number of EGF receptors per cell did not correlate with the type of growth response evoked by EGF. These results are consistent with those from a recent detailed analysis of variant A431 cells in which no consistent differences in EGF receptor concentrations were found between stimulated and null clones.[5] Furthermore, Rizzino et al.[6] recently isolated a clonal variant of A431 cells which retained a high EGF binding capacity and responded to EGF by growth stimulation.

It is also interesting to note that the introduction of a eukaryotic vector-containing human EGF receptor cDNA into NIH3T3 cells resulted in an increase in the number of EGF receptors to levels comparable to those observed in some human carcinomas, and conferred an EGF-dependent transformed phenotype to NIH3T3 cells. The presence of high levels of the EGF receptor in NIH3T3 cells did not result in growth inhibition by EGF.[7–9] Thus, the cellular growth responses evoked by the action of EGF are not simply determined by the number of EGF receptors but might also be influenced by the differences in the signal transduction system distal to EGF-receptor binding.

Anchorage-independent growth is a property closely associated with the transformed state in vivo, and EGF significantly increases the number of colonies of various neoplasms in soft agar.[10] Recently the dose-dependent stimulatory effects of EGF on the growth of A431 cells in soft agar assay have been described.[11] Our results in soft agar assay also revealed that cells whose monolayer growth were inhibited by EGF were dose-dependently stimulated by EGF in soft agar. It is possible that the production of endogenous growth factors could bring about colony formation in soft agar. However, the mechanisms underlying these different responses have not yet been elucidated.

References

1. Kamata N, Chida K, Rikimaru K, et al: Growth-inhibitory effects of epidermal growth factor and overexpression of its receptors on human squamous cell carcinomas in culture. Cancer Res 46:1648–1653, 1986.
2. Banks-Schlegel SP, Quintero J: Human esophageal carcinoma cells have fewer, but higher affinity epidermal growth factor receptors. J Biol Chem 261:4359–4362, 1986.
3. Kawamoto T, Mendelson J, Le A, et al: Relation of epidermal growth factor receptor concentration to growth of human epidermoid carcinoma A431 cells. J Biol Chem 259:7761–7766, 1984.
4. Buss JE, Kudlow JE, Lazar CS, et al: Altered epidermal growth factor (EGF)-stimulated protein kinase activity in variant A431 cells with altered growth responses to EGF. Proc Natl Acad Sci 79:2574–2578, 1982.
5. Lifshitz A, Lazar CS, Buss JE, et al. Analysis of morphology and receptor metabolism in clonal variant A431 cells with differing growth responses to epidermal growth factor. J Cell Physiol 115:235–242, 1983.
6. Rizzino A, Ruff E, Kazakaoff P: Isolation and characterization of A431 cells that retain high epidermal growth factor binding capacity and respond to epidermal growth factor by growth stimulation. Cancer Res 48:2377–2381, 1988.
7. Riedel H, Massoglia S, Schlessinger J, et al: Ligand activation of overexpressed epidermal growth factor receptors transforms NIH3T3 mouse fibroblasts. Proc Natl Acad Sci 85:1477–1481, 1988.
8. Velu TJ, Beguinot L, Vass WC, et al: Epidermal growth factor-dependent transformation by a human EGF receptor proto-oncogene. Science 238:1408–1410, 1987.
9. Di Fiore PP, Pierce JH, Fleming TP, et al: Overexpression of the human EGF receptor confers an EGF-dependent transformed phenotype to NIH3T3 cell. Cell 51:1063–1070, 1987.
10. Humburger AW, White CP, Brown RW: Effect of epidermal growth factor on proliferation of human tumor cells in soft agar. J Natl Cancer Inst 67:825–830, 1981.
11. Lee K, Tanaka M, Hatanaka M, et al: Reciprocal effects of epidermal growth factor and transforming growth factor β on the anchorage-dependent and independent growth of A431 epidermoid carcinoma cells. Exp Cell Res 173:156–162, 1987.

6

Tumor-Derived Immunosuppression in Esophageal Squamous Cell Carcinoma

Gerald O'Sullivan, Aine Corbett, Chariya Hahnvajanawong, Maurice O'Donoghue, John K. Collins

Introduction

Squamous cell carcinoma of the esophagus is an aggressive tumor with a high metastatic potential. Despite recent advances in diagnostic techniques and improvements in surgery, radiation, and chemotherapy, the prognosis remains dismal with a 5-year survival rate of less than 10%. The majority of these patients are incurable because of tumor metastases and require an effective systemic therapy which is, as yet, unavailable.

Recent techniques in biotechnology permit detailed study of tumor immune system interactions and provide adequate quantities of biological substances including biological response modifiers for cancer therapy.[1] The pharmacological efficacy of these agents, however, is predetermined by the tumor type and stage, tumor antigen strength, and heterogeneity, as well as the immune repertoire of the

Ferguson MK, Little AG, Skinner DB: Diseases of the Esophagus, Vol. I: Malignant Diseases. Futura Publishing Company, Inc., Mount Kisco, NY, © 1990.

patient. It is now well established that cancer patients, particularly those with head and neck and esophageal malignancy, exhibit both in vitro and in vivo evidence of immune suppression. This immune suppression results from the development of the tumor, progresses with the expanding tumor burden, and to date is refractory to therapeutic immune modulation.[2,3] The pathogenesis of this immune failure requires further investigation.

During the initial phase of cancer development, most patients are immunocompetent. Whether there is tumor containment by the effector immune system or subsequent growth facilitation through immune failure depends on the strength of the initial antitumor immune responses. The question arises why tumor growth progresses in the immunocompetent hosts who are capable of mounting antitumor immune responses. Possible answers include: (1) evasion of immune surveillance because of absence, weakness, or modulation of tumor surface antigens; (2) production by the tumor of soluble suppressor factors which block the proliferative and cytotoxic responses of responding lymphocytes; or (3) tumor growth and development results in production of suppressor T lymphocytes which are tumor antigen-specific and suppress specific immune responses.[3] In this context little is known regarding immunogenicity or biological responses of human squamous carcinoma of the esophagus.

If immunology is to play a role in prevention, detection, or therapy of human esophageal squamous carcinoma, a fundamental understanding of the host–tumor relationship is essential. The biological pathways and mechanisms of these bidirectional immune responses (host versus tumor and tumor versus host) unique to this tumor must be clarified. Successful immunotherapy will need to augment the effector responses and negate or neutralize immunosuppressive influence from the tumor.

In this chapter we focus on two questions. (1) Is there an immune response to esophageal squamous cell carcinoma? Implicit in this question is whether there are tumor-associated antigens specifically expressed in esophageal tumors. (2) What is the influence of the esophageal tumor on immune function?

Methods and Materials

The population studied included 12 patients who underwent esophagectomy for squamous cell carcinoma, 11 patients who underwent esophagogastrectomy for adenocarcinoma of the distal esophagus or esophagogastric junction, 16 patients who underwent partial colectomy for adenocarcinoma of the colon, and three patients with benign disease who had surgery of the esophagogastric junction.

Materials were obtained from each patient for study, including tumor and control tissues from the freshly excised organs and a lymph node near the tumor and a control or reference lymph node well distal to or if possible outside the lymph draining field of the tumor, usually at the base of the mesentery. These were obtained immediately on resection and transferred to the laboratory. Lymphocytes were harvested from the lymph nodes after extrusion through a fine wire mesh. Both lymph node lymphocytes and peripheral blood lymphocytes were banded in Ficoll Hypaque and subsequently washed three times. Lymphocyte mitogenic responses were evaluated by measuring the incorporation of tritiated thymidine after treatment of the cells with PHA, Con-A, or co-culture with irradiated donor lymphocytes (mixed lymphocyte culture).[4]

Esophageal Tumor Characteristics

Frozen sections of squamous cell cancer were labeled with monoclonal antibodies for MHC class 1 antigens (MHC-1), T lymphocyte subsets, and B lymphocytes. Appreciable levels of MHC class 1 antigens were found in the tumor cells of only one of the 10 studied patients (Table I). Similarly, these were absent from tumor-derived tissue culture cell lines which were re-expressed on treatment with α2 interferon (see Collins et al., Chapter 1 of this volume).

A moderate T lymphocyte infiltration, which was mainly confined to the stromal areas, was seen in all tumors. The predominant lymphocyte subset was the T helper inducer (Th/i) rather than cytotoxic suppressor (Ts/c). Low numbers of B lymphocytes were seen in all cases, although tumor-reacting immunoglobulins were scarcely detectable by immunofluorescent techniques.

Evaluation of T Lymphocyte Mitogenic Responses

The components of the immune system directly influenced by tumors are likely to be in the draining lymphatic tissue. We therefore compared the responses of lymphocytes from paratumor lymph nodes (tumor nodes) with those of distal lymph nodes (reference

Table I
Tumor Infiltrating Lymphocyte Subsets and HLA (MHC Class 1) Status of Squamous Cell Carcinomas

Case No.	*Age*	*Sex*	*Degree of Differentiation*	*HLA-1*	*PAN T**	*Th/i**	*Ts/c**	*B**
17	58	F	SCC moderate	−	1325	1021	323	208
36	61	F	SCC moderate	+	1127	810	321	422
25	82	F	SCC poor	−	991	962	69	208
42	72	F	SCC moderate	−	777	364	88	135
54	75	F	SCC moderate	−	2029	595	—	334
45	67	F	SCC well	−	1264	400	—	29
51	80	M	SCC well	−	764	42	—	40
68	66	M	SCC poor	−	718	724	—	34
82	41	M	SCC —	−	706	699	—	—

Th/i = Helper inducer
Ts/c = Suppressor/cytoxic
* Lymphocyte counts/mm^2

nodes). In a few cases we also evaluated the responses of lymphocytes from peripheral blood and from venous blood draining the tumor. A typical result from an individual patient is seen in Figure 1. Lymphocytes from the tumor node and from the tumor vein show impaired responses to lectin stimulation by comparison with those from the reference node or peripheral blood. This suggests a lymphocyte-suppressing influence by the squamous cell cancer which is predominantly a local phenomenon and may not be evident after blood or lymph dilution. Similar suppression effects were found on Con-A stimulation and in mixed lymphocyte culture assays. We consistently found the tumor node lymphocytes to be less responsive (reference tritiated thymidine incorporation = 100%); suppression in all tumor node lymphocytes ranged from 30% to 90%, $n = 12$, $P < .001$ (Fig. 2). This lymphocyte suppression was not reversed by interleukin 2 (IL2) treatment in vitro. Regional lymph node lymphocyte suppression was not seen for adenocarcinoma of the esophagogastric region or colon or in benign esophageal disease.

Alteration of B Lymphocyte Function

Human IgG-secreting hybridomas were generated by fusing tumor node lymphocytes with a mouse myeloma cell line. The re-

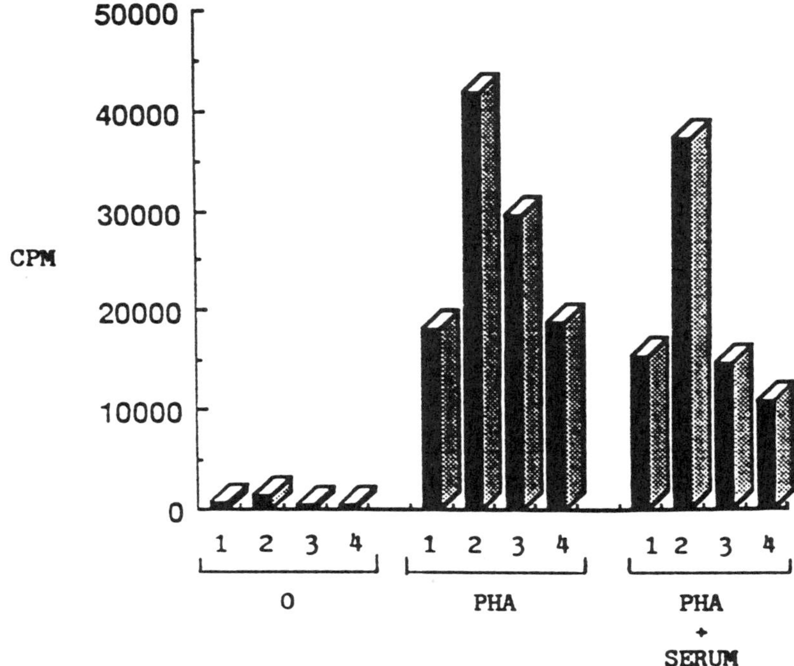

Figure 1: The proliferative responses of lymphocytes from a patient with squamous cell carcinoma as measured by tritiated thymidine incorporation after stimulation by lectins. The tumor node lymphocytes respond poorly to lectin stimulation by comparison with reference lymphocytes. 1 = lymphocytes from tumor node, 2 = lymphocytes from reference lymph nodes, 3 = lymphocytes from peripheral blood, 4 = lymphocytes from venous effluent of tumor, CPM = counts per minute of tritiated thymidine, 0 = baseline, PHA = phaseolus vulgaris agglutinin.

sulting human monoclonal antibodies were screened against normal tissue and tumor from each patient. In two patients with absent tumor or reacting serum immunoglobulins, patient-specific human monoclonal antibodies were produced which reacted individually to their tumors but not to control tissues. This indicates previous sensitization of B lymphocytes to esophageal tumor-associated antigens and suppression of potential responses prior to the fusion. We also looked for tumor-infiltrating immunoglobulins in each tumor using immunofluorescent staining of frozen sections. In esophageal squamous cell carcinoma, tumor-associated or tumor-reactive serum IgG was not

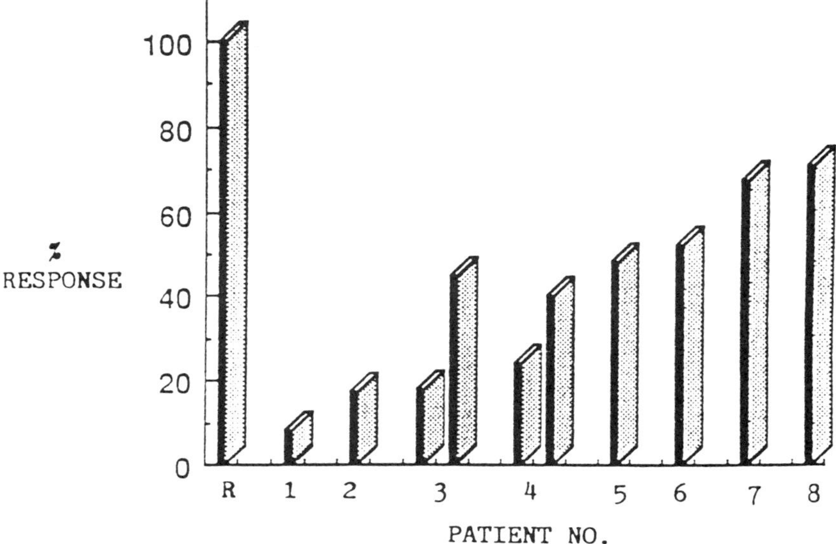

Figure 2: Response of reference and tumor lymph node lymphocytes to lectin stimulation in eight patients with squamous cell carcinoma. In all cases there is an impaired response of tumor node lymphocytes. R = reference = 100%; note for patients 3 and 4, proximal and distal tumor lymph nodes were studied and show impaired responses.

detectable. This was in sharp contrast to the finding in gastrointestinal (GI) adenocarcinomata where there was a strong antibody infiltrate. These findings provide further evidence of B lymphocyte suppression by the esophageal tumor.

Tumor-derived Immune Suppressive Activity

Potential immune suppressive activity was assayed by measuring suppression of donor lymphocyte responses to lectins and mixed lymphocyte culture reactions. Culture media conditioned by fresh tumor explants or tumor cell extracts resulted in lymphocyte suppression to basal levels (Fig. 3). In addition, serum-free medium conditioned by culture of tumor cell lines was profoundly suppressive. Immune suppression was not found in normal esophageal tissue explants or

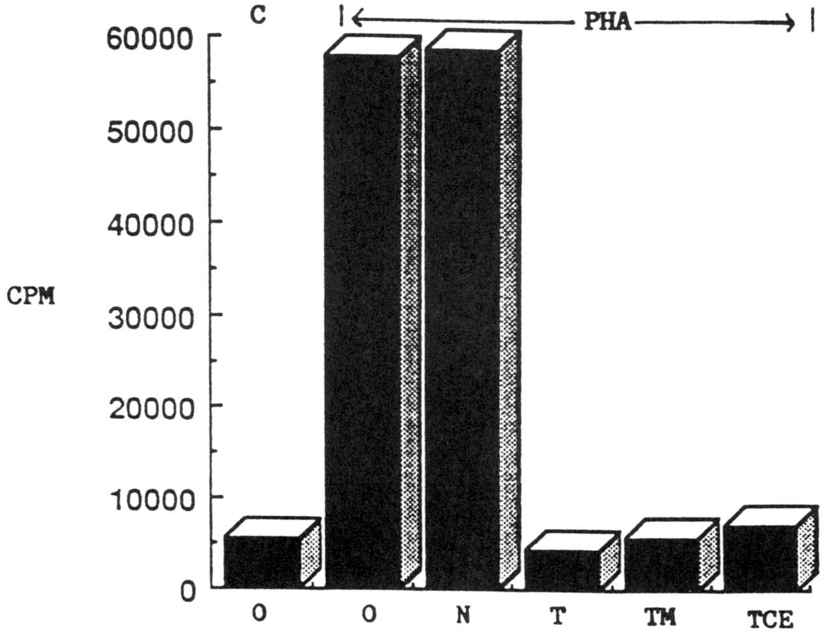

Figure 3: Baseline (C) and lectin responses of peripheral blood lymphocytes showing the influence of conditioned medium from explants of normal esophageal tissue (N), esophageal squamous cell tumor (T), tumor metastatic deposit (TM), and tumor cell extract (TCE). Note profound suppression of responses by tumor-conditioned media and extract only.

in culture media from normal epithelial or fibroblast cells in tissue culture.

Interleukin 2 treatment in vitro did not reverse the influence of the immunosuppressor (Fig. 4). This is in contrast to suppression found associated with colon adenocarcinomata which is reversible by IL2 stimulation.

We have also observed that a soluble mediator derived from esophageal tumor explants and tissue culture cell lines blocks the formation of functioning lymphokine-activated killer (LAK) cells in response to IL2. We also found that the suppressor inhibited the cytotoxic activity of preformed LAK cells. However, in the absence of suppressor activity, esophageal cell lines were effectively killed by allogenic LAK cells.

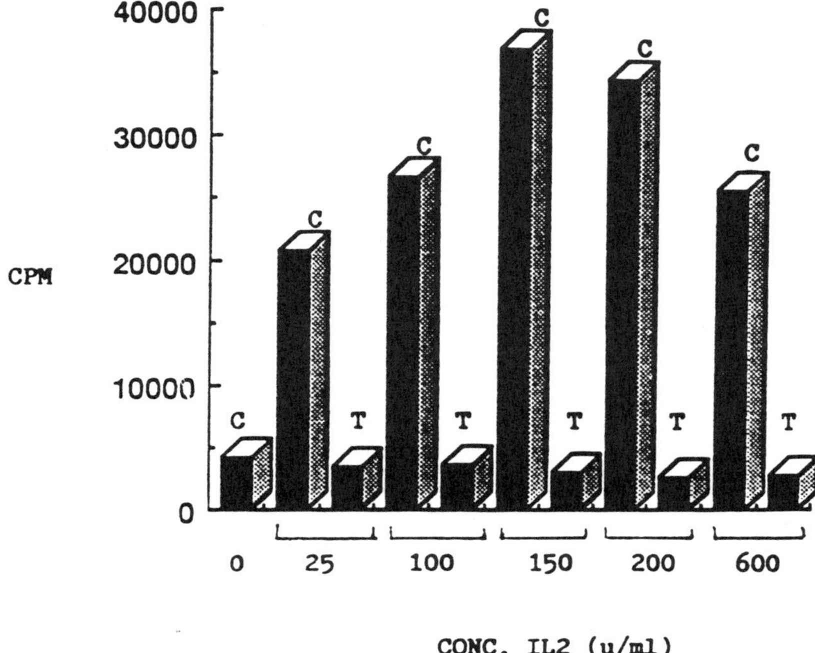

Figure 4: Response of peripheral blood lymphocytes to varying doses of interleukin 2 with and without treatment by immunosuppressor agent from esophageal squamous carcinoma; note failure of response of treated lymphocytes. C = control lymphocytes, T = lymphocytes treated with immunosuppressor factor.

Discussion

The finding of a T lymphocyte infiltrate in all esophageal carcinomas but not the control tissues indicate a T cell immune response against putative tumor antigens. Despite this, these T lymphocytes are, unquestionably, functionally ineffective as evidenced by the growth and metastatic spread of the tumors. Our data suggest that a soluble mediator derived from the tumor profoundly suppresses local lymphocytes. This could play a significant role in tumor escape as both the afferent and efferent limbs of the immune system would be rendered ineffective. Although few suppressor T lymphocytes were identified in the tumors, a tumor-specific T effector–suppressor cell switch response cannot be excluded, as the suppressor cell compartment and function is most likely to be the spleen and lymph node regions. It is noteworthy that most of the esophageal squamous cell tumors do not express MCH class 1 antigen. Modulation of MHC-1 from the cell surface could be another mechanism by which the tumor escapes immunosurveillance.

A notable finding was the paucity of tumor-reacting IgG-immunoglobulin from all squamous cell tumors and their sera. This is in sharp contrast to our findings for GI tract adenocarcinomas. A possible explanation for the difference between both types of tumor may be the relative strength of the surface antigens on the tumors. The generation of hybridoma-secreting human IgG monoclonal antibodies from two patients which reacted with their individual tumors but not with control tissues suggests prior sensitization of the B lymphocyte to tumor antigens. The proliferative capacity of the antibody-forming cells was most likely suppressed at the memory cell stage. It seems, therefore, that a tumor-derived suppression rather than a weak antigenic stimulus is the most likely cause of the poor humoral response. Indeed, the findings of tumor-specific human monoclonal antibodies and T cell infiltrates in the tumor are compelling evidence for the presence of tumor-associated antigens in esophageal squamous cell carcinoma, some of which may be specific to the individual patient.

A consistent observation was the profound persistent suppression of the tumor node lymphocyte responses. In contrast, lymphocytes from reference lymph nodes, and in most cases peripheral blood from the same patients, responded well to lectins and lymphokines, thus excluding age and nutritional or technical variations as potential explanations for the observed differences. We did not observe variations in lymph node responses from the corresponding anatomical regions in patients with benign disease. A similar tumor node versus reference node suppression was not found for GI tract adenocarcinomas. However, we have found that explants of colon carcinoma are lymphocyte suppressive, and our failure to demonstrate tumor node suppression in the adenocarcinomas may be due to loss of a suppressing agent during preparation and culture of these lymphocytes.

The only satisfactory explanation for our findings is that there is a profound local tumor-derived lymphocyte suppression in esophageal squamous cell carcinoma. This suppressing influence is effective against both B and T lymphocytes and should provide an advantage for metastasizing tumor cells to the regional lymph nodes. The mediator demonstrated in the tissue culture fluid is most likely the same agent of immunosuppression at the local tumor level in vivo. A soluble immune suppressing factor with similar biological properties is seen in the serum of patients with advanced squamous cell carcinoma of the esophagus.

Interleukin 2 therapy in vitro did not reverse the suppressor influence on lymphoproliferative responses, LAK cell generation, or preformed LAK cell cytotoxic killing activity. Extrapolating from these studies to the in vivo situation, it seems that an effective antitumor immune response is not possible for squamous cell carcinoma due to the powerful immunosuppressing influence of the tumor.

LAK cells are capable of killing esophageal carcinoma cells with high efficiency in the absence of the soluble suppressor (unpublished observation). If adaptive immunotherapy using ex vivo generated LAK cells or biological response modifiers is to achieve clinical reality for this tumor, negation or reversal of tumor-derived immunosuppression is a prerequisite. Debulking therapy may therefore have a primary role as the most effective way of removing the suppressor source—the tumor.

ACKNOWLEDGMENTS: This work was supported by grants from the Irish Health Research Board, The Cancer Research Fund at Mercy Hospital, Cork, and PARC Hospital Management. R-Interleukin 2 was a gift from Eurocetus, Amsterdam.

References

1. Oldham RK: Developmental therapeutics and the design of clinical trials. In: Principles of Cancer Biotherapy, Oldham RK (ed), New York, River Press Ltd, 1987, p 49.
2. Schulof RS, Goldstein AL, Sztein MB: Immune suppression: Therapeutic alterations. In: Principles of Cancer Biotherapy, Oldham RK (ed), New York, River Press Ltd., 1987, p 93.
3. North RJ: Suppressor cells: T cells and macrophages. In: Immunity to Cancer, Reif AE, Mitchell MS (eds), New York, Academic Press Inc., 1988, p 239.
4. Hoon PSB, Bowker RJ, Cochran AJ: Suppressor cell activity in melanoma: Draining lymph nodes. Cancer Res 47:1529, 1987.
5. Clayberger C, Wright A, Medeiros LJ, Loller TW, Link MP, Smith SD, Warnke RA, Krensky AM: Absence of cell surface LFA-1 as a mechanism of escape from immunosurveillance. Lancet 2:8558:533–536, 1987.

7

DNA Histogram in Esophageal Carcinoma Measured by Flow Cytometry

Taizo Minami, Hideaki Yamana, Genzan Shirozu, Kazuyoshi Sakamoto, Hiromasa Fujita, Teruo Kakegawa, Mitchel Mitsuo Yokoyama

Introduction

Flow cytometric technology enables us to investigate a large number of cells for their nuclear constituents. The automated mechanical analysis has the advantages of being more objective, rapid, and accurate than microspectrophotometric analysis. Numerous investigations of a variety of solid human carcinomas have been carried out by flow cytometric analysis.[1–3] Few studies on esophageal carcinomas using this technique have been reported to date. The aim of this study is to determine whether measurement of nuclear DNA contents by flow cytometry can be of value for the assessment of the degree of malignancy in esophageal carcinoma.

Materials and Methods

Techniques of Flow Cytometry

Five patients with early esophageal carcinoma and 45 patients with advanced esophageal carcinomas who had not received pre-

Ferguson MK, Little AG, Skinner DB: Diseases of the Esophagus, Vol. I: Malignant Diseases. Futura Publishing Company, Inc., Mount Kisco, NY, © 1990.

operative combined immunochemotherapy and radiotherapy were selected for cell nuclear DNA measurement. The samples, which included not only carcinoma cells but also cells taken from the macroscopically unchanged esophageal mucosa, were investigated in 10 patients. Peripheral blood lymphocytes from each patient were used as standards for measuring DNA Index (DI) value.

DNA Flow Cytometry

Fresh tissue samples were placed in RPMI 1640 culture medium and minced into small pieces and the tissues were treated by 1000 units/mL Protease (Godo Shusei Co., Ltd.) for 2 to 4 hours at 37°C with continuous agitation. The cell suspension obtained was passed through a stainless steel mesh filter (40 μm) and subsequently treated with 2 mL of Triton X-100 (pH 9.5) to disrupt the cell membrane. The disrupted materials were resuspended in 200 mL of 1% RNase solution and cell nuclear DNA was stained with 20 μL of 0.02% ethidium bromide. The measurement of nuclear DNA content was undertaken by flow cytometry (Spectrum III, Ortho Diagnostic Systems, Raritan, NJ).

The G_0/G_1 peak of cancerous stem cells in relation to that of lymphocytes is defined as the DI value. In cases where there was less than 20% pure carcinoma cells, the measurement of DI value was difficult and unreliable, and consequently the DNA analysis was stopped.

Statistical Analysis

DNA ploidy patterns and DI values were analyzed in comparison to pathologic staging and histologic assessment using Student's *t*-test and chi-squared test.

Results

DNA Ploidy Pattern of the Tumor

Figure 1 shows a representative DNA histogram obtained from fresh cases of esophageal squamous cell carcinoma. Twenty-four (48.0%) carcinoma samples contained a single G_0/G_1 peak and were

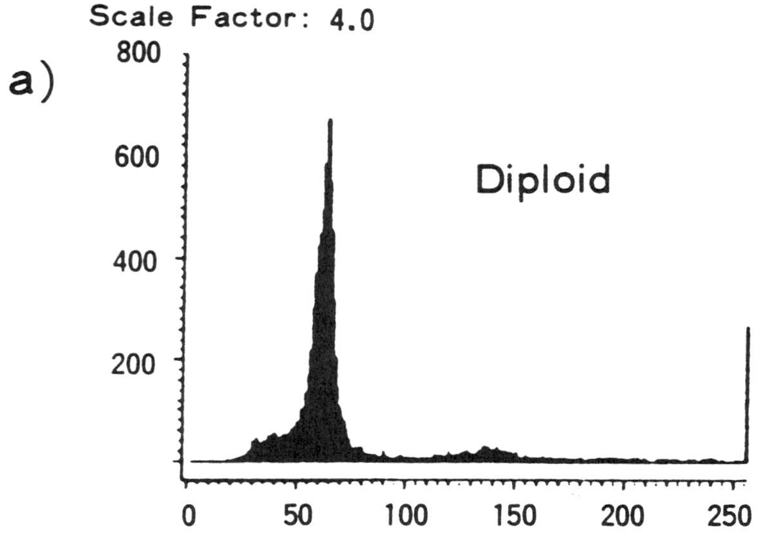

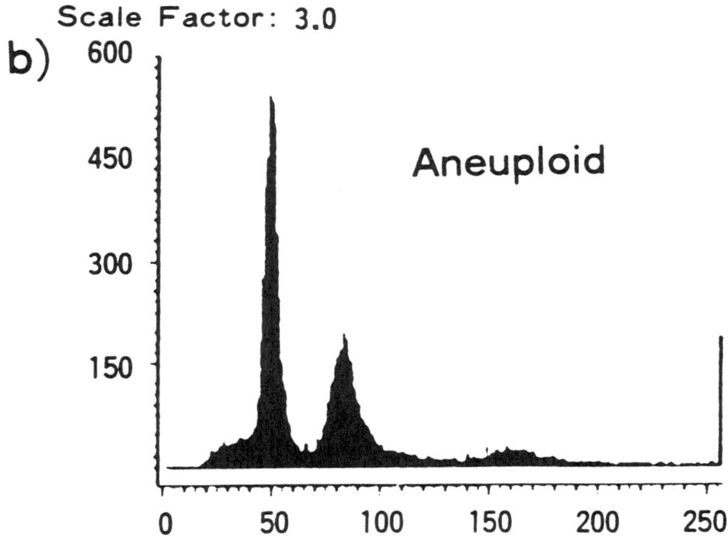

Figure 1: DNA histograms of esophageal carcinoma. (a) A 69-year-old female, with poorly differentiated squamous cell carcinoma showing no aneuploid peaks. (b) A 69-year-old male, with a moderately differentiated squamous cell carcinoma, and a distinct aneuploid G_0/G_1 peak with a DI of 1.6.

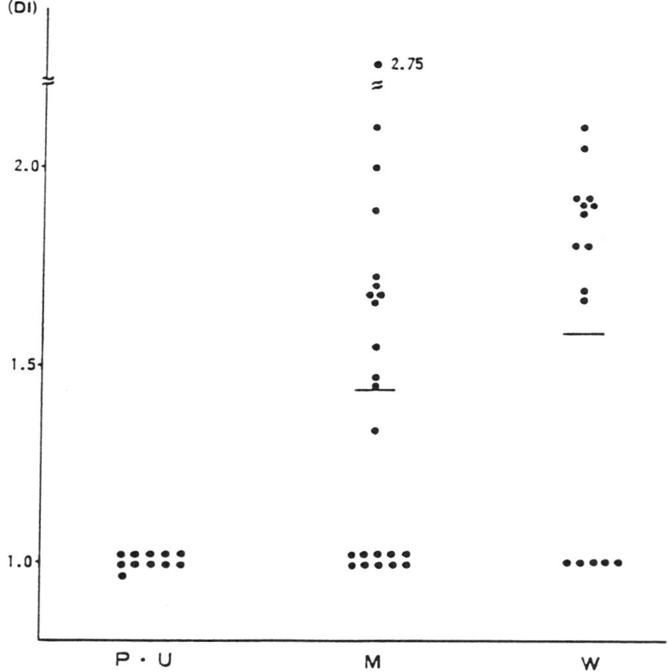

Figure 2: DNA index values according to histologic tumor grade. P = poorly differentiated squamous cell carcinoma, U = undifferentiated carcinoma. M = moderately differentiated squamous cell carcinoma. W = Well-differentiated squamous cell carcinoma.

classified as diploid. Aneuploidy, as shown by a second G_0/G_1 population, was found in 26 (52.0%) samples.

DNA Index Value in Measured Materials

All 10 samples of normal esophageal mucosa had diploid DNA histograms. In contrast, 26 of 50 esophageal carcinomas were aneuploid. Only one of five early carcinomas was aneuploid and the remainder of them were diploid. The DNA ploidy patterns based on the histologic type of the carcinoma are shown in Figure 2. Ten poorly differentiated squamous cell carcinomas and one undifferentiated carcinoma were all diploid. Ten of 23 (43.5%) moderately differentiated

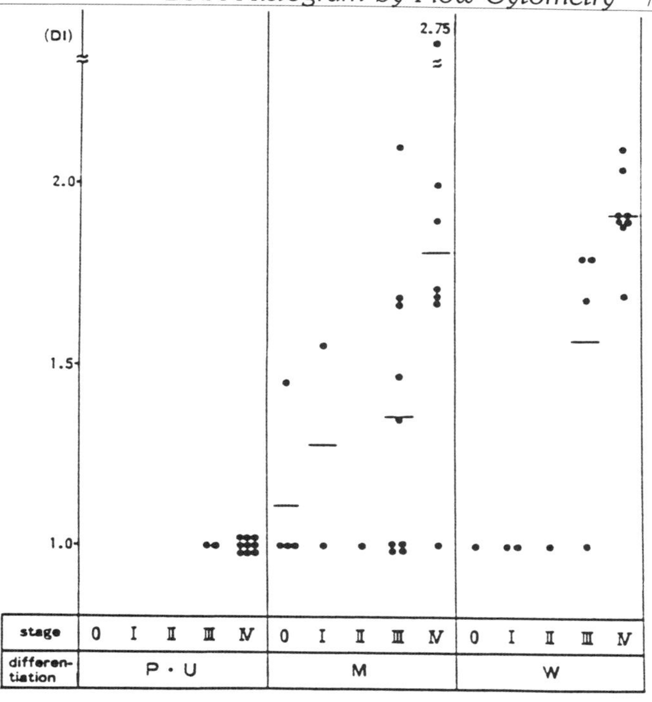

Figure 3: Correlation between DNA index values and histologic stage.[4] P = poorly differentiated squamous cell carcinoma, U = undifferentiated carcinoma. M = moderately differentiated squamous cell carcinoma. W = well-differentiated squamous cell carcinoma.

carcinomas were diploid and the others were aneuploid. The mean DI value in these cases was 1.4 ± 0.5. Five of 16 (31.3%) well-differentiated carcinomas were diploid and the other 11 cases were aneuploid with a mean DI value of 1.6 ± 0.4.

The relationship between the pathological stage of the carcinoma and the DI values is shown in Figure 3.[4] In the moderately differentiated groups, the DI value of stage 0 carcinomas was 1.1 ± 0.2, stage 1 was 1.3 ± 0.3, stage 2 was 1.0, stage 3 was 1.4 ± 0.4, and stage 4 was 1.8 ± 0.5. In well-differentiated groups, stages 0–2 were all 1.0, stage 3 was 1.6 ± 0.3, and stage 4 was 1.9 ± 0.1. DI values in carcinomas with advanced pathological stage tend to be greater than those of the earlier stage carcinomas. DI values in correspondence to the degree of lymph node metastases and depth of invasion showed a tendency similar to the pathological staging.

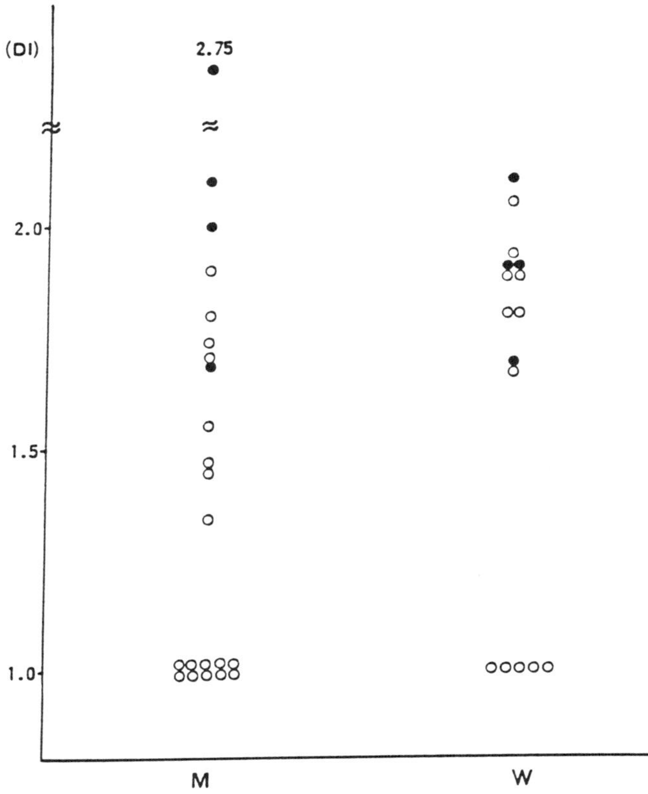

Figure 4: Postoperative prognosis of 39 esophageal carcinomas. ● = death from early recurrence within 1 year.

The relationship between postoperative death associated with recurrent cancer and the DI value was interesting. Thirty-seven of 50 cases treated by radical surgery survived for more than 1 postoperative year. Of the remaining patients, 11 died with lymph node and/or organ metastasis and two died following pulmonary arterial rupture due to carcinoma invasion, all within 1 year of surgery. Five of 11 (45.5%) patients with poorly or undifferentiated carcinomas, 4 of 23 (17.4%) in the moderately differentiated group, and 4 of 16 (25.0%) in the well-differentiated group died after early recurrence. Interestingly, 6 of 16 patients with moderately or well-differentiated carcinomas (37.5%) with DI ≧ 1.7 died after early recurrence, while only

2 of 23 carcinomas (8.7%) with DI < 1.7 died from recurrent cancer (Fig. 4).

Discussion

Flow cytometric analysis of nuclear DNA content has been developed as a means of identifying and characterizing tumor cell populations. In the present study, measurement of the nuclear DNA content in fresh specimens of esophageal carcinoma using flow cytometry was carried out. Aneuploidy in esophageal carcinoma was found in 26 of 50 (52.0%) cases, while the ploidy of normal esophageal mucosa was normal. Thus, nuclear DNA content of esophageal carcinoma was found to be distinctly different from that of the normal mucosa. These results suggest the activation of oncogenes or alteration of chromosomes during the course of initiation or progression in cancer cell growth.

Aneuploidy seemed to prevail in the groups of moderately and well-differentiated squamous cell carcinomas, while the group of undifferentiated and poorly differentiated carcinomas showed diploidy pattern alone. These results are different from those in carcinomas of the uterus and squamous cell carcinoma of the cervix,[5] in which diploid pattern is seen mainly in well-differentiated carcinomas. On the other hand, aneuploidy seems to prevail in well-differentiated gastric adenocarcinomas, while undifferentiated carcinomas have been shown to be diploid.[6]

The technique of flow cytometry does not allow absolute correct determination of diploid patterns, though it gives a good estimate. Thus, correlations between the histological type and the ploidy pattern must be viewed with some caution, taking into consideration the methodology used, the number of cases investigated, the heterogeneous composition of tumors, and the differences among organs being studied.

In the group of well-differentiated esophageal carcinomas, there was a fair correlation between the DI value and the degree of lymph node metastasis, the depth of invasion and the histologic stage. Furthermore, early death due to recurrence after radical esophagectomy was noted in cases with high DI value (DI $\geqq$ 1.7). The present results, therefore, demonstrate that determination of DI is useful in estimating the prognosis of patients with well-differentiated esophageal cancers. Other specific parameters are needed for evaluating the prognosis in poorly and undifferentiated carcinomas.

References

1. Macartney JC, Camplejohn R, Powell G: DNA flow cytometry of histological material from human gastric cancer. J Pathol 148:273, 1986.
2. Helio H, Karahar E, Nordling S: Flow cytometric determination of DNA content in malignant and benign bone tumors. Cytometry 6:165, 1985.
3. Ljungberg B, Stenling B, Roos G: DNA content and prognosis in renal cell carcinoma. Cancer 57:2346, 1986.
4. Japanese Society for Esophageal Disease: Guidelines for the clinical and pathologic studies on carcinoma of the esophagus. Jpn J Surg 6:70–86, 1976.
5. Atkin NB: Prognostic significance of ploidy level in human tumors: Carcinoma of the uterus. J Natl Cancer Inst 56:909, 1976.
6. Petrova AS, Subrichina GN, Tschistjakova OV, et al: Flow cytofluorometry, cytomorphology and histology in gastric carcinoma. Oncology 37:318, 1980.

8

Studies on the Growing Time of Esophageal Cancer

Satoshi Okura, Kin-chi Nabeya, Tateo Hanaoka, Kimio Onozawa, Shigen Ri, Tetsuya Nyumura

Introduction

Studies on the growing time of esophageal cancer, in spite of remarkable progress made in various examination methods for gastroenterologic tumors, are still unsatisfactory. Evaluating radiographic images retrospectively is an effective method in detecting the course of cancer growth. Significant progress has been made in gastric and colon cancers, but in esophageal cancer, the radiographic material is scarce. One reason for this is that the developing rate of esophageal cancer is relatively fast. In addition to this, opportunities for patients to undergo examination for this disease are rare, while from the physician's side, x-ray examinations require a certain skill to elicit subtle signs of early cancer. We performed a retrospective radiographic study to determine tumor volume growing time and the developing time of depth of invasion through the esophageal wall.

Materials and Methods

The subjects for investigation were 336 patients with esophageal cancer treated at the Second Department of Surgery at Kyorin Uni-

Ferguson MK, Little AG, Skinner DB: Diseases of the Esophagus, Vol. I: Malignant Diseases. Futura Publishing Company, Inc., Mount Kisco, NY, © 1990.

versity School of Medicine from 1973 to April 1989. Of this total, both curative and noncurative resected cases numbered 254, for a resection rate of 75.6%.

The investigation utilized patients who had been diagnosed as having esophageal squamous cell carcinoma in the past, and in whom x-ray films were available. Radiographic examinations were made on the rate of cancer growth in patients in whom follow-up was possible. The doubling time (DT) was calculated from the formula of Kusama[1] for estimating ideal growth rates of tumor length:

$$DT = \frac{t}{3}\left(\frac{\log 2}{\log d_2 - \log d_1}\right)$$

where the time interval needed for tumor length d_1 to develop to d_2 is t (months). To calculate the developing time of depth of invasion, measurements were made of the estimated depth of invasion in patients who had at least one radiograph made prior to the time of diagnosis. The final radiographic estimated depth of invasion was compared with the histologic depth of invasion on the resected specimen, based on a current classification of depth of invasion.

Cancer Developing Time

Radiographically, the average DT of 19 lesions in 18 patients in whom retrospective study was possible was 6.4 months. There were three cases in which the DT was less than 1 month and, contrarily, there were three cases in which the DT was more than 12 months (Table I). The majority of lesions were located in the middle thoracic esophagus. The x-ray taken at the time of diagnosis showed the spiral type of advanced cancer to be most frequent. There were four lesions of the superficial type, and of these, the DT of two cases was comparatively long.

Developing Time of Depth of Invasion in the Esophageal Wall

The developing time of depth of invasion in the esophageal wall was investigated in 19 lesions in 18 patients in whom radiographs prior to the time of diagnosis allowed depth of invasion estimation

Table I
Doubling Time of Esophageal Cancer

Case No.	*Age at Time of Diagnosis*	*Sex*	*Radiographic Pattern*	*Tumor Length*	*Doubling Time (DT) (months)*
1	65	M	funnelled	4.2	0.54
2	63	M	serrated	4.6	0.55
3	56	M	spiral	7.3	0.82
4	67	M	spiral	10.5	1.07
5	63	M	spiral	8.5	1.94
6	70	M	spiral	8.5	3.11
7	49	M	spiral	5.6	3.20
8	48	M	spiral	7.5	3.38
9	74	F	tumorous	3.4	3.43
10	63	M	spiral	9.7	4.86
11	56	M	superficial	3.4	4.98
12	68	M	serrated	4.6	5.56
13	50	M	spiral	7.0	6.74
14	75	M	spiral	4.8	4.69
			superficial	1.8	7.83
15	70	M	superficial	3.5	9.66
16	68	M	spiral	6.5	15.24
17	57	M	funnelled	3.3	17.67
18	70	F	superficial	1.8	25.40
					6.35 ± 6.38

$$DT = \frac{t}{3}\left(\frac{\log 2}{\log d_2 - \log d_1}\right)$$

d_1 = initial tumor length
d_2 = secondary tumor length
t = time interval for d_1 to develop to d_2 (months)

in the esophageal wall. Measurement of the histologic depth of invasion was made on the resected specimen (Table II).

The retrospective estimated depth of invasion and histologic depth of invasion in the resected specimens are shown in Table III. From m (mucosa) to sm (submucosa), the time interval was 16.0 ± 7.8 months; from sm to a_2, a_3 (invasion beyond muscularis propria) was 6.6 ± 3.8 months; and from m to a_2, a_3 was 21.1 ± 6.8 months. The interval from m to sm, and from sm to a_2, a_3 when added, is approximately 23 months. This is quite close to the interval of 21.1 ± 6.8 months of m to a_2, a_3. The case illustrated in Figure 1 is a 56-

Table II
The Depth of Invasion Estimation Standard of the Retrospective Radiograph

1. With double contrast method, superficial cancer was suspected and definite changes were acknowledged.
   - a. shallow niche
   - b. irregular low protuberance
   - c. shallow ulcer

   } (sm)

2. With double contrast method, no definite change acknowledged.
   - a. spots from barium residue
   - b. light and shade differentiations
   - c. sclerosis and irregularities of wall margins

   } (m)

3. Definitely advanced cancer
4. Filled image (excluded)

year-old male with a shallow ulcer that was presumed to be an sm cancer which in 5 months' time advanced to a_3.

Discussion

In order to study the growth course of gastroenterologic cancers, it is useful to perform retrospective radiographic evaluations. In stud-

Table III
Developing Time of Depth of Invasion in Esophageal Cancer

Initial Time	Resected Time	Number of Lesions	Duration (months)
1. (m) → sm		4	16.0 ± 7.8
2. (sm) ———	→ a_2, a_3	3	6.6 ± 3.8
3. (a_1, a_2)	→ a_2, a_3	4	4.5 ± 1.8
4. (m) ———	→ a_2, a_3	8	21.1 ± 6.8

( ) = Assumed initial depth of invasion
m = mucosal cancer
sm = submucosal cancer
a_1 = invasion barely reaching the adventitia
a_2 = definite invasion to the adventitia
a_3 = invasion into the neighboring structures

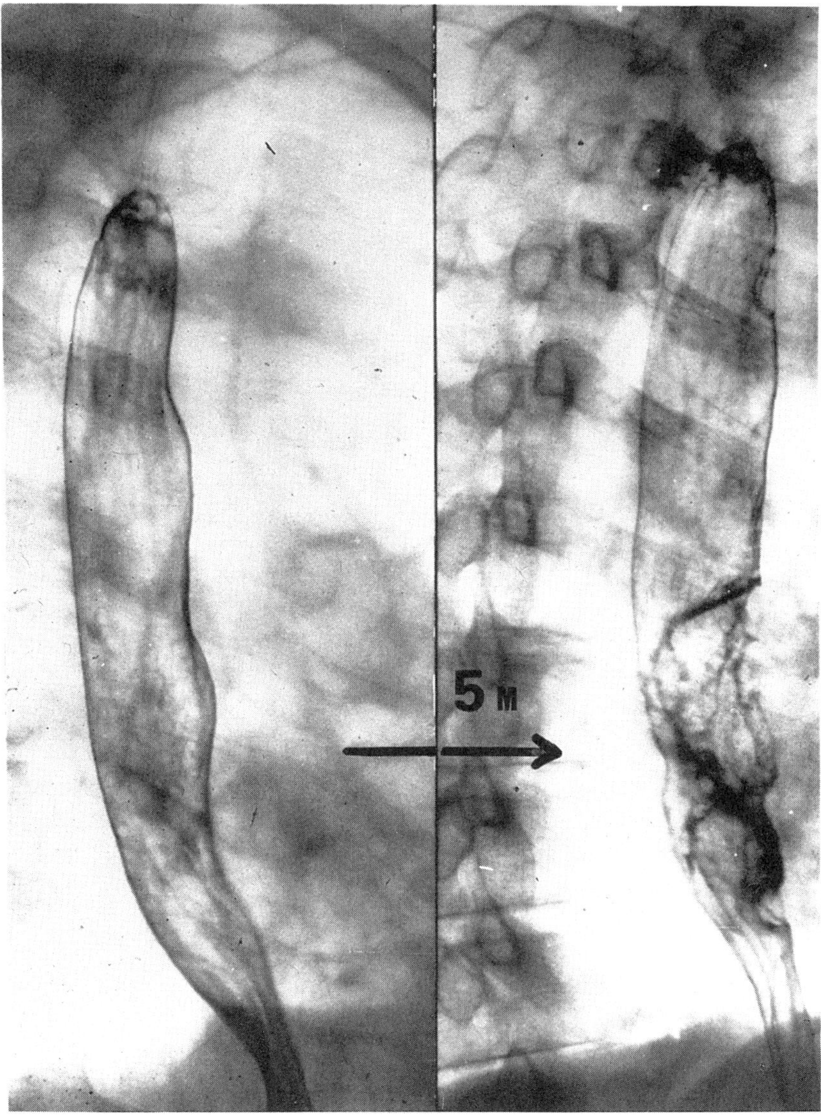

Figure 1: Estimated sm cancer progressing to a_3 cancer within 5 months.

ies on esophageal cancer in particular, the correct diagnosis of radiographic images of minute lesions is essential. This requires taking measures to ensure a high quality image. Techniques for creating double contrast radiographs have been reported.[3] It is thought that comparisons of the filled image, the double contrast picture, and mucosal fold wall image are important.[4]

A technique for estimating the developing time of cancer was proposed by Collins[5] in 1956. The development of a tumor is similar to index functioning. If one assumes that the growing rate of a tumor is constant, then the concept of DT can be introduced. This concept is now being used in the observation of growth processes of various organs and, in Japan, has become an index for determining the degree of malignancy and treatment methods.[1]

Nakamura et al.[6] have calculated a growth curve for gastric cancer. According to Kohri et al.[7] and Kawai et al.,[8] in early cancer the DT has a long duration, from 2 to 6 years, but in advanced cancer the DT is only 3 to 10 months. In colon cancer, according to Ushio et al.[9] and Matsuura et al.,[10] the DT of early cancer was 4 years, 4 months, and 2 years, respectively, which is quite long. In advanced cancer, the DT was 1 year and 7 months, respectively. It is apparent that in gastric and colon cancers, the DT of early cancer is lengthy, in advanced cancer the DT is short, and the difference between the two is great. Considering the growth of esophageal cancer, there are retrospective evaluations made radiographically by Fujita et al.[11] and Ogino et al.[12] that, in comparison with gastric and colon cancers, show the growth of esophageal cancer to be far more rapid.

The DT in our study was, on average, 6.4 months. There were extremely short cases doubling within 1 month and lengthy cases that took more than 1 year. The DT of the superficial type of early cancer tended to be long.

This result corresponds with the calculation of the developing time of depth of invasion in the wall: m to sm taking a rather long 16 months, while sm to a_2, a_3 (advanced cancer) took a rather short 7 months.

Momma[13] made an estimation from a clinical pathological viewpoint that the developing time of early esophageal carcinoma is slow.

The evaluations of cases in one study show that the m to sm cases took approximately 70% of the entire interval time of 16 months; and sm to a_2, a_3 (advanced lesions) took approximately 20% to 30% of the entire interval time, the latter progressing rapidly.

Evaluations of the growth of early cancer show that these can be divided into cancer cases that grow inward (the inner cavity type) and another type that progresses on the esophageal wall (the wall type).[14] Superficial type cancers that are thought to be the wall type have symptoms which are usually quite mild. Therefore, opportunities for x-ray examinations during this period are rare, and even if there is an opportunity, the delineation of the radiographic picture is poor and the cancer is often overlooked. Until the lesion is detected, it obviously continues to develop. It is most desirable to educate people regarding esophageal cancer. The public should undergo mass screening in areas where this disease is endemic. Such examinations should be made once every 6 months, preferably with first-class diagnostic techniques that permit the diagnosis of esophageal cancer in its earliest stage.

References

1. Kusama S: Chronology of the cancer. In: Clinical Tumorology, Japan, Nankodo Publishing Co., 1982, p 129.
2. Japapese Society for Esophageal Diseases: Guidelines for tbe clinical and pathologic studies on carcinoma of the esophagus. Jpn J Surg 6:69, 1976.
3. Shirakabe H, Nishizawa M: Diagnosis of intramucosal carcinoma of the esophagus. Stomach and Intestine 20:1311, 1985.
4. Nabeya K, Okura S, Hanaoka T, et al: Radiological studies of esophageal cancer development with emphasis on serial esophagography and Fuji computed radiography. Dis Esoph 1:23, 1988.
5. Collins VP, Laeffler RK, Tivey H: Observations on growth rates of human tumors. Am J Roentogenol 76:988, 1956.
6. Nakamura K, Ashizawa S, Takada H, et al: Correlation of time interval and gastric cancer size: so-called growth curve of gastric cancer (in Japanese). Stomach and Intestine 13:89, 1978.
7. Kohri T, Yamashita S, Shimamoto K, et al: The growth and propagation of gastric cancer in the human body (in Japanese). The Saishin-Igaku 24:471, 1969.
8. Kawai K, Takekoshi T, Ida K, et al: The course of gastric cancer: An opinion on two to three retrospective clinical cases (in Japanese). The Saishin-Igaku 24:909, 1969.
9. Ushio K, Shima Y, Gotoh H, et al: Growth and progression of colorectal cancer: Retrospective study based on roentgenologic findings. Stomach and Intestine 20:843, 1985.
10. Matsuura A, Kobayashi S, Kasugai T: Growth of colorectal cancer based on review of follow-up cases. Stomach and Intestine 20:859, 1985.
11. Fujita H, Hashimoto T, Shimazu H, et al: Retrospective study on cases of unsuspepted esophageal carcinoma. Jpn J Gastroenterol Surg 14:1, 1981.
12. Ogino T, Mai M, Akimoto R, et al: Growth of esophageal cancer by ret-

rospectlye follow-up study of esophagographies. Jpn J Gastroenterol Surg 17:2109, 1989.
13. Momma K: Clinico-pathological study on the mode of deeper infiltration of the esophageal cancer. Jpn J Gastroenterol Surg 7:93, 1974.
14. Nabeya K, Takigawa H, Ri S: Early esophageal cancer: Definition, pathology, present status and prognosis. Stomach and Intestine 11:285, 1976.

II.

Diagnosis and Staging: Editors' Overview

Early detection of esophageal cancer is thought to be the primary means by which the overall prognosis for this disease can be improved. Using a variety of cytologic techniques mass screening studies conducted in provincial regions of China where esophageal cancer is endemic demonstrate improved survival. The major difficulties in applying these methods to other populations include problems in identifying high-risk patient groups and socioeconomic issues such as cost-effectiveness. Similar difficulties attend other early identification techniques discussed in this section. In Chapter 9, Yamaki and his co-workers illustrate the utility of high resolution double contrast radiography in the diagnosis of early invasive cancers, particularly those which are morphologically of the elevated type. Nishizawa and Okada describe endoscopic techniques for detecting early esophageal cancer in Chapter 10. Their methods, which combine careful analysis of even slight changes in mucosal color and architecture with intravital staining to facilitate directed biopsy, are particularly useful for patients identified by cytologic screening studies. In Chapter 11, a similar approach to one high-risk group is discussed by Shiozaki et al., who demonstrate the utility of endoscopy with intravital staining in screening patients with a previous head and neck cancer.

Numerous staging systems currently exist for esophageal cancer. The Japanese efforts in establishing a clinically useful system have been particularly fruitful due to the high incidence of this disease in Japan as well as to their typically careful means of investigation. Nevertheless, further refinements are necessary to maximize the utility of clinical and pathological staging. In Chapter 12, Akiyama and his co-workers demonstrate that gross tumor morphology as determined radiographically or endoscopically can serve as an independent determinant of prognosis. In addition to appearance, tumor location can influence the applicability of standard TNM staging. For example, it is often difficult to apply the TNM system to cancers of the gastroesophageal junction. Similarly, Ruol et al. in Chapter 13 show that cervical esophageal cancers do not lend themselves to accurate prognostic staging based on the current TNM methodology, and suggest that superior mediastinal nodes be included as regional nodes for such cancers.

Computed tomography is the primary investigation currently used for clinical staging of esophageal cancer. A variety of new techniques have recently been introduced, among them endoscopic ultrasonography (EUS) and magnetic resonance imaging (MRI). Chapters 14, 15, and 16 discuss the utility of EUS, particularly in comparison to computed tomography. EUS is very accurate in determining gross depth of penetration, and has the remarkable ability to assess metastatic involvement of regional lymph nodes irrespective of their size. The primary problem with this technique at present is its limited usefulness in examining patients with highly obstructing lesions. Current efforts aimed at miniaturizing the ultrasound probe should overcome much of this difficulty. Finally, in Chapter 17, Maas et al. evaluate MRI as a staging tool. Even using ECG-gating to eliminate loss of resolution due to cardiac motion, MRI does not appear to have any advantage over CT except when sagittal and coronal images are used to evaluate aortic involvement. For regional staging, EUS appears to be the most accurate technique currently available.

9

Radiographic Detection of Early Esophageal Carcinoma

Goro Yamaki, Isamu Yamamoto, Kyooo Nanaumi, Hiroshi Akiyama, Masahiko Tsurumaru, Yoshimasa Ono, Harushi Udagawa, Hikoo Shirakabe, Hisao Hayakawa

Introduction

Early carcinoma is defined as one whose invasion is limited to the submucosal layer (sm-carcinoma) and which has no metastasis.[1] Present statistics compiled in Japan on a nationwide scale of the 5-year survival rate after operation for early carcinoma (Fig. 1) show that this is dependent upon differences in depth of invasion. Patients who had esophageal intraepithelial carcinoma (ep-carcinoma) survived at a rate of 100%, patients who had carcinoma whose invasion had reached the muscularis mucosae (mm-carcinoma) survived at a rate of 85.3%, and patients who had sm-carcinoma survived at a comparatively low rate of 69.2%. This means that, if our aim in diagnosis is limited only to finding sm-carcinoma, we will not obtain the most desirable prognosis. Our aim should be extended to finding not only sm-carcinoma, but also ep-carcinoma and/or mm-carcinoma. To this end, we have studied the following questions:

Ferguson MK, Little AG, Skinner DB: Diseases of the Esophagus, Vol. I: Malignant Diseases. Futura Publishing Company, Inc., Mount Kisco, NY, © 1990.

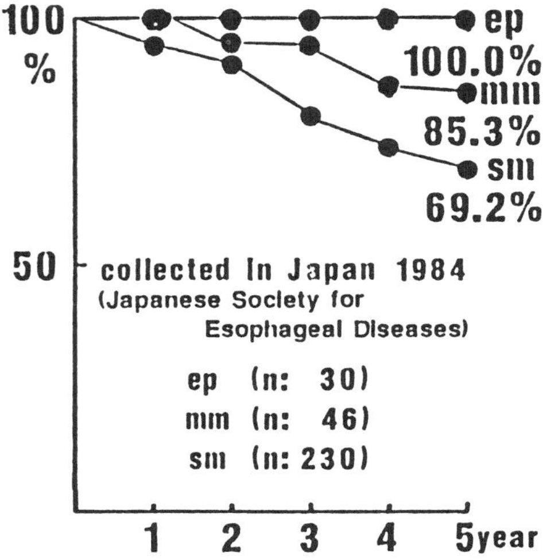

Figure 1: Postoperative 5-year survival rate of early esophageal carcinoma.

(1) With what accuracy is it possible for us to interpret initial x-ray examinations as suspicious for ep-carcinoma and/or mm-carcinoma, compared with the accuracy rate of finding sm-carcinoma?

(2) At what rate can we attain x-ray findings by magnified x-ray examinations?

(3) How can we obtain clearer pictures of carcinomatous lesions?

Material

We studied 126 patients (165 cancers) with untreated ep-carcinoma, mm-carcinoma, and sm-carcinoma during the 15 years from 1973 to 1988. The results are shown in Table I, classified into two main categories: single carcinoma and multiple carcinoma. Each of them is again classified by their degree of invasion.

Single Contrast Versus Double Contrast Radiographs

It is said that at x-ray examination, early lesions of carcinoma are frequently overlooked. Therefore, we have closely studied the like-

Table I
Materials Used in this Study: Toranomon Hospital, 1973–1988

	ep	*mm*	*sm*
single	16 (16)*	21 (21)	63 (63)
multiple	3 (9)	3 (6)	20 (50)

* Number of cases (number of lesions)
ep = Intraepithelial carcinoma
mm = Invaded to muscularis mucosae
sm = Invaded to the submuscoal layer

lihood of successful depiction of lesions using magnification radiographs. We have studied them in view of the macroscopic shape, degree of invasion, and size of lesion.

In the case of elevated-type lesions (IIA), single contrast pictures enabled us to locate a lesion of sm-carcinoma whose size was 3.5 cm in diameter in two pictures out of eight (25%), and those of mm-carcinoma whose size was 3.0 cm in four pictures out of 13 (31%). It was not possible for us to locate any carcinomas smaller than these, including the lesions of sm-carcinoma, as shown in Figure 2a. However, the double contrast pictures, as shown in Figure 2b, enabled us to located the lesions of sm-carcinomas larger than 1.4 cm at a rate of almost 100%, and those of sm-carcinoma whose size was 3.0 cm in 27 pictures out of 29 (93.1% success rate). The lesions of ep-carcinoma were identified in 21 pictures out of 48 (43.8% success rate). These results lead us to conclude that if double contrast pictures are taken of suspicious cases, there is a high possibility that cancerous lesions will be identified.

In the case of depressed-type lesions (IIc), single contrast pictures enabled us to locate the lesion of sm-carcinoma whose size was 3.0 cm in diameter in two pictures out of nine (22.2% success rate), as shown in Figure 3a. However, it was impossible for us to locate the lesions of mm-carcinoma and ep-carcinoma. On the other hand, the double contrast pictures enabled us to locate the lesions of sm-carcinoma larger than 2.5 cm in diameter at a rate of 100%, and the smaller mm-carcinomas were detected in 38.0% to 58.0%. We could locate a lesion of ep-carcinoma whose size was 2.5 cm in diameter in only four pictures out of 26 (15.4% success rate). This means that if the double contrast pictures are taken, even the lesions of mm-car-

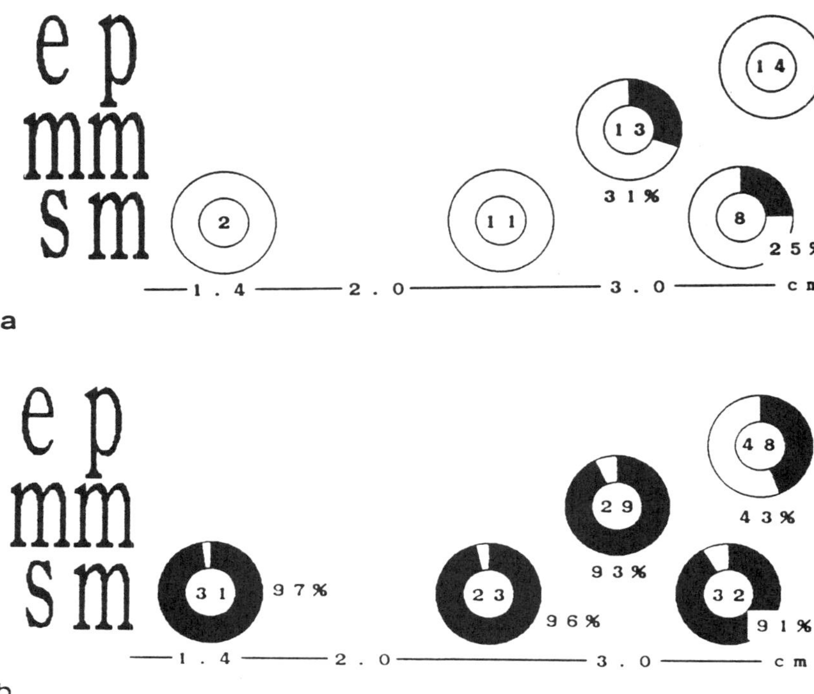

Figure 2: (a) The ratio of successful depiction of elevated-type lesions using single contrast x-ray techniques. (b) The ratio of successful depiction of elevated-type lesions using double contrast radiographs.

cinoma will be successfully found in one out of two patients. However, we cannot say anything for certain about the lesions of ep-carcinoma.

Diagnosis According to Depth of Invasion

Figure 4 shows the results of the initial x-ray examinations, classified by depth of invasion. There was only one case out of 16 that we could interpret as suspicious for ep-carcinoma (6.3% success rate), while in the case of sm-carcinoma, 57 out of 63 cases were successfully interpreted (90.5% success rate). There were a variety of reasons why we failed to correctly interpret the lesions in the other six cases with

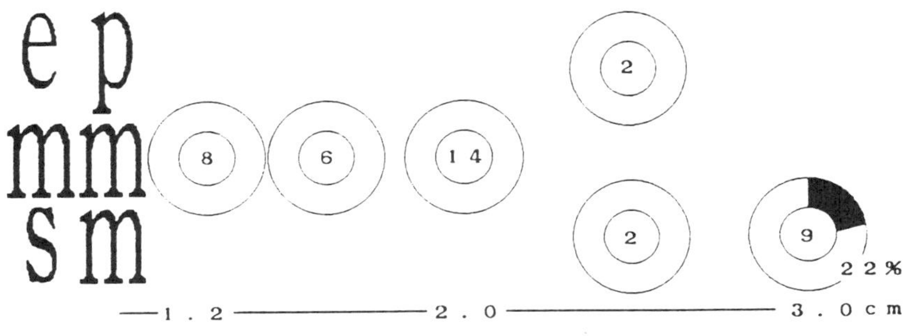

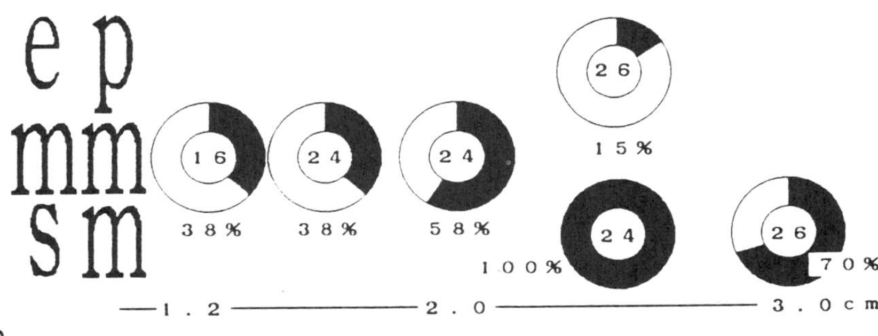

Figure 3: (a) The ratio of successful depiction of depressed-type lesions using single contrast techniques. (b) The ratio of successful depiction of depressed-type lesions using double contrast radiographs.

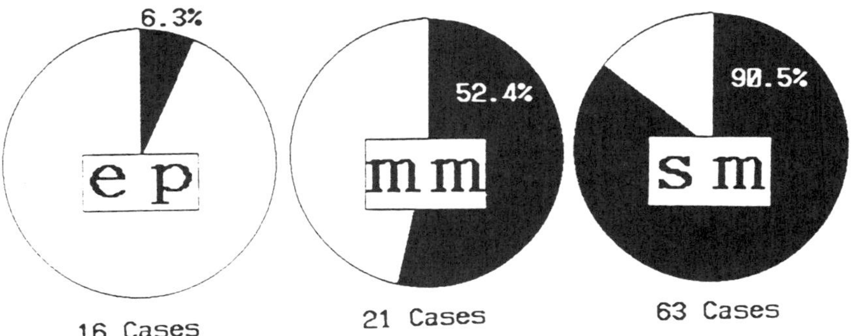

Figure 4: The results of the diagnostic ability of initial radiographic examination.

sm-carcinoma. In some cases, the sites of the lesions were hidden within the single contrast views. In other cases, the lesions were depicted but were overlooked when we interpreted the pictures. In summary, it was difficult to interpret the pictures as suspicious for ep-carcinoma in the initial x-ray examinations, but it was possible for us to locate about half of the lesions of mm-carcinoma.

Figure 5 is a double contrast picture of sm-carcinoma which was located in the middle esophagus. One can clearly see irregularity of the muscosal pattern 2 cm in length along the margin. In the case of sm-carcinoma, double contrast pictures will almost always allow us to diagnose lesions of sm-carcinoma having this much irregularity, providing we interpret the pictures carefully.

Diagnosis According to Morphology

Figure 6 shows the results of our interpretation of 16 lesions of ep-carcinoma, at the initial x-ray examination, based on their macroscopic shapes and sizes. There was only one case of an elevated-type lesion (IIa), but we did interpret it as suspicious for cancer. However, in the 15 cases of depressed-type lesions (IIc), it was totally impossible to interpret the pictures as suspicious for carcinoma regardless of their size. Even in the case of the elevated type of ep-carcinoma (IIa), it is possible to interpret the pictures as suspicious for the existence of cancerous lesions. The problem, however, remains as to the depressed type of lesions (IIc) as to how we can develop more accurate radiographic interpretation. Figures 7a and 7b show double contrast pictures of an ep-carcinoma in the lower part of the esophagus measuring 3.0 × 2.1 cm. Figure 7a shows the double contrast pictures of the specimen taken after resection, while Figure 7b is the one taken before the operation. In the area indicated by arrows, one can see a vague irregularity in the margin and some slight shade of barium covering the mucosa. In the case of IIc-type ep-carcinoma, very slight changes of this kind are often found. Our best efforts are required in interpreting such slight findings in these radiographs.

Figure 8 shows the examples of 21 cases of mm-carcinoma at the initial x-ray examination, examined in the same way as the ep-carcinoma lesions mentioned above. There were eight cases of elevated-type lesions (IIa) and five of them were interpreted as suspicious for cancer (62.5% success rate). The reasons why three cases were overlooked include failure to take double contrast pictures in two, and in

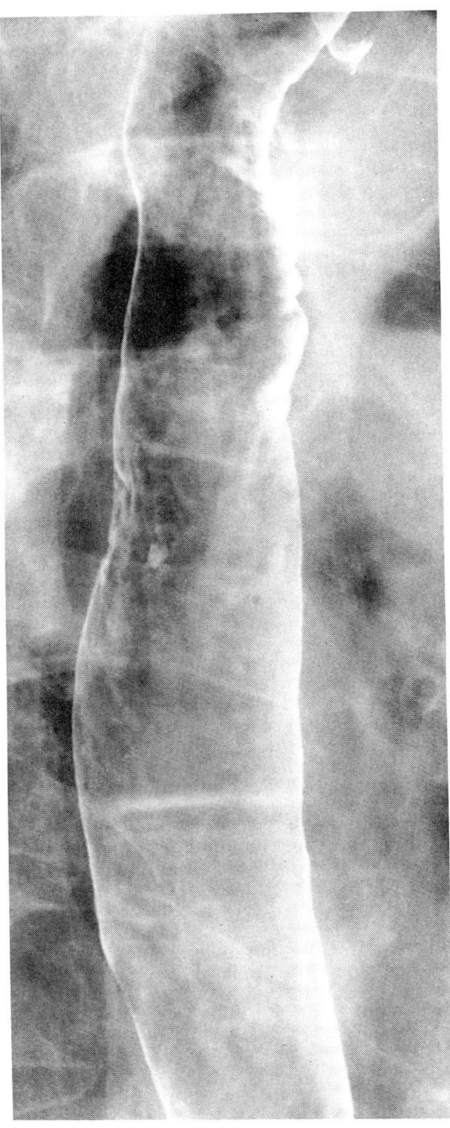

Figure 5: Preoperative double contrast picture of sm-carcinoma in the middle part of the esophagus.

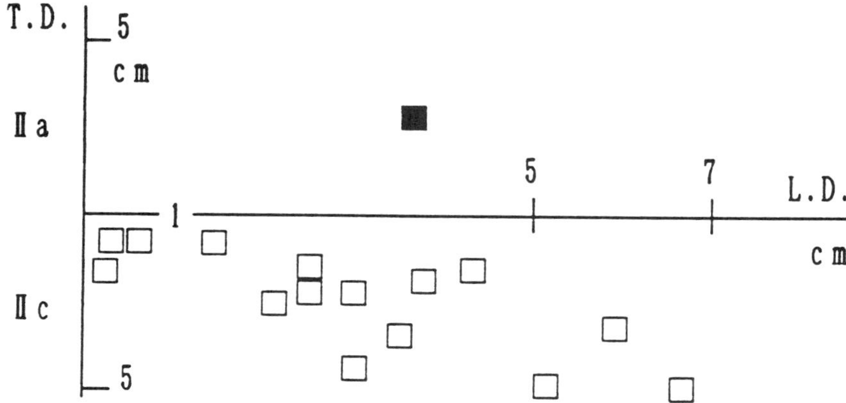

Figure 6: The results of our interpretation of ep-carcinoma according to their macroscopic shapes and sizes (initial x-ray examination). T.D. = transverse diameter; L.D. = longitudinal diameter (length); closed box = possible to interpret as suspicious for cancer; open box = impossible to interpret as suspicious for cancer.

one case the lesion was ep-carcinoma from a clinical viewpoint, although it invaded as deep as the musclaris muscosae in some areas. This tells us that if we employ double contrast radiographs routinely, we will rarely overlook elevated-type lesions (IIa).

There were 13 cases of the depressed-type lesions but we could interpret only three cases as suspicious for carcinoma (23.1% success rate). Even in the case of mm-carcinoma, we still have problems in interpreting the depressed-type lesions (IIc).

Figures 9a and 9b show a case of mm-carcinoma measuring 2 × 2 cm. In Figure 9a, a fully distended double contrast picture, there is unsatisfactory distension and a vague shadow of barium in the mucosal pattern (arrows). In the slightly distended double contrast picture shown in Figure 9b, however, we can see the same lesions far more clearly (arrows). Thus, slightly distended double contrast pictures are more effective for locating shallow depressions.

To sum up, there is no problem in locating elevated-type lesions of ep-carcinoma and mm-carcinoma (IIa). But in the case of the depressed-type lesions (IIc), it is totally impossible at present to locate the lesions of ep-carcinoma while there is some possibility of finding the lesions of mm-carcinoma. What are the reasons for this difference?

In trying to solve this problem, we have studied macroscopic

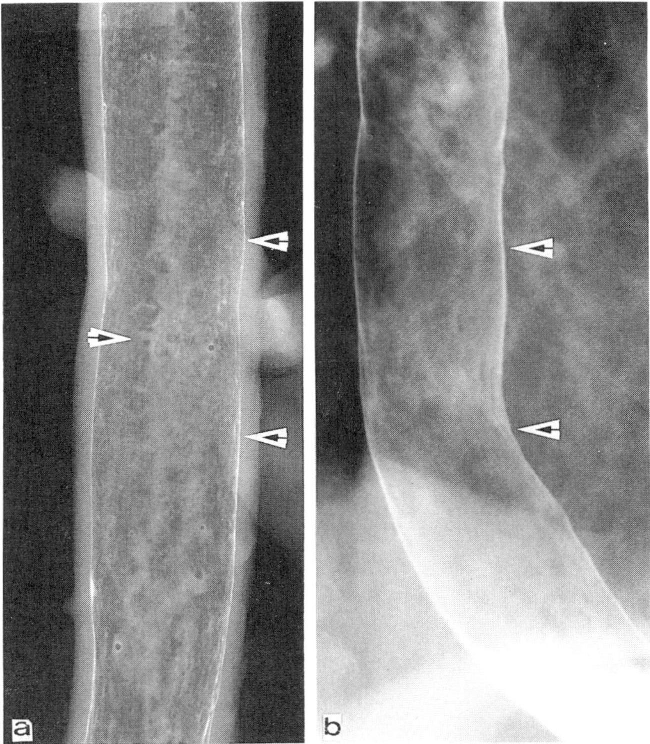

Figure 7: (a) Double contrast picture of ep-carcinoma in a resected specimen at the lower part of the esophagus. (b) Preoperative double contrast picture of the lesion.

appearances of ep-carcinoma and mm-carcinoma. The degree of depression of ep-carcinoma is very slight, close to flat. The margins of depression descend very gently, and almost no roughness on the surface can be recognized. The depth of depression, observed using a microscope, is 0.1 mm on the average. On the other hand, the lesions of mm-carcinoma are of the so-called "erosive type," and the margins of the depression can be clearly differentiated from the normal mucosa. Also, granularity and granular protrusion can be recognized at the bottom of the depression. The depth of depression observed using a microscope is from 0.2 to 0.4 mm on the average. That is, the lesions of ep-carcinoma are slighter in the degree of depression and less granular than the lesions of mm-carcinoma.

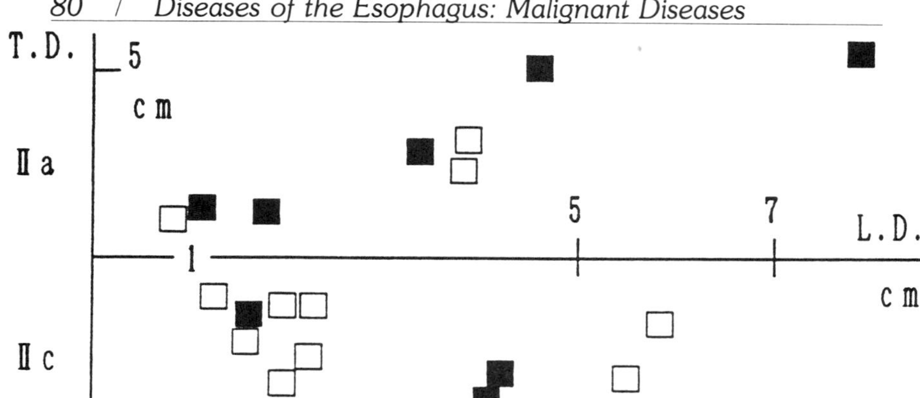

Figure 8: The results of our interpretation of mm-carcinoma according to macroscopic shapes and sizes (initial x-ray examination).

Therefore, it would be difficult not only to identify but to differentiate lesions of ep-carcinoma and mm-carcinoma, unless slightly distended double contrast radiographs are used routinely.

Multiple Cancers

As a result of pathological study, three cases of multiple ep-carcinoma in 19 cases (15.8%), three cases of multiple mm-carcinoma in 24 cases (12.5%), and 20 cases of multiple sm-carcinoma in 83 cases (24.1%) were found (Table I). In cases where one obvious lesion is diagnosed, we need to suspect other lesions of ep-carcinoma in the surrounding area. Figure 10 shows a case of multiple ep- and mm-carcinoma. In area A there is a shade of barium whose marginal lines are of irregular shape. Most of this lesion was dysplastic and an ep-carcinoma measuring 0.5 × 0.5 cm was found in the distal part of the lesion. A second area of irregular barium shading (B) proved to contain an mm-carcinoma measuring 0.5 × 0.5 cm. It is obvious that these changes can be quite subtle, and very careful interpretation is required when we diagnose multiple carcinomas.

Epithelial Spread

The nature of esophageal carcinoma is characterized by the spread of carcinoma into the intraepithelial mucosa, known as epi-

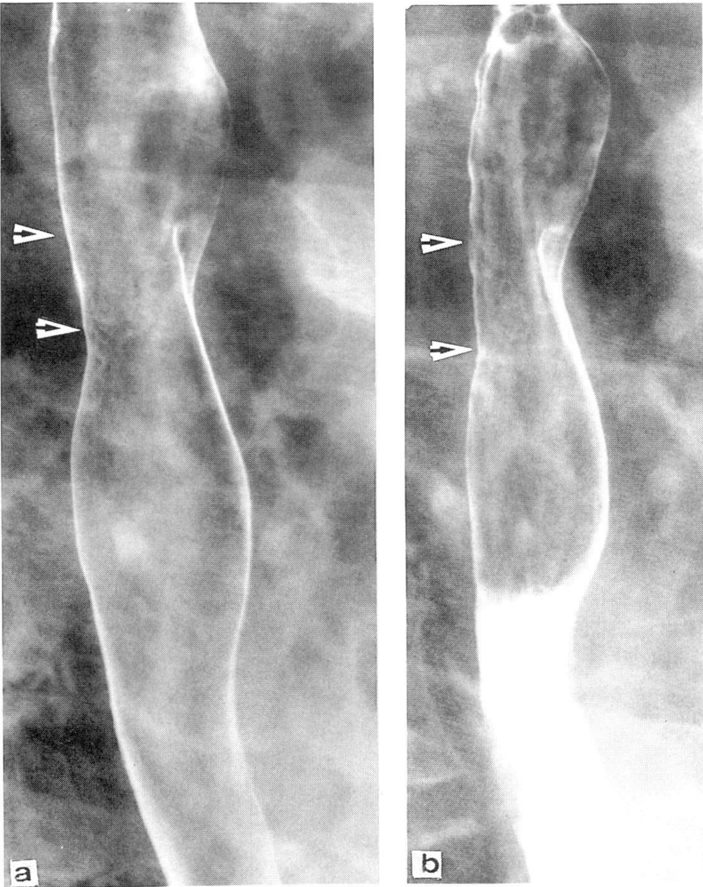

Figure 9: (a) A fully distended double contrast picture of mm-carcinoma. (b) The slightly distended double contrast picture.

thelial spread. Whether we give patients surgical treatment or x-ray therapy, it is important to clarify the margin of the proximal and distal spread.

The percentage of occurrence of lesions having ep-spread surrounding the main lesions throughout the esophagus was: mm-carcinoma, 10 lesions out of 32 (31.3%), and sm-carcinoma, 64 lesions out of 84 (76.2%). Figure 11 shows the sizes of the main lesions (the ones with the most marked elevation or depression, and the deepest

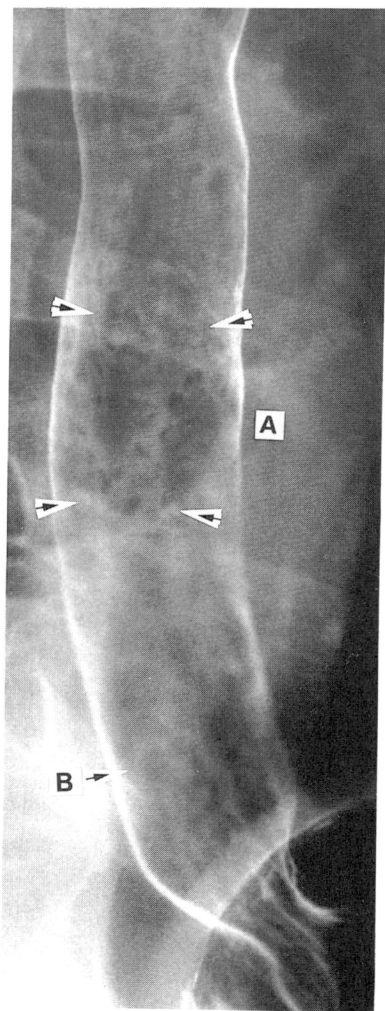

Figure 10: Preoperative double contrast picture of a case of multiple lesions. A = ep-carcinoma; B = mm-carcinoma.

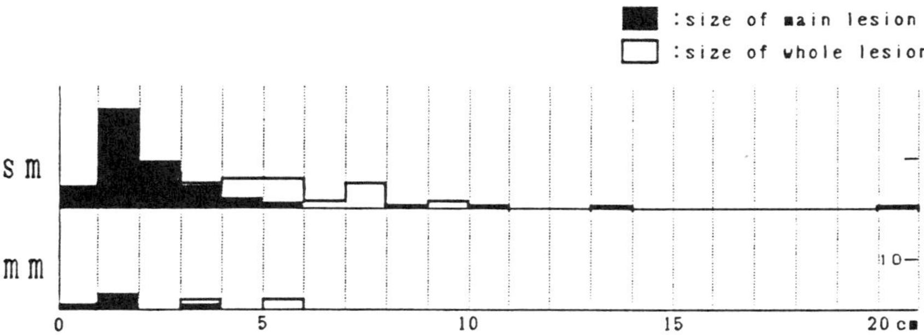

Figure 11: Relation between the size of the main lesion and the size of the whole lesion.

invasion), and the sizes of areas including intraepithelial spread. The mm-carcinoma main lesions were usually from 1.0 to 2.0 cm, and the sizes of lesions including epithelial invasion were about 5.0 cm. In the cases of sm-carcinoma, the sizes of the main lesions were from 1.0 to 3.0 cm, but the sizes including epithelial invasion measured from 5.0 to 10.0 cm. In radiographic examinations, it is easy to locate the lesions with marked elevation or depression, but from the clinical view it is necessary to consider the full extent of the lesions, including epithelial invasion.

Figures 12a and 12b show a lesion of sm-carcinoma, the size of which is 6.5 × 4.7 cm and which includes intraepithelial spread. Figure 12a is a double contrast picture of the resected specimen. In the area outlined by arrows, one can recognize granularity, and surrounding the granularity, a shading of barium. Figure 12b is a double contrast picture taken before the operation. In an area of about 2 cm in length (arrows), one can see some shades of barium on both proximal and distal sides. In the area where granularity is evident, there was sm-carcinomatous invasion, and in the surrounding area there existed ep-carcinoma.

Figures 13a and 13b show an ep-carcinoma whose size is 6.0 × 3.2 cm. Figure 13a is a double contrast picture of the resected specimen in which one can see a vague shade of barium whose marginal lines are irregular (arrows). Figure 13b is a double contrast picture taken before the operation. In the area outlined by arrows, one can recognize a vague shade of barium and some mucosal folds leading to the shade. The length of the area was 4.5 cm. It is necessary for us to keep lesions of this kind in mind when we examine lesions with little mucosal granularity which are larger than 5.0 cm in diameter.

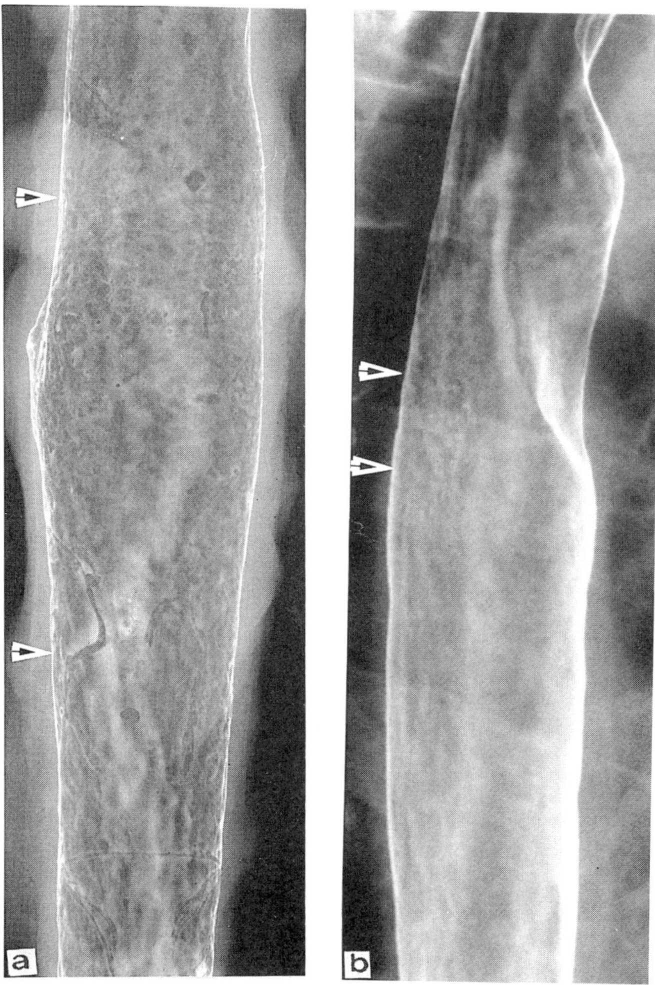

Figure 12: (a) Double contrast picture of sm-carcinoma from a resected specimen with intraepithelial spread. (b) Preoperative double contrast picture of the lesion.

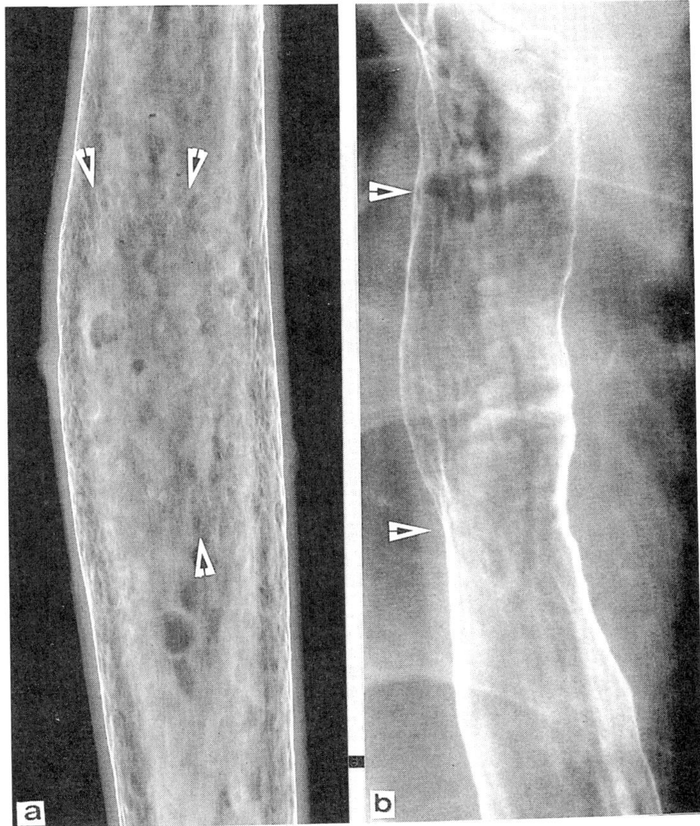

Figure 13: : (a) Double contrast picture of a widely spread ep-carcinoma in a resected specimen. (b) Preoperative double contrast picture of the lesion.

Conclusion

From these data and the discussion regarding the x-ray diagnoses of early esophageal carcinoma, we can conclude the following:

(1) There is almost no problem in interpreting lesions of sm-carcinoma.

(2) There is also little problem in diagnosing the lesions of elevated-type carcinomas (IIa).

(3) There are still problems in diagnosing depressed-type lesions (IIc). At present, it is evident that double contrast pictures are effective

in defining these lesions, and we should pay our utmost attention to even the slightest changes found in them.

(4) Little additional information is provided by overdistended double contrast pictures.

References

1. Japanese Society for Esophageal Disease: Guidelines for the clinical and pathologic studies on carcinoma of the esophagus. Jpn J Surg 6:70–86, 1976.

10

Endoscopic Diagnosis of Early Esophageal Cancer: Establishing an Effective Detection System

Mamoru Nishizawa, Toshikuni Okada

Introduction

Early detection of esophageal cancer has been extremely difficult. It has recently become feasible to detect cancer of the esophagus limited to the mucosa and without metastasis by the combined use of a small-diameter endoscope and intravital staining. The establishment of an early detection system is important, not merely to detect early cancers, particularly mucosal cancers, but also to improve the percentage of cancers detected at an early stage. To this end, high-risk individuals were selected for evaluation from among an otherwise healthy patient population. Endoscopy was carried out with a small-diameter scope, resulting in a highly effective means for detection of early esophageal cancer.

Methods and Results

A high-risk group of patients cannot be identified on the basis of symptoms. An analysis of 206 cancers showed that 63% of asymp-

Ferguson MK, Little AG, Skinner DB: Diseases of the Esophagus, Vol. I: Malignant Diseases. Futura Publishing Company, Inc., Mount Kisco, NY, © 1990.

Table I
Relationship Between Stage and Presence of Complaint (Nov. 1972–Mar. 1987)[1]

	Early	*Advanced*
No. of cases	57	149
Complaint-free	36 (63%)	23 (37%)
Complaint-positive	21 (15%)	126 (85%)
Dysphagia	1 (1%)	105 (99%)

tomatic patients had early stage cancers, while 85% of patients with symptoms related to their cancers had advanced disease. Most of the patients with symptoms complained of dysphagia (Table I).[1] Gender is an important consideration as well. According to a group of 7,409 esophageal cancer patients registered in Japan during the period 1976–1981, over 75% of patients over the age of 50 were male (Table II). In the Japanese population, cancer is most commonly found in the middle thoracic and lower thoracic esophagus, comprising 77% of all esophageal cancers (Table III).[1]

Once a high-risk population of individuals is identified, one must select the best means for diagnosing early cancers. Seventeen mucosal cancers detected at our center were all negative for lymph node metastasis, including ep (confined to the epithelium) and mm (extending only to the muscularis mucosa) cancers. We found that many of these cancers were missed by standard contrast radiographs but were detected by careful endoscopy using Olympus GIF-P3, GIF-P10, or GIF-P20 endoscopes. Major findings of early esophageal cancer endoscopically were discoloration, coarse unevenness, or a white plaque.

Table II
Incidence by Sex and Age According to Nationwide Statistics 1976–1981[1]

Age	*25–29*	*30–39*	*40–49*	*50–59*	*60–69*	*70–79*	*80–*	*Total*
Male		41	511	1,648*	2,317*	1,461*	166*	6,144
Female	3	12	92	269	502	342	45	1,265
Total	3	53	603	1,917	2,819	1,803	211	7,409

* corresponds to 75.5% of the total cancer cases

Table III
Location According to Nationwide Statistics 1976–1981[1]

Site	Male	Female	Total
Cervical	220	132	352
Upper thoracic	629	88	717
Middle thoracic*	3,394	673	4,067
Lower thoracic*	1,391	213	1,604
Abdominal esophagus	299	81	380
Cardia	166	57	233

* corresponds to 77% of the total

These findings were not conclusive for malignancy, however, unless confirmed by intravital staining with Lugol's solution or biopsy (Table IV). Endoscopy combined with intravital staining is considered crucial in detecting esophageal cancer at the earliest possible stage.

Mass screening has been shown to be feasible for select groups of high-risk patients. Males over the age of 50 were selected randomly from among the examinees entered in a gastric mass screening program, and endoscopy was carried out to evaluate the entire esophagus and stomach (Table V). Sixteen cases (0.19%) of esophageal cancers were detected from among 8,663 males, consisting of 11 (69%) early cases (eight of which were limited to the mucosa) and five advanced cancers. In contrast, females over the age of 50 were examined

Table IV
Comparison of Mucosal Cancer Between X-ray and Endoscopy

Case No.	1	2	3	4	5	6	7–10	11	12	13	14–17
depth	ep	ep	ep	ep	ep	ep	ep	mm	mm	mm	mm
ly-meta	–	–	–	–	–	–	–	–	–	–	–
x-ray	*	skip	*	*	*	skip	*	*	skip	*	skip
ordinary Endo.	**	**	**	**	**	**	**	***	*	**	**
Lugol Endo.	***	**	***	***	***	***	***	***	***	***	***

* missed
** spotted
*** concluded

Table V
Esophagus Cancers Detected through Mass Screening of Upper GI Tract

Age Group		50–54	55–59	60–64	76–69	70–	Total	Detectability
No. Examinees	*Male*	*2,614*	*1,981*	*2,251*	*1,197*	*620*	*8,663*	
	Female	*2,626*	*2,238*	*1,537*	*458*	*132*	*6,991*	
Cancers Detected	Male		ep 1		ep 2	ep 2	ep 5	0.19%
		mm 1			mm 2		mm 3	
		sm 1	sm 1	sm 1	sm 1		sm 4	
			adv 1	adv 1	adv 2		adv 4	
	Female	sm 1					sm 1	0.014%
							adv 0	

Examinees over 50, 1975–1987.
Mass Screening X-ray → Ordinary X-ray → Endoscopy.

in a similar manner, resulting in the detection of only one esophageal cancer (0.014%).

The diagnostic process can be illustrated by two representative cases. *Patient #1:* A 51-year-old male had no symptoms but was diagnosed on routine endoscopy as having a squamous cell cancer limited to the muscularis mucosa without metastasis (Fig. 1). During ordinary endoscopy, only a very subtle grainy appearance was evident 35 cm from the incisors. Lugol staining brought the area of concern into high contrast, permitting accurate diagnosis of the malignancy. *Patient #2:* A 51-year-old asymptomatic male was diagnosed as having a squamous cell cancer limited to the mucosa accompanied by no lymphatic metastasis (Fig. 2). During ordinary endoscopy, a slightly discolored area with some erythema was evident 30 cm from the incisors. Again, staining with Lugol's solution brought this region into good contrast, permitting an accurate diagnosis.

(Note: Figs. 1 and 2, color illustrations, are between pages 98 and 99.)

Discussion

The death rate for esophageal cancer is highest at France at 17.5 per 100,000 population, and is relatively high among females in Great Britain at 7.3 per 100,000. In Japan, corresponding rates are 8.5 for males and 1.9 for females per 100,000, an incidence that is relatively low compared to rates found for cancers of other digestive organs.[2]

Despite this, esophageal cancer is one of the most difficult malignancies to cure, largely because of its relatively advanced stage at the time of diagnosis.

The detection rate of cancer limited to the mucosa (ep + mm) is extremely low. Using Japanese nationwide statistics from 1984, a total of 25,077 esophageal cancers were recorded. Of these, 14,999 cancers (58.8%) were resected, of which only 43 cases of ep cancer (0.17%) and 102 cases of mucosal cancer (0.41%) overall were detected.[3] In contrast, data from a radiographic mass screening effort among healthy individuals performed in 1986 revealed only 16 cases of esophageal cancer detected out of a total of 223,479 examinations, of 0.007% of the total.[4] Therefore, using mass screening techniques based on radiographic findings, the likelihood of a useful cost-effective program being developed is quite low.

On the other hand, choosing high-risk patients as previously outlined and screening them using panendoscopy combined with intravital staining did result in a suitable detectability rate of 0.19%. In addition, the ratio of early cancer to all cancers was 69%, much higher than that reported previously. Therefore, in order to detect curable esophageal cancers, we should strive to develop screening programs aimed at males over the age of 50, whether or not they have symptoms, employing panendoscopy combined with mucosal staining using Lugol's solution as the primary diagnostic tool.

References

1. Annual Report of Nationwide Survey of Esophagus Cancer Registration (No. 1–8), fiscal 1979–1986, Japanese Research Society for Esophageal Disease, Toyko.
2. World Health Statistics, WHO, 1986.
3. Nakayama T, Mitomi T: Questionnaire Survey of the Esophagus Disease, 37th Japanese Research Society for Esophagus Disease, 1984.
4. Nationwide Statistics of Gastroenterological Mass Survey, Journal of Gastroenterological Mass Screening, 1988.

11

Endoscopic Examination of the Esophagus in Patients with Head and Neck Cancers

Hitoshi Shiozaki, Kenji Kobayashi, Tokiharu Yano, Hiroshi Yano, Shigeyuki Tamura, Hideaki Tahara, Takesada Mori, Kinji Nishiyama

Introduction

Esophageal cancer, because of its aggressive character, has a poor prognosis despite radical surgical treatment combined with radiotherapy and/or chemotherapy. However, cases with no lymph node metastases have a good prognosis after simple resection. This indicates that the prognosis of this condition could be improved if lesions were detected at an early stage. For early detection of small and superficial esophageal cancers, it is best to perform an endoscopic examination and biopsy of the esophagus following application of a modified Lugol's solution to the esophageal epithelium (EEBL).[1] We performed endoscopic examinations in patients who suffered from or had previously been treated for head and neck malignancies and were regarded as being at high risk for synchronous or metachronous esophageal cancer,[2–4] and found cases of synchronous and metachronous esophageal cancers at an extremely early stage. Clinicopathological analysis of these cases revealed that this type of examination

Ferguson MK, Little AG, Skinner DB: Diseases of the Esophagus, Vol. I: Malignant Diseases. Futura Publishing Company, Inc., Mount Kisco, NY, © 1990.

Table I
Endoscopic Findings and Histological Diagnosis of USLs

Site	Number	Number of Cases with USLs	Histological Diagnosis	
			Dysplasia	Carcinoma
Tongue	16	5	4	0
Oral Cavity	6	3	1	1
Pharynx	19	11	4	2
Larynx	15	4	4	0
Total	56	23	13	3

may improve the prognosis of esophageal cancer. This is a preliminary report of a successful trial of screening for esophageal cancer.

Materials and Methods

Patients

Fifty-six patients with head and neck malignancies who were treated at Osaka University Hospital entered this study. The sites of the primary head and neck tumors are indicated in Table I. All primary tumors were treated by radiation with or without chemotherapy or surgical resection. Each patient gave informed voluntary consent before the endoscopic examination. The patients ranged in age from 40 to 80 years (mean age = 59.3), and the male to female ratio was 4:1. The mean interval between diagnosis of the first malignancy and the endoscopic examination was 3 years and 3.6 months.

Endoscopic Examination

The endoscopic examination was performed with a video-endoscope (V-10, Olympus, Tokyo, Japan) or an optical pan-endoscope (P-10, Olympus, Tokyo, Japan). Following initial endoscopic appraisal and photography of the esophagus, stomach, and duodenum, half-strength glycerol-free Lugol's solution was instilled via a polyethylene tube under direct vision to coat the entire epithelium of the esophagus using the method reported previously.[1,5] The Lugol's solution dyes the lesions of benign and malignant disorders in a different manner from normal mucosa which is colored greenish brown. Most of the lesions are not stained and show as white or yellow regions (unstained lesions = USLs), while some are stained more deeply than normal mucosa. USLs include malignant lesions.[2] If suspicious USLs were detected, biopsy was performed and the specimens obtained were examined histologically to make a definite diagnosis.

Clinical and Histological Evaluation

The histological features of the specimens obtained by biopsy and resection were assessed using H&E stained sections. The terminology used in this report for location, staging, and histology is derived from the TNM (tumor node metastasis) staging system,[6] except for the depth of invasion of primary tumor.[7] The abbreviations ep, mm, and sm indicate that primary tumor invasion was limited to the epithelium, muscularis mucosa, and submucosa, respectively.

Results

Endoscopic Examination

Endoscopic findings of the screened patients are shown in Table I. USLs were detected in 23 of the 56 patients examined in this series, and the number of USLs related to the site of the primary cancer is also indicated in Table I. In three patients, the USLs were proven to be cancers by histological examination of biopsy specimens. Two of them were synchronous with head and neck cancer, and the other was detected metachronously by EEBL 2 years and 10 months after the primary cancer. The histological diagnoses of mild, moderate, and severe dysplasia were given to 13, 0, and 1 case among the 23 cases with USLs.

Endoscopic and Clinicopathological Features of the Esophageal Cancer Patients

The clinical findings and the pathological features are shown in Table II. There were multiple esophageal lesions in the two synchronous esophageal cancer patients. Of the five cancerous lesions in these

Table II
Clinical and Pathological Features of the Cases with Esophageal Cancer

No.	*Age*	*Sex*	*Primary Cancer*	*Timing*[a]	*Location of e.c.*[b]	*Gross Type*[c]	*Depth*[d]	*Operation*[e]
1	49	F	Hypopharynx	Syn.	Middle	Flat	mm	Lary. + Eso.
					Lower	Flat	ep	
2	49	M	Hypopharynx	Syn.	Middle	Sl. Dep.	ep	Lary. + Eso.
					Lower	Flat	ep	
3	54	M	Oral Cavity	Meta.	Lower	Flat	mm	Eso.

[a] Syn. = synchronous, Meta. = metachronous
[b] e.c. = esophageal cancer, Middle = middle esophagus, Lower = lower esophagus
[c] Sl. Dep. = slightly depressed
[d] Depth = depth of invasion, ep = limited to the epithelium, mm = confined to muscularis mucosa
[e] Lary. = laryngectomy, Eso. = esophagectomy

three cases, only one could be detected by barium studies and ordinary endoscopy due to the fact that it was slightly depressed. However, the rest of the lesions could not be detected by these two examination methods since they were completely flat. All the lesions were classified into the T1 or Tcis categories of the TNM classification, and there was no evidence of lymph node metastases. All of the detected lesions were treated surgically with or without radiotherapy.

Case Report

This patient (patient no. 3, male, 54 years old) had a past history of having been treated for cancer of the floor of the mouth by radiation in December 1985. Two years and 10 months later, he was examined by EEBL. No abnormal findings were detected by ordinary endoscopic observation (Fig. 1A), but well-defined irregularly shaped USLs were visible after the application of Lugol's solution (Fig. 1B). The lesions proved to be malignant on histological examination of biopsy specimens. He underwent subtotal esophagectomy and the resected esophagus was histologically examined in detail. The depth of tumor invasion was mm in a small area and ep in the rest of the lesions. The cancerous lesions were surrounded by multiple dysplastic regions.

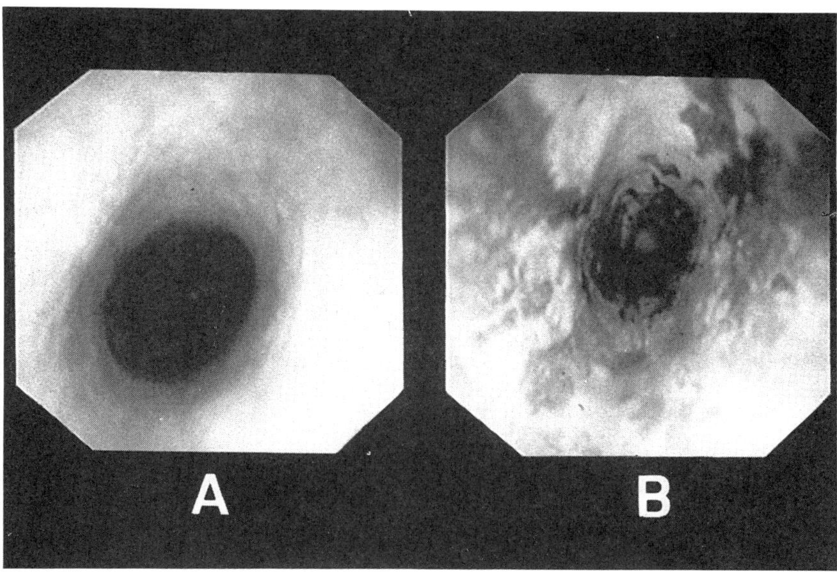

Figure 1: Endoscopic appearance of esophagus without (A) or with (B) application of Lugol's solution. No abnormal findings were detected by ordinary observation (A), but well-defined irregularly shaped USLs were visible after application of Lugol's solution. The lesions proved to be cancerous on histological examination of biopsy specimens.

Discussion

We have demonstrated the value of screening with EEBL. In the present study, we found three cases of esophageal cancer, for a frequency of second primary esophageal cancers in patients with head and neck cancer of 5.4% This percentage is far higher than the spontaneous occurrence of esophageal cancer. The etiology of the high rate of occurrence of second primary esophageal cancers is still unknown, although the existence of multiple cancerous lesions together with multiple dysplastic lesions implies that the esophageal mucosa of these patients might have an abnormal proliferative potential. Careful examination of the esophagus should be recommended during evaluation for the treatment of head and neck cancer. It should also be noted that all the cases detected in this study were diagnosed at an extremely early stage when the esophageal cancer could still be controlled by simple resection.

Clinicopathological analysis revealed that these cancers were too small and flat to be detected either by barium studies or by ordinary endoscopic examination. This indicates the value of EEBL for detecting early esophageal cancers, emphasizes the need for its use in head and neck cancer, and implies its applicability for detecting esophageal cancer in the general population.

References

1. Sugimachi K, Ohno S, Matsuda H, Mori M, Kuwano H: Lugol-combined endoscopic detection of minute malignant lesions of the thoracic esophagus. Ann Surg 208:179, 1988.
2. Goodner JT, Watson WL: Cancer of the esophagus: Its association with other primary cancers. Cancer 9:1248, 1956.
3. Shaha AR, Hoover EL, Mitrani M, Marti JR, Krespi YP: Synchronicity, multicentricity, and metachronicity of head and neck cancer. Head Neck Surg 10:225, 1988.
4. Kawamoto S, Ikeda H, Nishiyama K, Miyata Y, Masaki N, Shigematsu Y: Occurrence of multiple primary cancers in patients with head and neck cancers. Gan No Rinsho 28:1, 1982 (in Japanese).
5. Brodmerkel GJ Jr: Shiller's test: An aid in esophagoscopic diagnosis. Gastroenterology, 60:813, 1971.
6. UICC (International Union Against Cancer): TNM Classification of Malignant Tumors, 4th ed, Berlin, Springer-Verlag, 1987.
7. Japanese Society for Esophageal Diseases: Guidelines for the Clinical and Pathologic Studies on Carcinoma of the Esophagus, 7th ed. Tokyo, Japan, Kanehara Co., 1989.

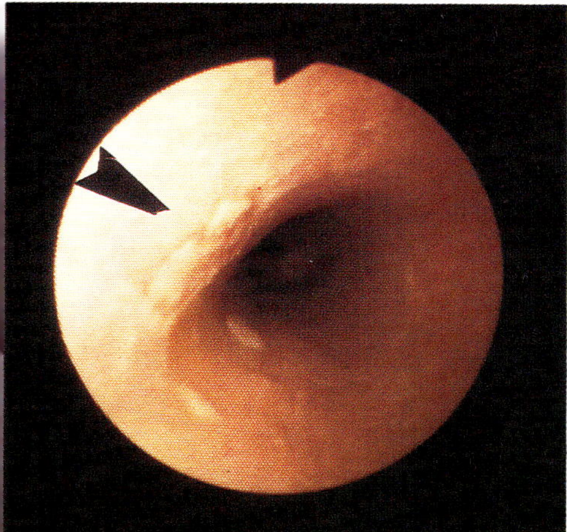

Figure 1: (a) An image taken through forward-viewing endoscope (GIF-P10). A very subtle grainy appearance is present 35 cm from the incisors.

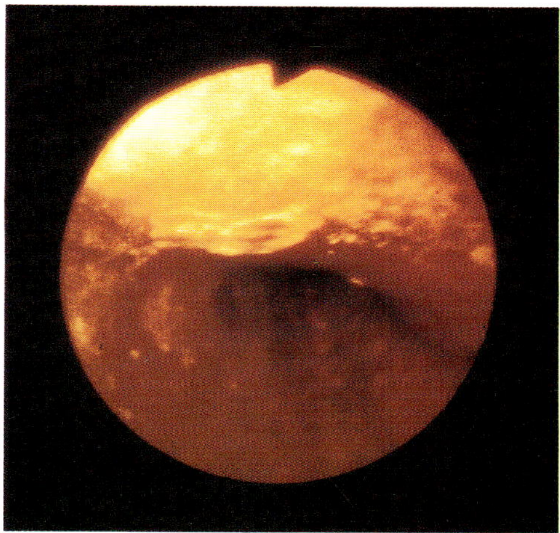

Figure 1: (b) The Lugol-stained image of the esophagus pictured in 1a. A stained area is surrounded by an unstained area showing a whitish hue.

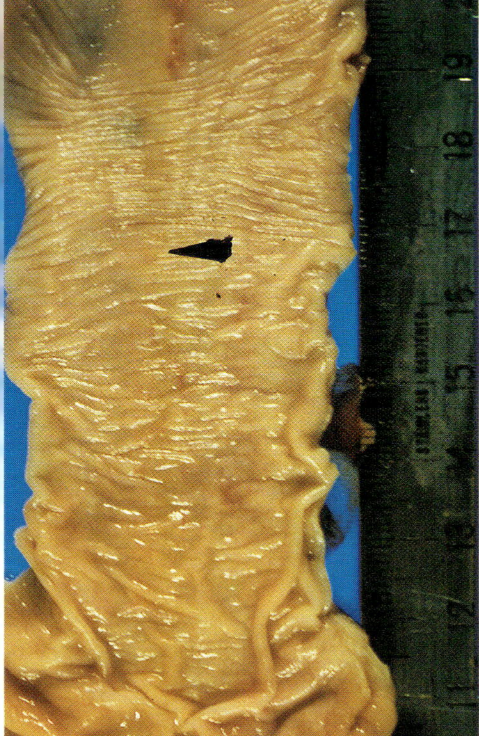

Figure 1: (c) In the raw resected specimen, it is difficult to detect the lesion by the naked eye.

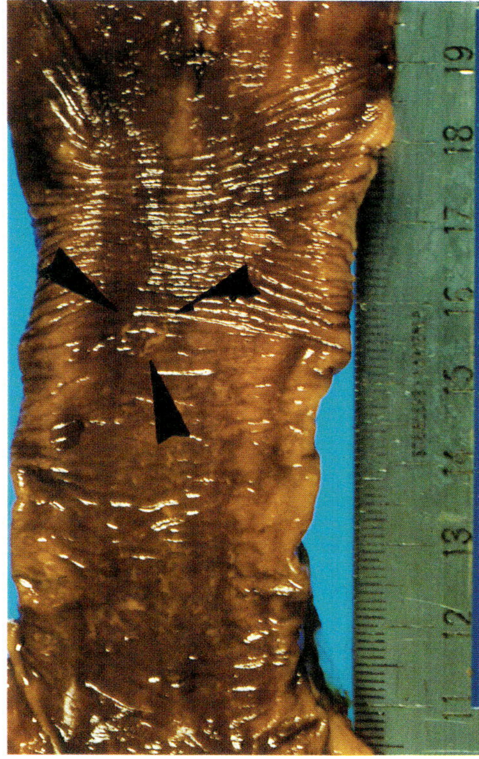

Figure 1: (d) A Lugol-stained image from the specimen in 1c, containing a circular unstained part with a well-stained 5 × 4 mm center. The unstained area was consonant with the cancer spread.

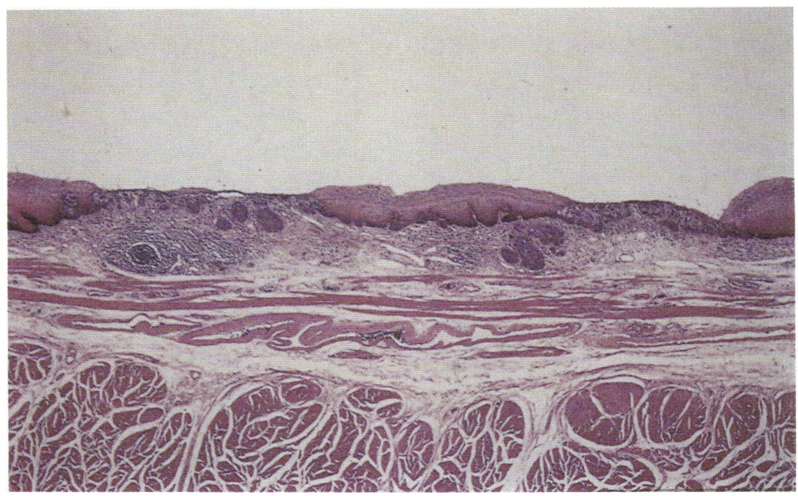

Figure 1: (e) Microscopic image. The cancer has slightly invaded the lamina propria.

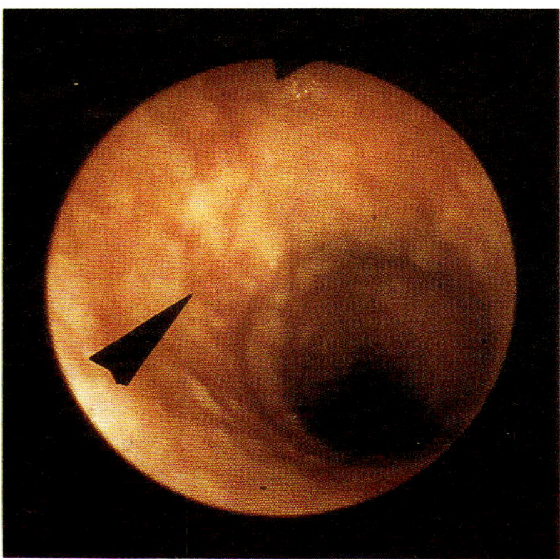

Figure 2: (a) An ordinary endoscopic image (GIF-XK10). A discolored area with accompanying redness is present 30 cm from the incisors.

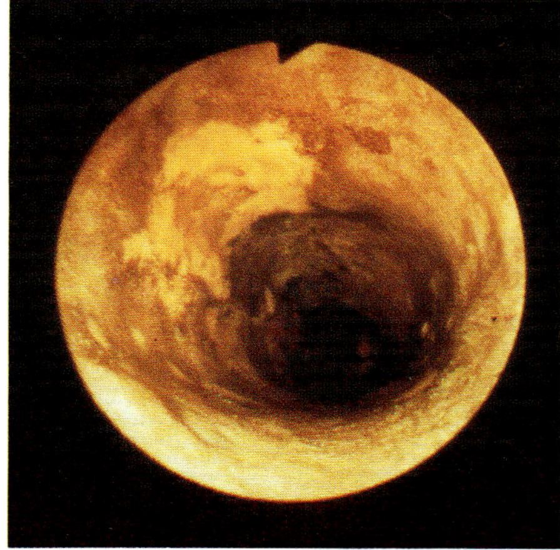

Figure 2: (b) The Lugol-stained endoscopic image. The lesion is discernible as unstained part.

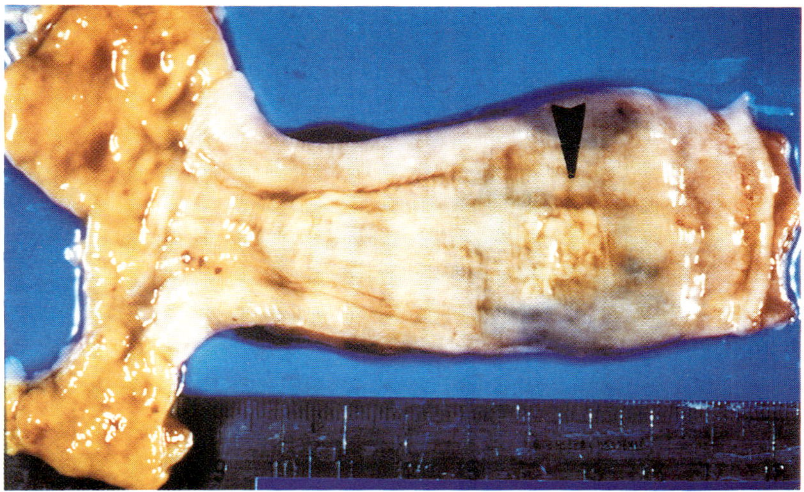

Figure 2: (c) In the resected specimen, a discoloration was present that was slightly raised.

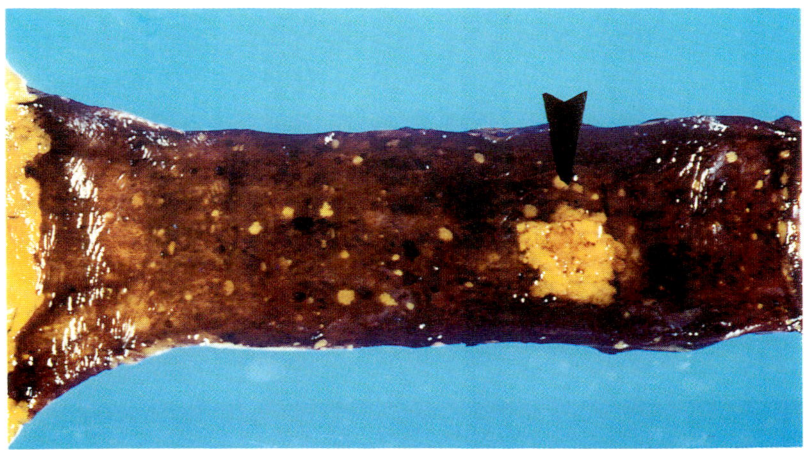

Figure 2: (d) The Lugol-stained specimen from Figure 2c demonstrates a clearly delineated unstained part measuring 20 × 17 mm.

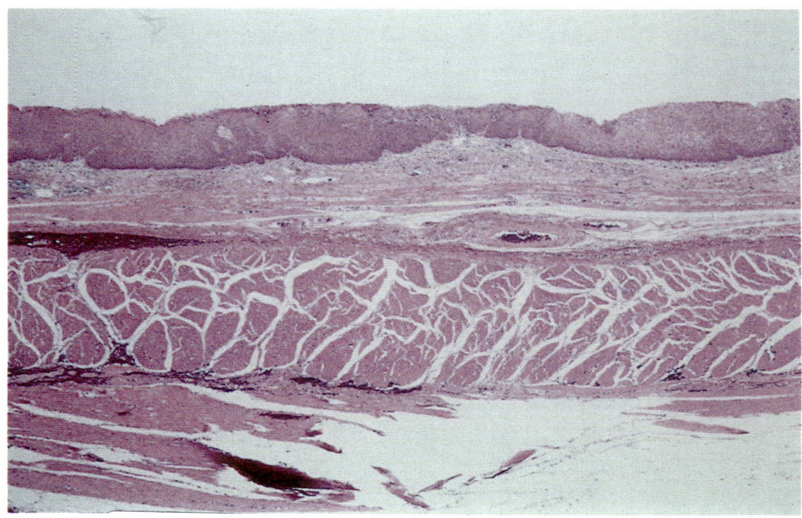

Figure 2: (e) The microscopic image showed a squamous cell cancer confined to the epithelial layer.

12

New Proposal for Preoperative Staging of Cancer of the Esophagus Based on Tumor Pattern and Malignancy

Hiroshi Akiyama, Masahiko Tsurumaru,
Yoshimasa Ono, Harushi Udagawa

Introduction

In squamous cell carcinoma of the esophagus, it is known that tumor size does not significantly correlate with survival.[1] Surgeons should not be discouraged from operating on patients with large tumors. However, surgeons frequently tend to be discouraged by the unexpectedly poor results obtained following operations on patients with small tumors. Taking this into consideration, any clinical staging or classification should include the tumor pattern as it is found to correlate with the clinical aggressiveness of the tumor. Such a classification is invaluable in clarifying indications for surgery and in predicting prognosis. By simply observing the gross appearance of the tumor, important information can often be obtained regarding its clinical behavior and prognosis.

Ferguson MK, Little AG, Skinner DB: Diseases of the Esophagus, Vol. I: Malignant Diseases. Futura Publishing Company, Inc., Mount Kisco, NY, © 1990.

Materials and Methods

It is of the utmost importance to determine the macroscopic appearance of a lesion by radiography and fiberoptic endoscopy before any therapeutic decisions are made. Tumor morphology is not always distinct, and there are often overlaps between tumor types, giving way to a wide range of possibilities. Consequently, evaluation of tumors is sometimes made arbitrarily and subjectively by surgeons or endoscopists. In fact, some tumors are too advanced to retain their original pathological features. Another difficulty in assessment worth considering is the presence of extensive esophageal narrowing that prevents a thorough gross examination. In addition, patients are often referred from other institutions, having first been treated with radiotherapy. Inflammation and reflux esophagitis, particularly with lower esophageal tumors, prevent a worthwhile appraisal. It is, therefore, expedient not to insist on categorizing all tumors into a specific classification, thus avoiding misinterpretation and error in clinical judgment.

Of 469 resected cases with squamous cell carcinoma of the thoracic esophagus (Department of Surgery, Toranomon Hospital, 1972–1987), accurate assessment of macroscopic pattern was possible in only 124 cases. It should be noted that these 124 cases do not represent all of the cases seen during this period. Advanced squamous cell carcinoma of the esophagus could be classified into the following types (Tables I and II): exophytic protuberant (low grade malignancy); ulcerative with a regular border; ulcerative with irregular border; superficial; endophytic; and endophytic with protuberance (high grade malignancy). To avoid any misunderstanding, early or minor carcinomas were excluded from the series.

Results

Exophytic Protuberant Type

The term *exophytic* applied in this description denotes intraluminal growth. The lesions tend not to be ulcerated but have a cauliflower appearance (Fig. 1a). Microscopically, they tend to be well-differentiated with an element of keratinization. They have a unique endoscopic appearance since this growth is exclusively intraluminal,

Table I
Frequency of Lymph Node Metastases According to Macroscopic Pathology of Primary Tumors

Macroscopic Pathology	*No. of Cases*	*Frequency of Metastases per No. of Dissected Nodes*		*Frequency of Metastases per No. of Cases*	
Exophytic, protuberant	7	1/203	(0.5%)	1/7	(14.3%)
Ulcerative with regular edges	15	12/353	(3.4%)	5/15	(33.3%)
Ulcerative with irregular edges	73	232/2450	(9.5%)	50/73	(68.5%)
Superficial	14	37/422	(8.8%)	10/14	(71.4%)
Endophytic	7	36/376	(9.6%)	7/7	(100%)
Endophytic, protuberent	8	32/352	(9.1%)	6/8	(75%)
Total	124	350/4156	(8.4%)	79/124	(63.7%)

and the small areas of surrounding epithelium are displaced by the expanding tumor growth. Usually, dysphagia is not a major problem.

These tumors are characterized by slow growth which is almost entirely intraluminal with little penetration into the wall. This is in contrast to their enormous size. Technically, resection of such tumors is therefore relatively easy. On microscopic examination of associated dissected lymph nodes, the frequency of involvement is exceedingly

Table II
Survival Rates of Different Types of Esophageal Tumors after Resection

Macroscopic Pathology	*No. of Cases with Minimum 5-Year Follow-Up*	*No. of 5-Year Survivors*	*5-Year Survival Rates*
Exophytic, protuberant	7	6	86%
Ulcerative with regular edges	15	13	87%
Ulcerative with irregular edges	73	11	15%
Superficial	14	4	29%
Endophytic	7	0	0%
Endophytic, protuberant	8	0	0%

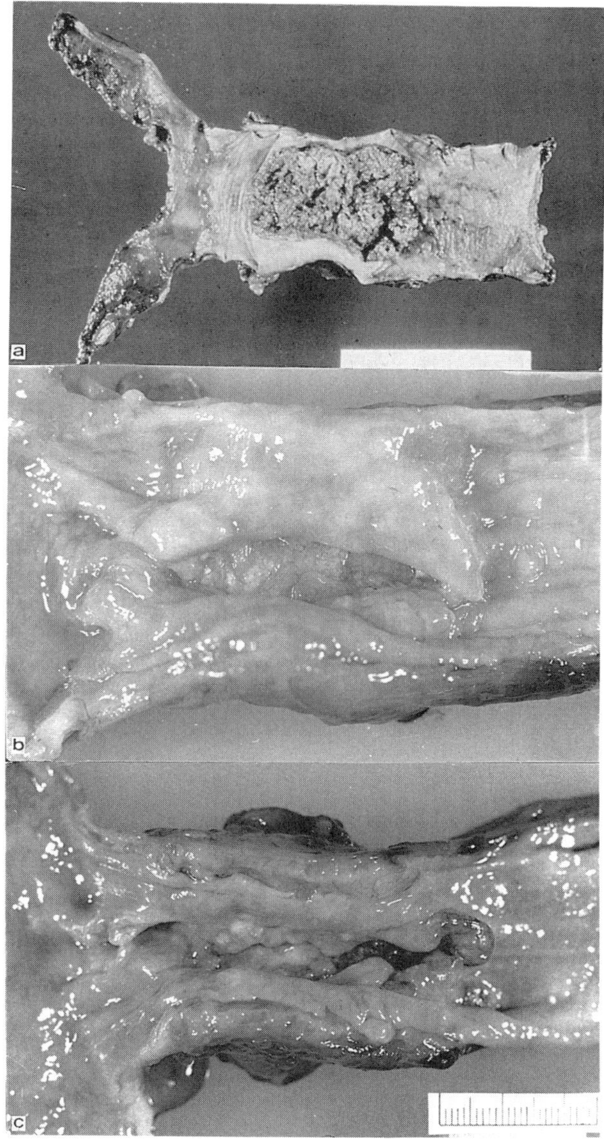

Figure 1: Macroscopic pathology of squamous cell carcinoma of the esophagus. (a) Exophytic protuberant. (b) Ulcerative with regular edges. (c) Ulcerative with irregular edges. (*Continued*)

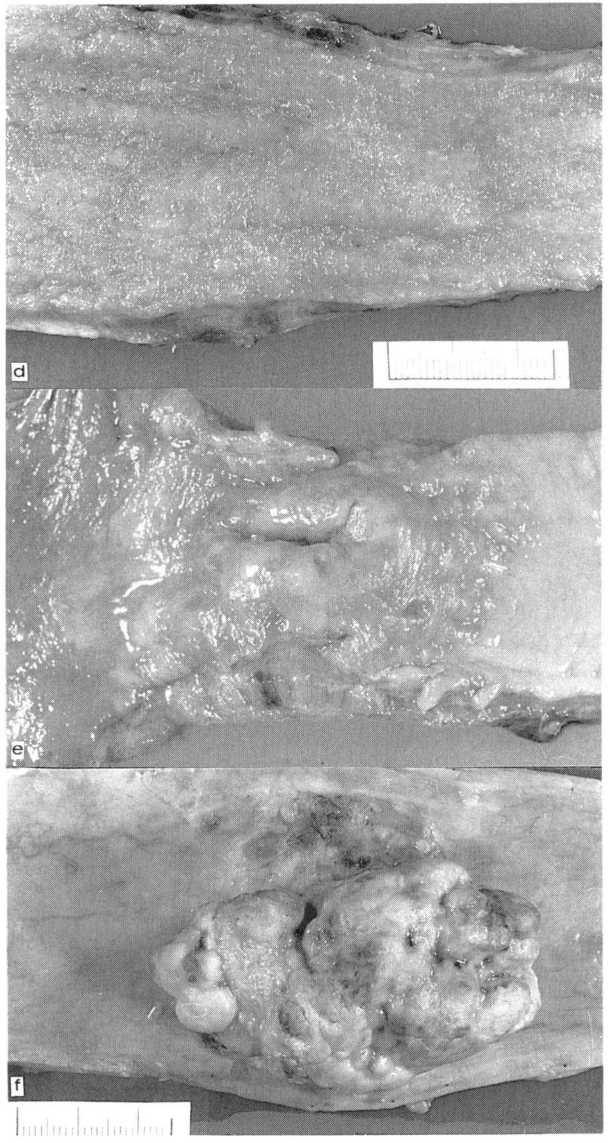

Figure 1: (*Continuation*) (d) Superficial. (e) Endophytic. (f) Endophytic, protuberant.

low compared to other types of tumors (Table I). If the tumor is resectable, the outcome is uniformly satisfactory. The 5-year survival rate for patients with this type of lesion after resection is 86% (Table II). Although some of these tumors eventually reach advanced stages infiltrating important structures, the lymph nodes often remain free of carcinoma or localized metastases. Naturally, in these latter patients, survival may not be prolonged.

Ulcerative Type with Regular Border

The concept of ulcerative tumors relating to their border appearance was first introduced by Kogure and his colleagues.[2] The ulcerative lesion with regular borders has a relatively shallow ulcer floor and regular high borders displacing normal epithelium (Fig. 1b). The overall appearance of the lesion tends to be exophytic with intraluminal growth.

The ulcerative tumor with regular borders has been shown to be less aggressive than those with irregular borders. This is supported by the fact that in the ulcerative lesion with regular borders, the rates of positive lymph nodes per number of lymph nodes examined and per case were 3.4% and 33.3%, respectively. These rates are comparatively much lower than those of the ulcerative tumors with irregular borders and those of superficial-type tumors. Intramural spread is rare. The 5-year survival rate after resection of this type of tumor is 87% (Table II).

Ulcerative Tumors with Irregular Borders

Tumors of this type are the most common lesions in our series. The margins of the ulcer are characteristically irregular with an uneven ulcer base. The edges of the lesion are usually low and occasionally undermining (Fig. 1c). Vascular invasion and intramural spread are common. The frequency of lymph node involvement per number of nodes examined and per number of cases is 9.5% and 68.5%, respectively. Both rates are higher than those of the ulcerative tumor with regular borders (Table I). The 5-year survival rate of patients with this lesion is disappointingly low (15%) (Table II). Since intramural spread is not uncommon with this lesion, satellite nodules and skip lesions are unfavorable signs.

Superficial Type

The major part of the tumor is confined to the superficial layers of the esophageal wall. These tumors either may be isolated in a small or wide area or may present as multifocal lesions disseminated widely through the mucosa, therefore being referred to as the superficial spreading type (Fig. 1d). Studies and observations of a number of superficial spreading tumors has led to the conclusion that these lesions arise separately in susceptible individuals and result from prolonged exposure of an already unstable mucosa to carcinogens. Eventually, with further tumor growth, the appearances change, and small elevated areas coalesce, followed by ulceration and invasion to deeper layers. Cellular or structural differentiation may not be easy since these lesions are often confined to the mucosal layer. Prognosis after resection of this type of tumor is variable since factors such as depth of growth and extent of spread generally determine the outcome. These tumors are, therefore, appropriately allocated within the scale of malignancy between tumors of low grade and those of high grade malignancy, with a 5-year survival rate of 29% (Table II).

Endophytic Type

The major part of tumor growth is found beneath the mucosa and often only a small part of the lesion is seen to erode through the mucosa. This type of carcinoma is further characterized by ingrowth of tumor (Fig. 1e). Biopsies taken from the surface are often negative and can be deceptive, hence leading to late diagnosis when the tumor is small. In general, the endophytic carcinoma is poorly differentiated or entirely undifferentiated, or may present as oat cell carcinoma with its characteristic invasivenss and poor outlook. Fortunately, this type of tumor is not too common, the incidence in our unit being 6% of all resected specimens (Table II).

A tumor of this type often presents with invasion into the wall and the surrounding mediastinal tissue. Evidence of vascular involvement is frequently demonstrated on histology. Dysphagia secondary to constriction is usually a problem. The rate of nodal metastases per number of nodes dissected and number of cases was as high as 9.6% and 100%, respectively. Unfortunately, there were no 5-year survivals in our series with this type of lesion (Table II).

Endophytic Proturberant Type

These are extremely malignant tumors. On microscopy, they reveal a poorly differentiated squamous cell or undifferentiated carcinoma. On gross appearance, they may be hard or fragile, and the major part of the surface of the lesion may be covered with normal squamous epithelium (Fig. 1f). Central necrosis may be present, causing it to resemble the ulcerative type. Extensive intramural and intravascular invasion occurs. Usually dysphagia is not an initial problem. The highly malignant nature of this tumor type predisposes to widespread blood-borne metastases and lymph node involvement. The rate of nodal metastases per number of dissected nodes and cases was 9.1% and 75%, respectively (see Table I). With this type of tumor, resection with the aim of prolonging survival offers little advantage, even though technically possible. Widespread vascular metastases predominate even before the tumor has penetrated the full thickness of the esophageal wall. Patients, therefore, succumb to the effects of secondary spread well before occurrence of invasion into vital structures in the mediastinum by the primary tumor.

Discussion

The grade of malignancy of a tumor is an important factor to be considered before determining the appropriate management of a patient. Accurate information regarding tumor malignancy, however, is not always easily available preoperatively. By simply examining the gross appearance of the tumor, important information can be obtained regarding its behavior. Any clinical classification should include not only the gross appearance of squamous cell carcinoma, but its correlated clinical significance. Such a classification is invaluable in clarifying the indications for surgery and in predicting its outcome. This, in addition to grading based on microscopic differentiation, provides a reliable overall impression of the degree of malignancy of such a lesion.

Carcinomas of the esophagus, as in other lesions within the gastrointestinal tract, often comprise a wide spectrum of cellular activity, and a single biopsy may not give representative information of the entire tumor. The gross pathological appearance of squamous cell carcinoma of the esophagus has been described by various authors.[2–7] Mostly, classifications derive from the distinctive features of such lesions in common with malignancies in other parts of the alimentary tract, such as protuberance, ulceration, infiltration, and their various combinations. However, the gross appearance of esophageal tumors is somewhat different from that of gastric or colonic carcinomas, and demands an entirely different pathological classification. Conventional parameters of the degree of malignancy, including tumor differentiation, Broder's, and other histopathological interpretations are still helpful, but the information is only available after completion of surgery. Another interesting and useful prognostic indicator, particularly in early tumors, is cytophotometric DNA analysis of mucosal and submucosal carcinoma of the esophagus as reported by Sugimachi et al.[8] Future studies may provide improved parameters for identifying accurately the grade of tumor malignancy.

Conclusions

Prognosis of esophageal cancer depends on several factors which are difficult to evaluate prior to surgery with the exception of endoscopic morphology and tumor histology. Histologic grade of malignancy and endoscopic morphological growth pattern were correlated with the survival rate after resection in 124 patients with squamous cell carcinoma. The results are the basis for a new effective preoperative staging of cancer of the esophagus. The 124 patients were divided into six groups according to the morphological growth patterns of their tumors observed on endoscopy and subsequently verified by gross examination of the resected specimens. They were: (1) exophytic protuberant; (2) ulcerative with regular edges; (3) ulcerative with irregular edges; (4) superficial; (5) endophytic; and (6) endophytic protuberant. Without regard to the extent of lymphatic spread at the time of the operation, 5-year survival rates after curative resection were: (1) 86%; (2) 87%; (3) 15%; (4) 29%; (5) 0%; and (6) 0%, respectively. Exophytic protuberant type and ulcerative type with regular edges were the least malignant. Ulcerative type with irregular edges and superficial type were moderately malignant. The highly malignant types were the endophytic and endophytic protuberant.

It is proposed that preoperative staging for cancer of the esophagus should be based on the endoscopic morphological growth of the tumor. Additional information on the depth of the growth can be determined by endoscopic ultrasonography and may further improve endoscopic staging of the disease.

References

1. Akiyama H, Tsurumaru M, Watanabe G, Ono Y, Udagawa H, Suzuki M: Development of surgery for carcinoma of the esophagus. Am J Surg 147:9–16, 1984.
2. Kogure T, Itai Y, Akiyama H: Gross pathology and prognosis in cancer of the esophagus. Jpn J Cancer Clin 22:227–233, 1976.
3. Tanner NC, Smithers DW: Tumors of the Oesophagus, Edinburgh, Livingstone, 1961, p 94.
4. Takahashi K: Squamous cell carcinoma of the esophagus: Stromal inflammatory cell infiltration as a prognostic factor. Cancer 14:921–933, 1961.
5. Ming SC: Tumors of the esophagus and stomach. In: Atlas of Tumor Pathology, Washington, DC, AFIP, 1973, pp 30–36.
6. Japanese Society For Esophageal Diseases: Guidelines for the clinical and pathologic studies on carcinoma of the esophagus. Part II. Pathologic classification. Jpn J Surg 6:79–86, 1976.
7. Postlethwait RW: Surgery of the Esophagus. Norwalk, CT, Appleton-Century-Crofts, 1986, pp 377–379.
8. Sugimachi K, Ide H, Okamura T, Matsuura H, Endo M, Inokuchi K: Cytophotometric DNA analysis of mucosal and submucosal carcinoma of the esophagus. Cancer 53:2683–2687, 1984.

13

Cancer of the Cervical Esophagus: Critical Analysis of the New TNM Staging System

Alberto Ruol, Romeo Bardini, Andrea Segalin, Surendra Narne, Carlo Castoro, Luigi Bonavina, Franco Cavazzini, Alberto Peracchia

Introduction

Tumors of the cervical esophagus and of the hypopharynx have long been considered together, despite their differing origins, since they pose similar clinical and therapeutic problems.[1–4] The new classification of cancer of the cervical esophagus[5] clears up this confusion by excluding definitively all the tumors involving the hypopharynx and the pharyngo-esophageal junction. Most studies analyzing the prognostic accuracy of the TNM staging system were performed on patients with tumors of the thoracic esophagus,[6] and even the study which served as the baseline for determining the prognostic classes of the new TNM system[7,8] did not take tumors of the cervical esophagus into account. Due to the lack of available studies in the literature, this analysis was performed in patients with squamous cell carcinoma of the cervical esophagus to verify the accuracy and the prognostic value of the new clinical and pathological TNM staging system.

Ferguson MK, Little AG, Skinner DB: Diseases of the Esophagus, Vol. I: Malignant Diseases. Futura Publishing Company, Inc., Mount Kisco, NY, © 1990.

Materials and Methods

Between 1980 and 1987, 202 patients with cancer of the cervical esophageal region were observed. In 129 patients the tumor was located in the cervical esophagus, in 56 the cervical esophagus was secondarily involved by a primary tumor of the hypopharynx, and in 17 a tumor of the cervical esophagus was detected during follow-up after laryngectomy for cancer. Our therapeutic attitude was to operate when a patient's general status and preoperative staging of the tumor were permissive. We did not undertake an operation when the preoperative work-up showed that only a palliative resection of the tumor was possible. Of 129 patients with primary cancer of the cervical esophagus, 66 underwent surgical resection, which was curative in 56 patients and palliative in 10. One-stage pharyngo-laryngo total esophagectomy and gastric pull-up was the standard operation; esophagectomy was performed using a transhiatal approach in most cases.

The study included 63 consecutive patients with a tumor confined to the cervical esophagus who underwent surgical resection, and in whom the comparison between clinical and pathological staging was possible. The other three patients underwent preoperative radiation and/or chemotherapy and were excluded.

Results

The comparison between clinical and pathological TNM staging in the 53 patients who underwent curative resection showed a clinical understaging in 20 patients (Table I); the T status was understaged in 19 cases and overstaged in 8; the N status was understaged in most cases. The 10 patients who underwent palliative resection were considered to be understaged clinically; the clinical and the surgical pathologic stages were stage II in 7 and 0 patients, stage III in 8 and 1, and stage IV in 0 and 9 patients, respectively.

Twenty-five of 53 patients who underwent curative resection had lymph node metastases in the operative specimen. The location of metastatic nodes was as follows: laterocervical in 10, supraclavicular in 3, paraesophageal in 11, along recurrent laryngeal nerves in 14, paratracheal in 2, posterior mediastinal in 4, and lower paraesophageal in 2. No metastatic nodes were found along the lesser gastric

Table I
Comparision Between Clinical and Pathological Staging of Cancer of the Cervical Esophagus According to T and N Status and Stage

	T1	*T2*	*T3*	*T4*	
pT1	3	2	—	—	5
pT2	—	1	5	1	7
pT3	—	—	16	—	16
pT4	—	1	18	6	25
	3	4	39	7	53

	N−	*N+*	
pH −	26	2	28
pN +	20	5	25
	46	7	53

	Stage I	*Stage II*	*Stage III*	*Stage IV*	
pStage I	3	—	—	—	3
pStage II	1	18	—	—	19
pStage III	—	19	12	—	31
pStage IV	—	—	—	—	—
	4	37	12	—	53

curvature or the celiac axis. Overall, positive mediastinal and abdominal nodes were found in 8 (32%) and 0 (0%) cases, respectively.

The mean survival after curative resection in 10 evaluable patients with metastatic paraesophageal, recurrent nerve, and/or paratracheal nodes was 22.4 months; for the 6 evaluable patients with positive mediastinal nodes it was 10.3 months; and for the 5 patients with deep laterocervical or supraclavicular nodes it was 5.8 months. A statistical analysis was not performed due to the small number of patients per each group of nodes involved. Only the cervical nodes are considered local-regional by the TNM guidelines; however, since our survival data contradicted the above prognostic criteria, we included among local-regional nodes both the cervical and the mediastinal ones. The 2-year actuarial survival rates after curative resection are reported in Table II.

Neoplastic recurrence after curative resection was diagnosed in 16 patients, and its exact location was documented in 13; it was in the neck in 8 cases (61%), both in the neck and at distance in 3 (23%), and only at distance in 2 (16%).

Table II
Two-Year Survival Rates After Curative Resection According to the pT and pN Status and p-Stage

pT1N0 (n = 3)	100%	pT2N+ (n = 3)	33%	p-Stage I (n = 3)	100%
pT2N0 (n = 6)	33%	pT3N+ (n = 5)	25%	p-Stage IIA (n = 17)	30%
pT3N0 (n = 11)	24%	pT4N+ (n = 17)	16%	p-Stage IIB (n = 3)	33%
pT4N0 (n = 8)	20%			p-Stage III (n = 30)	22%

Discussion

Tumors of the cervical esophagus and of the hypopharynx should be considered separately. In our experience, the actuarial 5-year survival rate after curative resection was 17% and 43%, respectively.[9] However, with the new definition of cancer of the cervical esophagus,[5] there are cases that are difficult to classify.[10] How should borderline tumors involving both the cervical esophagus and the hypopharynx be classified? How should we consider patients who have undergone laryngectomy for cancer and develop a new malignancy of the cervical esophagus during follow-up? In our experience,[11] these latter tumors should not be included among primary esophageal cancers since they have a very dismal prognosis independent of the disease-free interval after laryngectomy (mean: 3 years; range: 1–19 years). The 2-year and 3-year survival rate after resection of the new esophageal malignancy was 10%, and 0%, respectively.

In the present study, the clinical TNM stage of cervical esophageal cancer was discordant with pathological findings in nearly 50% of the cases (30 of 63 patients) and was therefore inaccurate and unreliable both for therapeutic planning and for prognostic evaluation. However, it should be noted that the study covered the period between 1980 and 1987 and that the most recent CT and ultrasonographic scanners are much more accurate than those used in the early 1980s. Furthermore, endoscopic ultrasonography (EUS) became available to us only during the last year. The evaluation of the T status is difficult since its new definition is based on pathological criteria which are not easily assessed by means of preoperative exams. At present, EUS is the most accurate exam to assess the degree of parietal involvement and should be used routinely.[12] The N status should be investigated by means of ultrasonography of the neck, EUS, and CT scan.

The prognostic value of pathological TNM staging was not confirmed in our study. Only the prognosis of p-stage I patients was better than that of patients in the other stages, while patients with a p-stage IIA, IIB, or III tumor had comparable survivals. This result may be related to one or more of the following causes: the small number of patients considered, the lack of prognostic significance of the TNM staging system, or lymph node understaging. In this regard, it should be pointed out that despite the fact that most patients did not undergo mediastinal lymphadenectomy through a thoracotomy or a sternotomy, recurrence after curative resection was located mainly in the neck (11 of 13 cases) and not inside the mediastinum.

An unsolved question concerns the classification of mediastinal lymph node metastases which are considered as M1 LYM (stage IV) by the TNM guidelines. Is it justified to consider paraesophageal, paratracheal, and recurrent nerve nodes which are located inside the mediastinum only a few centimeters distal to the corresponding cervical nodes as M1? The present N classification seems arbitrary to us and to other authors,[13] since the rate of metastatic mediastinal nodes found on the operative specimen was not negligible (32% of the N+ cases, 8 of 25), and the survival of these patients was comparable to that of patients with positive nodes only in the neck. Lamprecht[14] reported neoplastic involvement of the mediastinum in 44% of 79 patients with a tumor of the hypopharynx. Cancer of the cervical esophagus seems to have a similar tendency towards mediastinal infiltration.[15] Therefore, we think that the following mediastinal nodes, which are in direct continuity with the corresponding cervical ones, should be considered as local-regional: paraesophageal, paratracheal, and recurrent nerve. The number of metastatic nodes may also be considered a prognostic factor: one versus more than one according to Peracchia,[16] one or two versus more than two according to Ando,[17] and less than five versus five or more according to Skinner.[6]

To our knowledge, only two studies[18,19] analyzed the staging of cancer of the cervical esophagus separately from cancer of the hypopharynx and of the intrathoracic esophagus. The prognostic role of nodal status was evaluated by Kasai[18] in 45 patients undergoing esophagectomy. The 5-year survival rate of patients without node metastases was 46.3%, and no patients with positive nodes reached the 2-year interval. Collin[19] studied 35 patients who had undergone curative resection and demonstrated that the survival was comparable in patients with partial-thickness (T1–T2) and full-thickness tumors (T3), and only patients with a tumor invading adjacent structures (T4) had a significantly worse prognosis than patients with a T1–T3 tumor. The lymph node status was studied in 25 patients in whom paraesophageal and cervical nodes were metastatic in 21 patients (84%), but the preoperative diagnosis was correct in only 7. After curative resection, a local-regional recurrence, i.e., in the neck, was detected in 88% of the cases. One more paper dealt at least in part with the present topic: Kakegawa[20] studied 64 patients with a tumor of the cervical and cervico-thoracic esophagus who underwent esophagectomy. The following lymph nodes were metastatic: laterocervical in 2.9% of the patients, retropharyngeal in 2.9%, deep cervical in 14.3%, cervical paraesophageal in 14.3%, supraclavicular in 11.4%, mediastinal paraesophageal in 11.4%, and abdominal in 2.9%. Esophagectomy without thoracotomy was considered unsatisfactory due to the incomplete mediastinal lymphadenectomy.

The issue of cervical esophageal cancer staging was not specifically discussed even during the last meeting of the ISDE committee for the TNM staging of cancer of the esophagus. Most speakers presented studies performed on patients with cancer of the intrathoracic esophagus, and some presented even mixed data on esophageal and cardia cancers. Only Iizuka[21] proposed to grade the extent of lymph node dissection as follows: *class 0* = resection of the primary, without lymph node dissection; *class 1* = as in class 0 plus dissection of the cervical paraesophageal nodes; *class 2* = as in class 1 plus functional or radical neck dissection (paratracheal nodes, internal jugular vein lymph nodes, recurrent nerve lymph nodes, and supraclavicular nodes); *class 3* = as in class 2 plus dissection of mediastinal nodes. We think that the above proposal should be taken into account in future studies.

Conclusion

Clinical TNM staging of cancer of the cervical esophagus is inaccurate and is therefore unreliable for therapeutic decision-making and prognostic evaluation. The pathological TNM staging should be revised, especially as far as N status is concerned. Much work is still required to improve the accuracy and reliability of the TNM staging of cancer of the cervical esophagus.

References

1. Silver CE: Surgical treatment of hypopharyngeal and cervical esophageal cancer. World J Surg 5:499, 1981.

2. Schuller DE: Reconstructive options for pharyngeal and/or cervical esophageal defects. Arch Otolaryngol 111:193, 1985.
3. Lam KH, Wong J, Lim STK, et al: Pharyngogastric anastomosis following pharyngolaryngo-esophagectomy: Analysis of 157 cases. World J Surg 5:509, 1981.
4. Lam KH, Choi TK, Wei WI, et al: Present status of pharyngo-gastric anastomosis following pharyngolaryngo-oesophagectomy. Br J Surg 74:122, 1987.
5. UICC, International Union Against Cancer: TNM Classification of Malignant Tumors, Hermanek P, Sobin LH (eds), Berlin, Springer-Verlag, 1987, p 40.
6. Skinner DB, Little AG, Ferguson MK, et al: Selection of operation for esophageal cancer based on staging. Ann Surg 204:391, 1986.
7. Japanese Committee for Registration of Esophageal Carcinoma: A proposal for a new TNM classification of esophageal carcinoma. Jpn J Clin Oncol 14:625, 1985.
8. Iizuka T: New TNM classification for carcinoma of the esophagus. In: Diseases of the Esophagus, Siewert JR, Holscher AH (eds), Berlin, Springer-Verlag, 1988, p 355.
9. Peracchia A, Ancona E, Merigliano S, et al: Surgical strategy in therapy of cancer of the cervical esophageal region: Ten-year experience. In: Proceedings of the International Symposium on Cancer of the Esophagus, Sendai, Japan, 1985, p 67.
10. Harrison DFN, Thompson AE: Pharyngolaryngoesophagectomy with pharyngogastric anastomosis for cancer of the hypopharynx: Review of 101 operations. Head Neck Surg 8:418, 1986.
11. Peracchia A, Bardini R, Ruol A, et al: Terapia chirurgica dei carcinomi dell'ipofaringe e dell'esofago cervicale. In: Proceedings of the 11th Congress, SICO, Genoa, 1987, p 737.
12. Murata Y, Ide H, Fukui H, et al: The role of ultrasonography for preoperative staging in esophageal cancer. In: Proceedings of the Research Committee meeting on the TNM Classification of Esophageal Carcinoma of the ISDE, Tokyo, 1988.
13. Elias D, Lasser P, Eschwege F, et al: Etude retrospective de 88 cas de cancer de l'oesophage cervical et definition d'une nouvelle approche therapeutique. J Chir 120:243, 1983.
14. Lamprecht J, Lamprecht A, Kurten-Royhers R: Mediastinale beteilingung bei karzinomen der subglottis, des hypopharynx und des zervikalen oesophagus. Laryngol Rhinol Otol 66:88, 1987.
15. Gluckman JL, Weissler MC, McCafferty G, et al: Partial vs total esophageactomy for advanced carcinoma of the hypopharynx. Arch Otolaryngol Head Neck Surg 113:69, 1987.
16. Bardini R, Ruol A, Asolati M, et al: Comparison of different staging systems and prognostic factors for esophageal cancer. In: Proceedings of the Research Committee meeting on the TNM classification of Esophageal Carcinoma of the ISDE, Tokyo, 1988.
17. Ando N: Prognosis of the patients in terms of the number of positive nodes. In: Proceedings of the Research Committee meeting on the TNM classification of Esophageal Carcinoma of the ISDE, Tokyo, 1988.

18. Kasai M, Nishihira T: Reconstruction using pedicled jejunal segments after resection for carcinoma of the cervical esophagus. Surg Gynecol Obstet 163:145, 1986.
19. Collin CF, Spiro RH: Carcinoma of the cervical esophagus: changing therapeutic trends. Am J Surg 148:460, 1984.
20. Kakegawa T, Yamana H, Ando N: Analysis of surgical treatment for carcinoma situated in the cervical esophagus. Surgery 97:150, 1985.
21. Iizuka T: Proposal of grading of extent of lymphnode dissection. In: Proceedings of the Research Committee meeting on the TNM classification of Esophageal Carcinoma of the ISDE, Tokyo, 1988.

14

Prospective Study Comparing Endoscopic Ultrasonography and Computed Tomography in 56 Resected Esophageal Carcinomas

Brice Gayet, Laurent Palazzo, Valerie Vilgrain, Yves Menu, J.A. Paolaggi, François Fékété

Introduction

In order to select the best treatment for esophageal carcinoma (EC), it is necessary to assess very accurately the stage of the tumor.[1] As far as operable patients without metastases are concerned, surgical indications depend on paraesophageal spread and location of the tumor.[2] For this regional staging, several authors have suggested that endoscopic ultrasonography (EUS) is highly valuable,[3–5] while computed tomography (CT) continues to be recommended.[6,7] There are only a few studies with small numbers of patients that prospectively compare results of these tests with surgical and pathological findings.[8,9] This prospective study was undertaken to evaluate and compare the usefulness of EUS and CT in assessing the local and regional extension of EC, excluding cardia carcinoma.

Ferguson MK, Little AG, Skinner DB: Diseases of the Esophagus, Vol. I: Malignant Diseases. Futura Publishing Company, Inc., Mount Kisco, NY, © 1990.

Patients and Methods

Between March 1987 and March 1988, 85 patients with a proven EC had complete preoperative assessment of their tumors. Thirty-four patients had no exploration or resection and were excluded. Fifty-one patients, 46 males and five females, had 56 EC resected and were included in this prospective study. Their ages ranged from 35 to 75 years with a mean of 55 years. No patient received preoperative radiation therapy or chemotherapy.

The results of EUS and CT were prospectively and separately collected without knowledge of the results of other exams. The same detailed questionnaire filled in by the endoscopist for EUS and the radiologist for CT was compared to surgical and pathological findings. The parameters evaluated were: degree of parietal involvement; tumor invasion into adjacent structures; cervical, thoracic, or abdominal metastatic lymph node involvement (10 sites for each patient); and tumor staging according to the classification of the Japanese Society of Esophageal Diseases.[10] Two groups of 28 tumors were defined by whether the echoendoscope could (group I, 25 patients) or could not (group II, 26 patients) pass through the tumor. A carcinoma was defined as superficial when the invasion was limited to the mucosa or the submucosa with or without lymph node involvement. A so-called advanced tumor invaded into or beyond the muscularis propria.

CT scans were performed using a Siemens Somatom DR obtaining contiguous 8-mm sections from the upper thoracic outlet to the lower part of the liver. Oral and intravenous contrast material was routinely administered. The format followed was based on criteria already validated by a prospective controlled study on 250 previously resected patients.[11]

For the tracheobronchial tree involvement, only two signs were considered: (a) extrinsic growth present between the aortic arch and the trachea or the aorta and the main left bronchus; and (b) thickening or intraluminal growth of the tracheobronchial wall. For aortic involvement, only two signs were used: (a) growth coming into contact with the vessel and distorting its lumen; and (b) extension of growth, and not the tumor itself, between the vertebrae and the aorta. A lymph node was considered metastatic if its largest diameter measured more than 6 mm in the posterior mediastinum, 10 mm in the celiac area, and 20 mm at the subcarinal level.

The EUS equipment consisted of an Olympus fiberscope (UM 2).

The apparatus displays five alternating hyper- and hypoechoic layers, of 3–4 mm in full thickness, representing the esophageal wall and interfaces between its anatomic layers. From superficial to deep, parietal invasion was defined as follows:

mucosal spread (a0 m): no abnormality of the third hyperechoic layer and either normal EUS or thickness of the second hypoechoic layer of less than 2 mm;

submucosal spread (a0 sm): thickness of more than 2 mm of the third hyperechoic layer;

muscle invasion (a0 mp): thickening within the fourth hypoechoic layer surrounded by a hypoechoic border;

adventitial spread (a1): continuous thickening reaching the fifth hyperechoic layer;

periesophageal spread (a2): thickening reaching the fifth hyperechoic layer which is interrupted;

adjacent structure involvement (a3): thickness within the structure without a hyperechoic border between the tumor and the organ concerned or with tumor growth inside it.

In the determination of metastatic lymph node involvement, we used the following criteria:

1. Any node deforming the esophageal adventitia was considered as metastatic; spindle- or triangular-shaped subcarinal and left paratracheal lymph nodes were considered benign as were nonvisualized nodes.

2. An oval- or spherical-shaped node was considered metastatic.

3. An uneven echo pattern with hyperechoic internal spots and/or a clear-cut border suggest a metastasis.

4. A node of less than 5-mm diameter was considered benign, while one with a diameter of more than 10 mm might be metastatic.

Results

The primary tumor was cervical in three cases and thoracic in 48 cases (7 upper third, 32 middle third, and 9 lower third); five patients had two tumors. Surgical findings were available in all cases through combined abdominal and right thoracic approach associated with a cervicotomy in 14 patients. Pathology revealed 51 squamous cell carcinomas, four adenocarcinomas in Barrett's esophagus, and one melanoma. No complications resulted from EUS or CT in this study.

In group I, in which examination of the whole tumor was done,

Table I
Accuracy of Endoscopic Ultrasonography (EUS) in Determining Depth of Parietal Invasion

		EUS-Group I						EUS-Group II						
		m	*sm*	*mp*	*a1*	*a2*	*a3*	*m*	*sm*	*mp*	*a1*	*a2*	*a3*	*NV*
Histology	m	9						1						
	sm	1	4											
	mp			2	1							1		
	a1										1			
	a2				2	6						11		1
	a3						3		1		1	4	5	2

Group I: 28 tumors completely examined in 25 patients; Group II: 28 tumors partially or not visualized in 26 patients.
m = mucosa; sm = submucosa; mp = muscularis propria; a1 = adventitia; a2 = mediastinal tissue; a3 = adjacent structure invaded; NV = upper extent of the tumor not visualized.

the accuracy for parietal spread assessment was 85.7% by EUS. Table I depicts the results of EUS compared to the actual depth of invasion. Discrimination between superficial EC and more advanced EC was 100%. Three patients had proven adjacent structure involvement, diagnosed three times by EUS and twice by CT (Table II). For nodal

Table II
Detection of Infiltration into a Contiguous Structure by Endoscopic Ultrasonography (EUS) and Computed Tomography (CT) Based on Surgical Findings

		Group I			Group II			Total*
		Surgery	*EUS*	*CT*	*Surgery*	*EUS*	*CT*	*EUS + CT*
Nonresectable structures	Left Bronchus	3	3	2	1	0	1	4/4
	Trachea				2	1	1	2/2
	Pulmonary Vein				1	1	1	1/1
	Aorta				1	0	0	0/1
Resectable structures	Pleura	1	0	0	6	2	1	3/7
	Pericardium	2	2	2	4	2	1	4/6
	Lung	1	0	0	4	0	1	1/5
	Diaphragm				1	0	0	0/1

* number of patients correctly assessed by the association of EUS and CT/number of patients presenting with involvement. Some patients had more than one organ involved.

Table III
Detection of Lymph Node Involvement by Endoscopic Ultrasonography (EUS) and Computed Tomography (CT)

	Group I		*Group II*	
	EUS	*CT*	*EUS*	*CT*
True positive	10	6	15	8
True negative	234	235	140	142
False positive	4	3	4	2
False negative	2	6	2	9
Sensitivity (%)	83	50	88	47
Specificity (%)	98	99	97	99
Accuracy (%)	98	96	96	93

Group II: anlaysis of sites proximal to the tumor only.

involvement, sensitivity was 83% by EUS and 50% by CT. Accuracy was very high at 88% versus 96%, respectively (Table III).

In group II, the accuracy of parietal spread assessment was only 64% by EUS. Local invasion into anatomical structures was confirmed by exploration for 16 tumors. The diagnosis was made in 11 cases equally by EUS and CT, better by EUS in eight cases and better by CT in six cases. For lymph nodes situated above the tumor, sensitivity was 88% using EUS and 47% using CT, but CT was able to realize a more complete assessment throughout.

Accuracy of staging, using the Japanese classification, was 84% and 61%, respectively, by EUS for patients of group I and group II (Table IV). The value of CT in the preoperative staging of EC was limited by its low sensitivity in determining parietal growth and lymph node involvement.

Discussion

The prognosis of EC is directly linked to the degree of parietal and lymphatic involvement.[1] For both, EUS had a very good accuracy (84%) and sensitivity and should be mandatory for clinical staging of esophageal carcinoma. On the other hand, when properly interpreted, CT is a good preoperative form of investigation to assess tumor spread beyond the esophageal wall and visceral metastases, two of the main factors upon which resectability depends.[9]

Table IV
Accuracy of Endoscopic Ultrasonography (EUS) in Determining the Preoperative Stage According to the Japanese Classification[10]

		EUS-Group I						*EUS-Group II*				
		0	*I*	*II*	*III*	*IV*		*0*	*I*	*II*	*III*	*IV*
	0	9		2			0					
	I		1				I					
Histology	II		1				II			1		
	III			1	8		III			1*	10	
	IV					3	IV	1*		2*	6	5

* The patients in whom the tumor was not visualized were staged accordingly to the findings of the supratumoral lymph nodes.

As far as lymph node metastases detection by CT was concerned, the high number of positive findings that turned out to be false at pathology resulted in a very low sensitivity (for the surgeon) even if it had a good accuracy. With respect to infiltration of the esophageal wall, the results were similarly disappointing. However, CT visualized extraluminal growth quite well and was able to predict operative difficulties. CT findings can be very valuable in planning a surgical approach.

This study suggests that EUS allows a very accurate discrimination between advanced and superficial esophageal carcinoma. However, for these latter tumors, it was unable to separate intraepithelial (in situ) from intramucosal cancer when the macroscopic lesion was flat or erosive, and mucosal from submucosal spread with certainty because the muscularis mucosa has no echoic signal. We use a 2-mm criteria which applies to flat tumors and never to polypoid ones. Microscopic involvement of the adventitia (the difference between a1 and a2 tumors) is also impossible to detect. Finally, for extension into surrounding structures, EUS is complementary to CT. For lymph node involvement, our results are impressive, especially because some misdiagnoses might be rectified. Four false-positives were due to very large but triangular-shaped subcarinal lymph nodes and should be logically interpreted as benign. The two false-negatives of group I were abdominal nodes not visualized, probably due to our inexperience.

In conclusion, EUS seems to be the best preoperative aid for regional assessment of EC without stenosis, while CT will remain necessary for stenosing carcinomas until miniaturization of the probes currently in use allows them to pass through an advanced cancer. Finally, CT might be necessary in all cases for the assessment of pulmonary and/or liver metastases.

References

1. Sugimachi K, Matsura H, Kai H: Prognostic factors of esophageal carcinoma: Univariate and multivariate analyses. J Oncol 31:108, 1986.
2. Fékété F, Gayet B, Favas A, et al: Indications et résultats du traitement chirurgical du cancer de l'oesophage thoracique. Ann Chir 42:185, 1988.
3. Murata Y, Muroi M, Yoshida M, et al: Endoscopic ultrasonography in the diagnosis of esophageal carcinoma. Surg Endosc 1:11, 1987.
4. Takemoto T, Ito T, Aibe T, et al: Endoscopic ultrasonography in the diagnosis of esophageal carcinoma with particular regard to staging it for operability. Endoscopy 18:22, 1986.
5. Tio TL, Denhartogjager FC, Tytgat GN: The role of endoscopic ultrasonography in assessing local resectability of esophagogastric malignancies: Accuracy, pitfalls and predictability. Scand J Gastroenterol 21:78, 1986.
6. Fékété F, Gayet B, Frija J: Contribution of computed tomography in the staging of cancer of the esophagus: A prospective study on 53 patients. In: Esophageal Disorders: Pathophysiology and Therapy, DeMeester TR, Skinner DB (eds), New York, Raven Press, 1985, p 73.
7. Quint L, Glazer G, Orringer M, et al: Esophageal carcinoma: CT findings. Radiology 155:171, 1985.
8. Souquet JC, Valette PJ, Berger F, et al: Endosonographie et staging tumoral des cancers epidermoïdes de l'oesophage. Gastroenterol Clin Biol 12:2, 1988.
9. Ziegler K, Sanft C, Semsch B, et al: Endosonography is superior to computed tomography in staging tumors of the esophagus and the cardia. Gastroenterology 94:517A, 1988
10. Japanese Committee for Registration of Esophageal Carcinoma: A proposal for new TNM classification of esophageal carcinoma. Jpn J Clin Oncol 14:625, 1985.
11. Gayet B, Frija J, Cahuzac J, et al: Intérêt de la tomodensitométrie dans le cancer de l'oesophage. Etude prospective et aveugle. Gastroenterol Clin Biol 12:23, 1988.

15

Endosonography Versus Computed Tomography for Determination of Loco-Regional Spread in Esophageal Cancer:
A Prospective Controlled Study

Horst Grimm, N. Soehendra, K. Hamper, R. Maas

Introduction

Survival of patients with esophageal cancer is mainly determined by the depth of tumor infiltration and lymph node involvement.[1,2] Thus an accurate staging of the tumor is mandatory for proper selection of the modality of treatment. There are several reports showing high accuracy of computed tomography (CT) in preoperative staging of esophageal malignancies, and this imaging method is currently routinely employed for this purpose.[3,4] However, the results of CT in detecting lymph node metastases have been shown to be poor, and in some recently published data its sensitivity for determining loco-regional spread of esophageal cancer was questioned.[5,6]

Endoscopic ultrasonography (EUS) is emerging as a new reliable method for preoperative staging of gastrointestinal tumors. It is re-

Ferguson MK, Little AG, Skinner DB: Diseases of the Esophagus, Vol. I: Malignant Diseases. Futura Publishing Company, Inc., Mount Kisco, NY, © 1990.

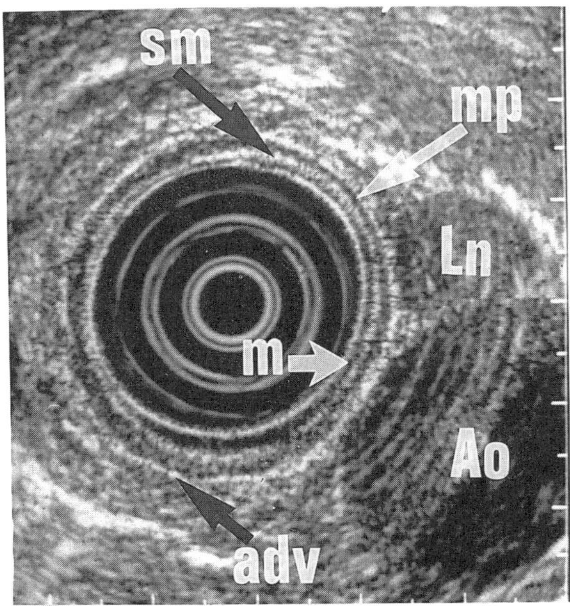

Figure 1: EUS picture showing the normal five-layered structure of the esophageal wall. m = mucosa, sm = submucosa, mp = muscularis propria, adv = adventitia, Ao = aorta, Ln = lymph node.

ported to have a high sensitivity not only in determining the depth of tumor infiltration, but even for detecting lymph node metastases.[7–9] The aim of this study was to assess the accuracy of EUS in preoperative staging of esophageal cancer and to compare its results with those of CT regarding invasion of adjacent organs and lymph node spread.

Materials and Methods

From January 1987 to February 1989, a total of 58 patients with histologically proven esophageal carcinoma were examined with EUS and CT as part of a preoperative staging protocol. Twenty-four patients who underwent surgery were included in this study. There were 19 men and 5 women whose ages ranged from 39 to 78 years (mean 55.4 years). The results of EUS and CT were compared to the histology of the resected specimens. When resection was not possible,

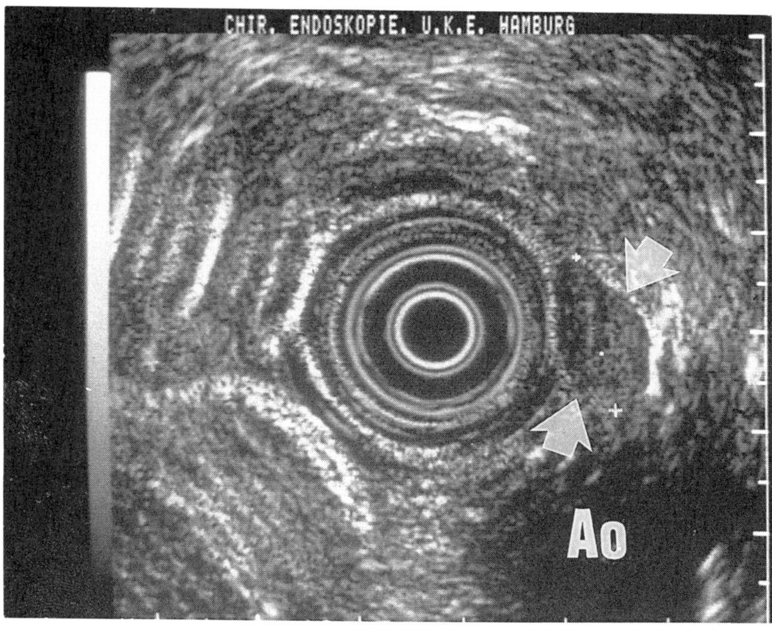

Figure 2: Metastatic paraesophageal lymph node (arrows) as seen by EUS. Ao = aorta.

the intraoperative findings as well as sample biopsies were taken for comparison.

EUS was performed with an Olympus echoendoscope (GF-UM2/EU-M2), 7.5 MHz; 5–10 mg of diazepam and 20–40 mg N-butylscopolaminiumbromid (Buscopan) were given intravenously as premedication. The depth of tumor infiltration was determined based on the five-layered structure of the esophageal wall[9,10] (Fig. 1). In evaluation of lymph nodes, clearly defined boundaries and a hypoechoic internal structure, either homogeneous or heterogeneous, were considered criteria for malignancy[9,11] (Fig. 2).

CT was performed either on the Somatom II, Siemens (256 × 256 matrix) or the Somatom Plus, Siemens (512 × 512 matrix). Contrast media was given for examination in 17 cases. Three patients had oral and 14 had oral plus additional IV administration. Contiguous slices, 8-mm thick through the thorax and upper abdomen, were used to determine the local tumor extension to adjacent structures, loco-regional and distant lymph node involvement, and distant spread to

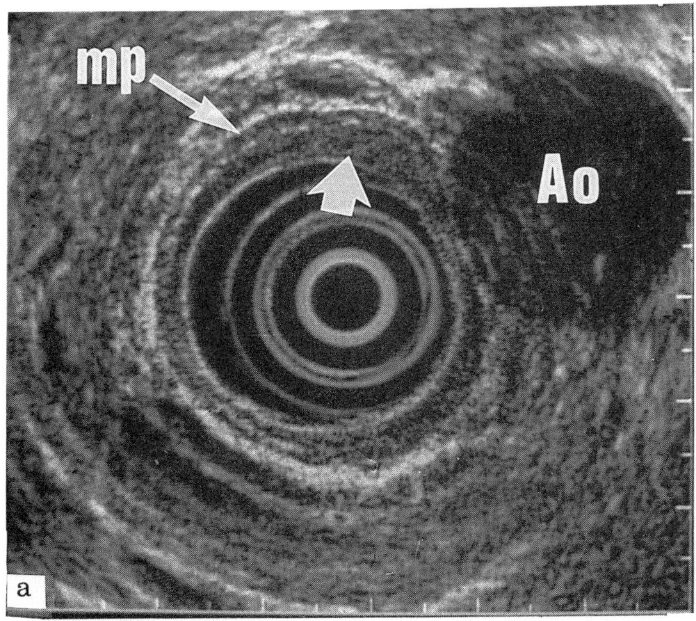

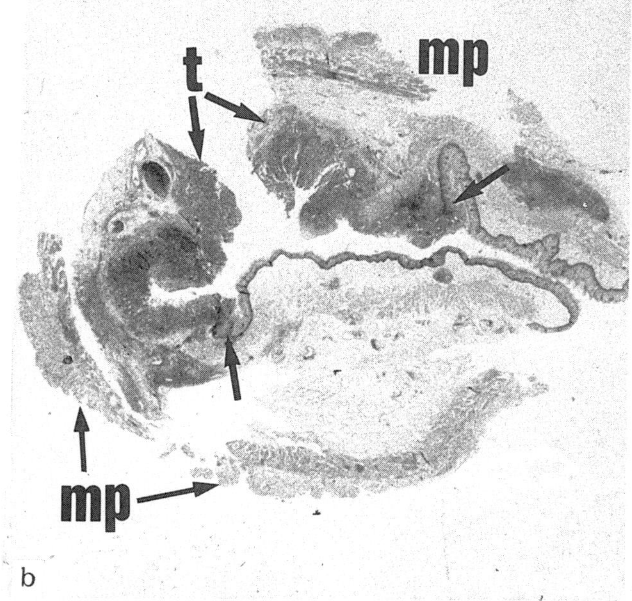

Figure 3: (a) Esophageal carcinoma (arrow) limited to the submucosa. mp = muscularis propria, Ao = aorta. (b) Histology of the resected specimen which confirms the diagnosis of early cancer. t = tumor, mp = muscularis propria. Arrows depict transition between tumor and normal tissue.

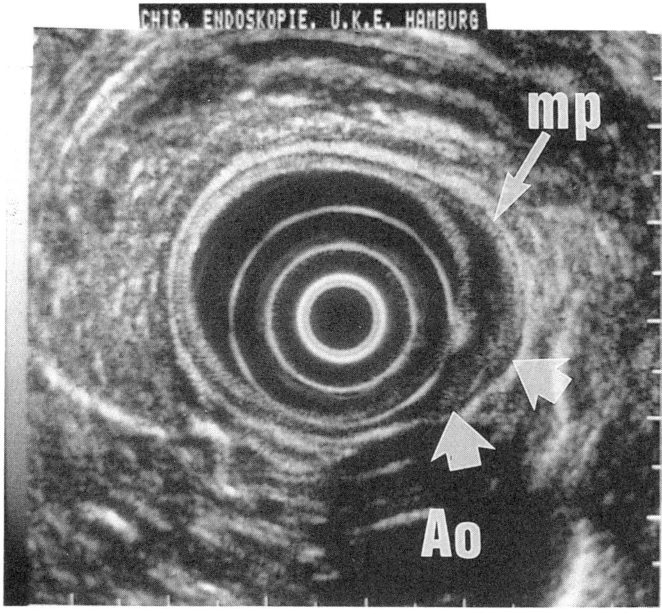

Figure 4: Esophageal carcinoma with superficial invasion of the muscularis propria (arrows). Ao = aorta, mp = muscularis propria.

other organs. Lymph nodes more than 1 cm in diameter were considered suspicious for metastases.

The histologic evaluation of tumor and lymph nodes was done according to the new TNM classification.[12] Statistical analysis was performed using the McNemar test.

Results

In the group of operated patients (N = 24), there was a total of 29 tumors (two patients had three tumors and one patient had two tumors). Twenty-two of these lesions were squamous cell carcinomas and seven were adenocarcinomas. Two tumors were located in the upper third of the esophagus, 15 in the middle third, and 12 in the distal third. Seven patients had a tight stenosis, and the echoendoscope could be passed in only two of these patients.

Eight tumors were limited to the submucosa (Fig. 3), 6 to the

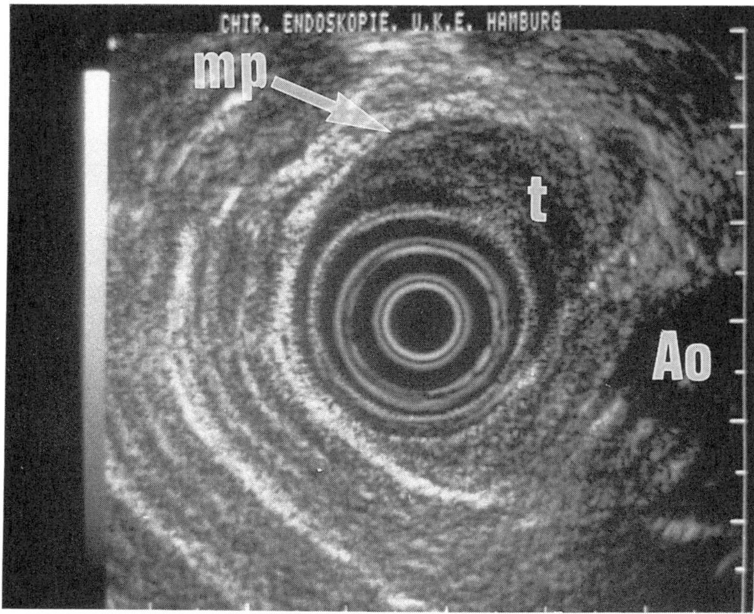

Figure 5: Esophageal carcinoma with extension through the muscular layer. t = tumor, Ao = aorta, mp = muscularis propria.

muscular layer (Fig. 4), and 12 had already infiltrated the adventitia (Fig. 5). In two cases there was an infiltration of adjacent organs by the tumor (Fig. 6).

One intramucosal cancer was not demonstrated by EUS but the correct stage was determined because no infiltration of the submucosa was seen. Thus, considering the different layers of the esophageal wall, the accuracy rate of EUS in determining the depth of tumor infiltration was 86% (Table I). According to the TNM classification, the accuracy of staging was 87% (21 of 24 patients). A proper histologic examination of lymph nodes was possible in 23 out of 24 patients. Loco-regional lymph node involvement was present in 15 patients. These were correctly diagnosed by EUS in 13 cases and by CT in only three (Table II). The overall accuracy rate of EUS was 83%, sensitivity 87%, and specificity 75%, whereas CT showed an overall accuracy rate of 48%, sensitivity 20%, and specificity 100%.

Comparing the accuracy of both methods in detection of involved loco-regional nodes, EUS was superior to CT, the difference being

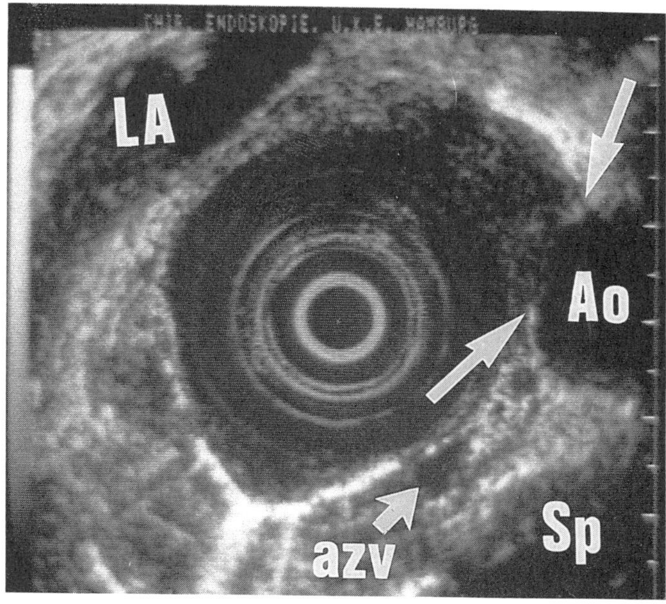

Figure 6: Advanced esophageal cancer with infiltration of the aorta (arrows). Ao = aorta, LA = left atrium, azv = azygos vein, Sp = spine.

Table I
Accuracy of EUS in Diagnosis of Tumor Invasion

	Histology/Intraoperative Findings				
EUS	*m*	*sm*	*mp*	*adv*	*adj org*
m	1				
sm		7	2		
mp		1	3		
adv			1	12	
adj org					2

Accuracy rate: 86% (25/29)

m = mucosa; sm = submucosa; mp = muscularis propria; adv = adventitia; adj org = adjacent organs

Table II
Evaluation of Regional Lymph Nodes: Comparison betweeen EUS and CT (n = 23 patients)

	EUS			*CT*		
Histology	*True*	*False +*	*False −*	*True*	*False +*	*False −*
pN0 (n = 8)	6	2	—	8	0	—
pN1 (n = 15)	13	—	2	3	—	12

Overall accuracy rate: EUS = 83%
CT = 48%

pN0 = no regional lymph node metastasis; pN1 = regional lymph node metastasis

statistically significant ($p < 0.002$). Seven patients had spread to celiac nodes, detected in two cases with CT. EUS evaluation of celiac nodes was possible in only four of these cases because of impassable stenosis in three. The correct diagnosis was made by EUS in two whereas the other two were wrongly classified as nonmetastatic. Two patients had distant metastasis to other organs (one lung, one liver), both detected by CT but not by EUS.

In the two patients with infiltration of adjacent structures (one aorta, one left atrium and aorta), the diagnosis was assessed correctly by EUS but not by CT.

Discussion

Our results show that EUS is an accurate method for assessing the depth of tumor infiltration. Pitfalls were mainly related to microscopic tumor invasion or accompanying inflammatory changes not distinguishable from the tumor itself on EUS. The current results do suggest superiority of EUS over CT, however, a definitive conclusion regarding local spread to other structures cannot yet be drawn due to the limited number of cases.

Concerning detection of loco-regional lymph node metastases, this study demonstrates the higher accuracy of EUS compared with CT, the difference being statistically significant. The main reason for this is the fact that most of the metastatic nodes had a diameter of less than 1 cm. Furthermore, possibility of proper assessment of the boundaries and internal echostructure gives EUS an added advantage for lymph node evaluation.

EUS had a clear limitation in the diagnosis of distant node metastases in patients with nonpassable stenoses, but CT failed to provide any further information. Due to the limited depth of penetration, EUS is generally not a suitable method for detecting distant metastasis to other organs. For this purpose, especially for pulmonary metastasis, CT plays an important role.

In our opinion, at present EUS is the method of choice for preoperative assessment of loco-regional spread of esophageal cancer. We hope that with further improvement of EUS equipment, the limitation imposed on this diagnostic modality can be overcome.

References

1. Skinner DB, Ferguson MK, Soriano A, et al: Selection of operation for esophageal cancer based on staging. Ann Surg 204:391, 1986.
2. Siewert JR, Roder JD: Chirurgische Therapie des Plattenepithelcarcinoms des Oesophagus-erweiterte Radikalität. Langenbecks Arch Chir 372:125, 1987.
3. Moss AA, Schnyder P, Thoeni RF: Esophageal carcinoma: Pretherapy staging by computed tomography. AJR 136:1051, 1981.
4. Grosser G, Wimmer B, Ruf G: Computertomography beim ösophaguskarzinom. Eine prospektive Studie. Fortschr Röntgenstr 143:288, 1985.
5. Quint LE, Glazer GM, Orringer MB, et al: Esophageal carcinoma: CT findings. Radiology 155:171, 1985.
6. Laas J, Scheller E, Haverich A, et al: How accurate is preoperative staging by computed tomography in esophageal carcinoma? In: Diseases of the Esophagus, Siewert JR, Hölscher AH (eds), Berlin, Springer Verlag, 1988, p 177.
7. Tio TL, Cohen P, Coene PP, et al: Endosonography and computed tomography of esophageal carcinoma, preoperative classification compared to the new (1987) TNM system. Gastroenterology 96:1478, 1989.
8. Kouzu T, Ogino Y, Isono K: Endoscopic ultrasonography in esophageal disease. In: Recent Topics of Digestive Endoscopy, Takemoto T, Kawai K (eds), Amsterdam, Excerpta Medica, 1987, p 54.
9. Murata Y, Muroi M, Yoshida M, et al: Endoscopic ultrasonography in the diagnosis of esophageal carcinoma. Surg Endosc 1:11, 1987.
10. Kimmey MB, Silverstein FE, Martin W: Ultrasound interaction with the intestinal wall: Esophagus, stomach and colon. In: Endoscopic Ultrasonography in Gastroenterology, Kawai K (ed), Tokyo, Igaku-Shoin, 1988, p 35.
11. Tio TL, Tytgat GNJ: Endoscopic ultrasonography in analysing periintes-

tinal lymph node abnormality. Scand J Gastroenterol 21(Suppl 123):158, 1986.
12. Hermanek P, Sobin LH: TNM-classification of Malignant Tumours: International Union Against Cancer, 4th edition, New York, Springer Verlag, 1987.

16

Preoperative Staging of Thoracic Esophageal Cancer by Ultrasonography According to the New TNM Classification

Yoko Murata, Misao Yoshida, Hiroko Ide, Shigeru Suzuki, Akiyoshi Yamada, Fujio Hanyu

Introduction

Precise estimation of the extent and stage of esophageal cancer should be made in order to select the appropriate treatment. Various diagnostic modalities have been used to obtain accurate information preoperatively, but satisfactory results have not yet been obtained. Endoscopic ultrasonography is a valuable method for diagnosis, not only of the depth of tumor invasion, but also in the detection of lymph node metastasis. The present study was undertaken to assess the value of ultrasonography for preoperative staging in thoracic esophageal cancer.

Methods and Patients

The endoscopic ultrasonographic system (Olympus Gastrofiberscope Model UMI,2,3 and the ultrasound observation unit EUM type

Ferguson MK, Little AG, Skinner DB: Diseases of the Esophagus, Vol. I: Malignant Diseases. Futura Publishing Company, Inc., Mount Kisco, NY, © 1990.

1,2) was used to diagnose thoracic lymph node metastasis and the depth of tumor invasion. The device at the tip of the scope is a radial scanner with an available frequency of either 7.5 or 12 MHz. A water-filled balloon was used as the coupler. Conventional ultrasonography (RT3600 linear type 7.5, 3.5 MHz, and 90A 3.75 MHz) was used for the diagnosis of cervical and abdominal lymph nodes and liver metastasis. Since 1983, endoscopic ultrasonography (EUS) and conventional ultrasonography (US) have been performed in 348 patients with thoracic esophageal cancer. All patients underwent surgery and the tumors were resected. In 204 patients, the scope passed beyond the tumor and total observation was possible. These cases were classified according to the new TNM system and the preoperative staging was verified by histopathological findings.[1]

Results

Depth of Tumor Invasion

A normal esophageal wall image by EUS consisted of five alternating hyperechoic and hypoechoic layers. The third layer, which is hyperechoic, corresponds to the submucosal layer. The fourth layer, which is hypoechoic, corresponds to the muscularis propria.[2] We also believe that the first layer might be the epithelial layer and the second the muscularis mucosa based on our in vitro experiments.[3]

The depth of cancer invasion was defined by the number of layers destroyed by the tumor. If, as shown in Figure 1a and b, the first and the second layers were occupied by a hypoechoic mass but the third layer under the tumor was preserved, then the tumor may be diagnosed as a mucosal cancer. Differentiation between an epithelial cancer and a cancer invading the muscularis mucosa in vivo was difficult, and they were included in a single category as mucosal cancer. Destruction as far as the third layer defines the tumor as submucosal (Fig. 1c). It is also possible to determine whether cancer has infiltrated an adjacent organ. If, for example, cancer has destroyed all layers and the thoracic aortic wall presents an ill-defined border, these findings suggest that the cancer has invaded the aorta (Fig. 2). In 204 patients with thoracic esophageal cancer, the accuracy of diagnosis of the depth of tumor invasion was 88% (Table I).

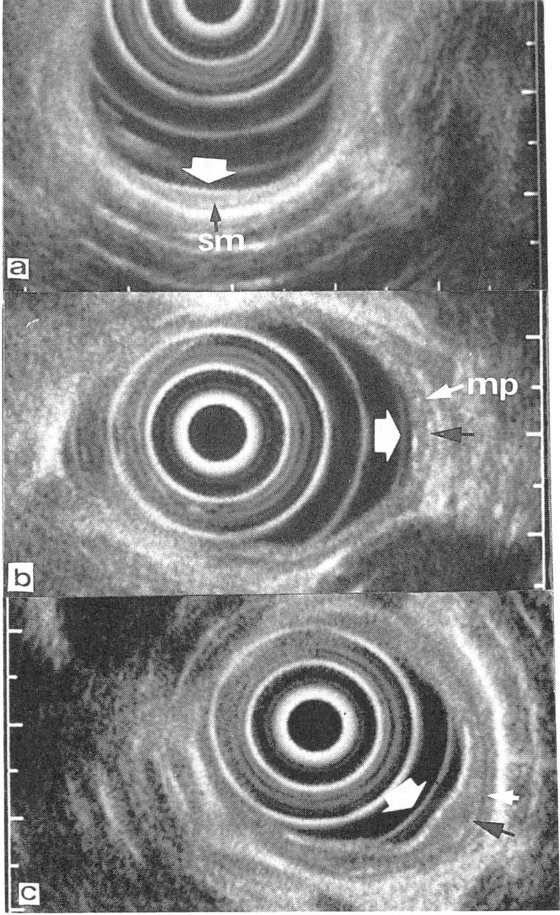

Figure 1: (a) Epithelial cancer. (b) Cancer limited to the muscularis mucosa. (c) Cancer limited to the submucosal layer. The thick arrows show the cancer, the black arrows (sm) indicate the submucosal layer, and the thin white arrows show the muscularis propria.

Diagnosis of Lymph Node Metastases

EUS can detect posterior mediastinal lymph nodes of more than 3 mm in the shortest dimension. US can indicate cervical lymph nodes of 3 mm in the shortest dimension or abdominal lymph nodes of more

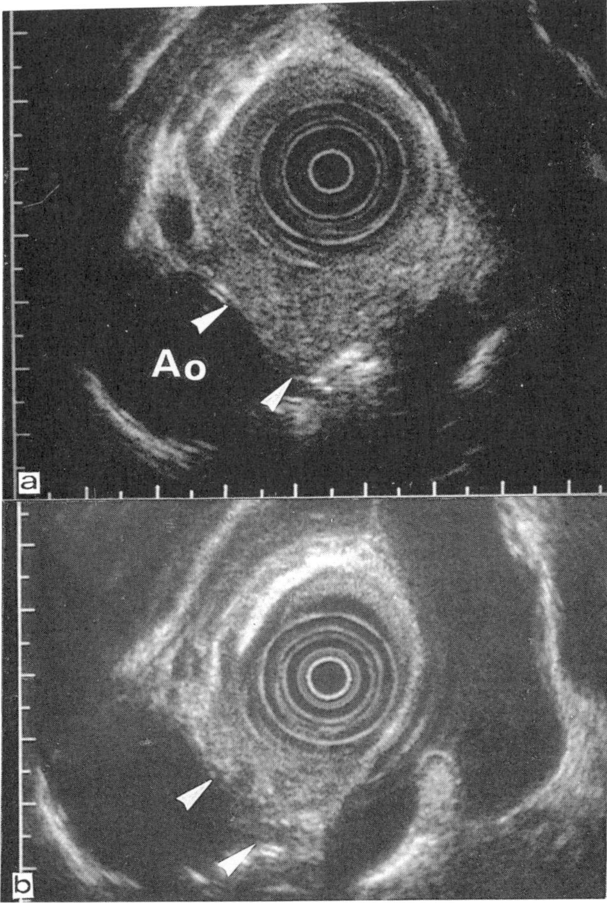

Figure 2: Cancer invasion of the aorta (Ao). The area of invasion of the descending aorta appears between the arrows (a). The size of the tumor decreased after radiotherapy (b).

than 5 mm in the shortest dimension. Since it was difficult to determine whether a metastasis was present, the gross appearance of the lymph nodes was retrospectively studied in resected specimens. The metastatic lymph nodes tended to have a spherical shape and were more than 5 mm in the shortest dimension.[3] The ultrasonographic features were also studied, demonstrating that the metastatic lymph nodes had a tendency to have a distinct border and a hypoechoic

Table I
Correlation of EUS Results with Pathological Findings in the Depth of Tumor Invasion[1]

EUS Diagnosis	*Pathology* T1 (m	sm)	T2	T3	T4	
—	1					
T1 (m)	15	4				
T1 (sm)	1	47	3			
T2		4	28	4		
T3		1	5	82		
T4				2	7	
Correct	15/17	47/56	28/36	82/88	7/7	179/204
%	88%	84%	78%	93%	100%	88%

T1 = Tumor invades lamina propria or submusoca
m = Tumor limited to the muscularis mucosa
sm = Tumor limited to the submucosa
T2 = Tumor invades muscularis propria
T3 = Tumor invades adventitia
T4 = Tumor invades adjacent structures

heterogeneous internal echo (Fig. 3).[3] On the basis of these results, the following diagnostic criteria for lymph node metastases were established: (1) spherical shape especially when more than 5 mm in the shortest dimension, (2) a distinct border, and (3) a hypoechoic heterogeneous internal echo. Based on the above criteria, lymph node metastases were correctly evaluated in 94% for neck, 88% for posterior mediastinum and 94% for abdomen (Table II).

Liver Metastasis

Liver metastases were represented as multiple hypoechoic or hyperechoic lesions by US. One out of 348 patients was misdiagnosed and a liver metastasis was found during operation. However, in the same period, liver metastases were detected by US in eight patients and were confirmed by computed tomography or angiography and an unnecessary operation was avoided. When these eight patients were included, sensitivity was 89% and specificity 100%. Excluding them, sensitivity was 0% and specificity 100%.

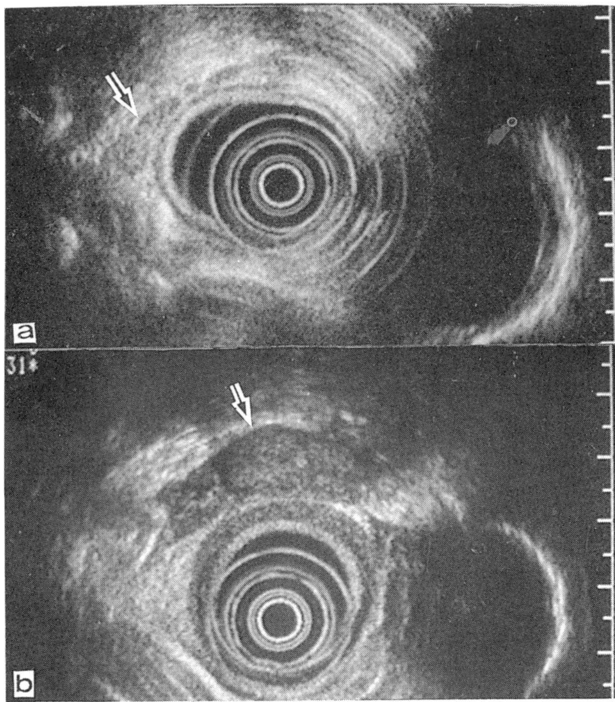

Figure 3: (a) Nonmetastatic lymph node. The arrow shows a subcarinal lymph node with an indistinct border and a homogeneous internal echo. (b) Metastatic lymph node. A subcarinal lymph node with a distinct border is indicated by the arrow. It has a hypoechoic heterogeneous internal echo.

Table II
Accuracy of EUS, US in Detection of Lymph Node Metastasis

Location	*Sensitivity*	*Specificity*	*Accuracy*
Cervical	95%	94%	94%
Posterior Mediastinum	85%	88%	88%
Abdomen	90%	95%	94%

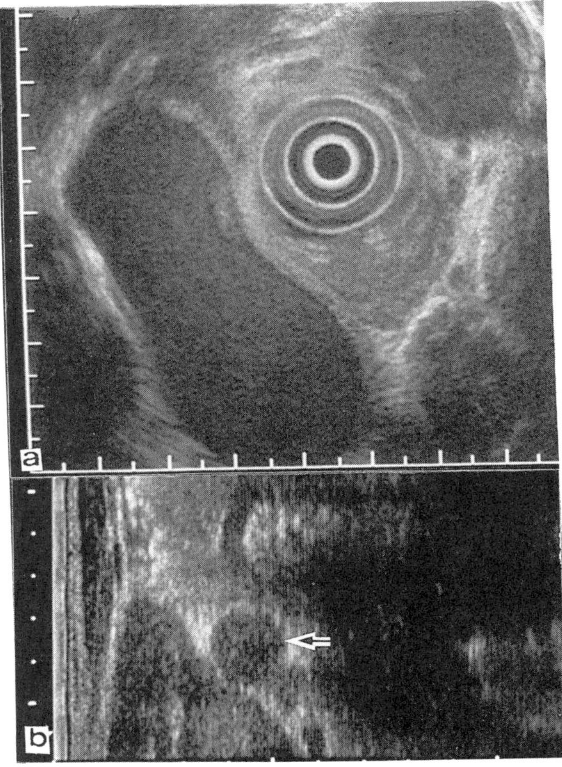

Figure 4: Stage IV cancer. A cancer invasion of the adventitia is diagnosed by EUS (a). Several celiac lymph nodes are detected by US and are suspected to be metastatic (b).

Staging of Esophageal Cancer According to the New TNM Classification

The above ultrasonographic findings were used to classify each stage according to the new TNM classification.[1] Each preoperative stage was verified by pathological analysis. The staging of esophageal cancer was accurately diagnosed in 0% of stage 0 patients, 67% of stage 1, 34% of stage 2A, 80% of stage 2B, 82% of stage 3, and 71% of stage 4 patients. The overall accuracy was 66% (Table III).

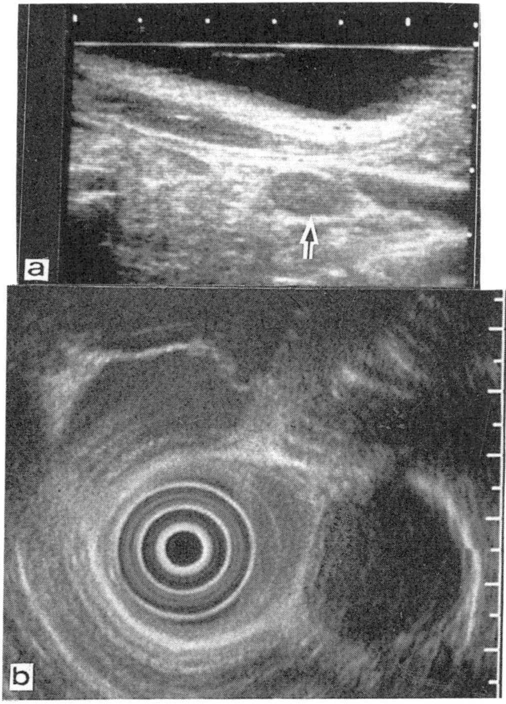

Figure 5: Stage IV cancer. A cancer invasion of the adventitia is indicated by EUS (a). A small cervical lymph node is detected by US and is metastatic.

Table III
Correlation of US, EUS Staging and Pathological Staging[1]

Stage		
0	0/7	(0%)
I	34/50	(68%)
IIA	20/58	(34%)
IIB	19/24	(79%)
III	72/88	(82%)
IV	85/120	(71%)
Total	231/348	(66%)

Discussion

This study describes the clinical value of EUS and US in the staging of esophageal cancer. It also outlines some of the difficulties involved in diagnosis. When diagnosing the depth of cancer invasion, differentiation of the epithelial cancer from cancer invading the muscularis mucosa was difficult, and Tis tumors could not be distinguished from T1 cancers. Another problem was that the scope was too big to pass through advanced tumors, giving a total observation rate of 60%. However, 69% of patients with T4 tumors in whom the scope could not be passed beyond the tumor could be accurately staged nevertheless.

When assessing the presence or absence of lymph node metastases, the size of the lymph node has been used as the primary criterion in various imaging modalities. However, accuracy rates are limited.[4] Normal lymph node size has also been measured to establish normal thresholds,[5,6] and our finding that a normal lymph node was less than 5 mm in the shortest dimension was similar to that reported in other papers. Metastatic lymph nodes have a tendency to be spherically shaped.[2,7] Moreover, ultrasonographic features such as a border and an internal echo were studied[3] and we were able to establish additional criteria. Using these criteria an overall accuracy of 88–94% was achieved. However, the sonographic patterns are not specific and the echo patterns of nodes of less than 5 mm in diameter are difficult to interpret. There were several exceptions, for example, lymph nodes with microscopic metastasis, tuberculosis, and idiopathic lymphadenopathy. We conclude that accuracy rate by EUS and US has limitations. However, excluding some special cases, if the sonographic readings of lymph nodes fit our criteria, the likelihood of the presence of lymph node metastasis is high.

References

1. Japanese Committee for Registration of Esophageal Carcinoma: A proposal for a new TNM classification of esophageal carcinoma. Jpn J Clin Oncol 14:625–636, 1985.
2. Murata Y, Muroi M, Yoshida M, et al: Endoscopic ultrasonography in diagnosis of esophageal carcinoma. Surg Endosc 1:11, 1987.
3. Murata Y: The evaluation of endoscopic ultrasonography and conventional ultrasonography for staging in superficial esophageal cancer: Assessment by histological and clinical course. JJSE 22:195, 1989.

4. Dooms GC, Hricak H: Radiologic imaging modalities, including magnetic resonance, for evaluating lymph nodes. West J Med 144:49, 1986.
5. Glazer GM, Gross BH, Quint IR, et al: Normal mediastinal lymph nodes: Number and size according to American Thoracic Society mapping. AJR 144:261, 1985.
6. Genereux GP, Howie JL: Normal mediastinal lymph node size and number: CT and anatomic study. AJR 142:1095, 1984.
7. Wiljasalo M: Lymphographic Differential Diagnosis of Neoplastic Diseases. Helsinki, Helsingfors, 1965.

17

Magnetic Resonance Imaging of Esophageal Carcinoma with ECG Gating at 1.5 Tesla:
Experience in 21 Patients with Correlation to Computed Tomography and Endosonography

R. Maas, V. Nicolas, H. Grimm, E. Meyer-Pannwitt, P. Franz, E. Bücheler

Introduction

Magnetic resonance imaging (MRI) has already been proven to have considerable diagnostic potential in the study of diseases of the brain and spine. During recent years, some interesting work has been done regarding MRI of the thorax[1,2] and the mediastinum.[3–5] There are only a few reports of examinations of esophageal diseases[6,7] with resistive magnets at low tesla (T) like Epstein: 0.12 T or with superconducting magnets at relatively low field strength like Quint: 0.3.5 T or Ross: 0.6 T. Therefore, we felt it would be interesting to summarize our experience in staging patients with esophageal cancer using a 1.5-T magnet under electrocardiogram (ECG) gating and to compare these results with computed tomography (CT) and endoscopic ultrasonography (EUS). Although CT is recognized as a di-

Ferguson MK, Little AG, Skinner DB: Diseases of the Esophagus, Vol. I: Malignant Diseases. Futura Publishing Company, Inc., Mount Kisco, NY, © 1990.

agnostic method for evaluation of the esophagus, some experts still feel the value of CT in preoperative tumor staging is very controversial.[8–10] Besides basic technical MRI problems of imaging in the mediastinum, the following questions were addressed:

1. How accurate can a classification be determined preoperatively?
2. How precisely can MRI diagnose tumor invasion of the aorta, tracheobronchial tree, and heart (T4 classification)?
3. What are the advantages of using a paramagnetic contrast agent (gadolinium-DTPA)?
4. What is the ability of MRI in the detection of metastatic lymph nodes?

Materials and Methods

From December 1987 to May 1989, 21 patients with a histologically proven esophageal carcinoma were investigated using MRI. There were 16 male and 5 female patients with an average age of 54.9 years. The location of the tumor was as follows: 1 in the upper third, 11 in the middle, and 9 in the lower third of the esophagus. Ten patients out of this group were operated on, in whom diagnostic statements could be proven surgically.

MRI was performed in a superconductive magnet (Gyroscan S 15, Philips), which was working at 1.5 T. All patients were examined by means of ECG gating. Multiple-slice technique was used with a body coil to create transverse and sagittal or coronal planes. T1-weighted images were obtained with a TE (echo time) of 20–30 msec (depending on the cardiac cycle) and a TR (repetition time) of 500–800 msec and a variation of read-out gradients as well as gradient-echo imaging (fast-field echoes = FFE). The thickness of the contiguous slices was 7–10 mm with two or four measurements. Gadolinium-DTPA was given intravenously as a paramagnetic contrast agent at a dosage of 0.1 mmol/kg of body weight.

Comparable CT examinations were obtained within 10 days of MRI, using various investigation parameters. In the majority of cases, the slice thickness was 8 mm in a contiguous mode and oral as well as intravenous contrast agent was given. Only CT scanners of the second or third generation were used.

EUS was performed with an Olympus echoendoscope (GF-UM 2/EU-M 2). This instrument is equipped with a rotating sector scanner of 7.5 MHz. The rigid portion of the tip is 42 mm, the depth of penetration is 8 cm, and the focal distance is 30 mm. The scanning examination technique was already described in detail.[11,12]

Results

MRI depicted all primary esophageal tumors (n = 21) except one case, which was a T1 stage confined to the mucosa. This case was also missed by CT. Artifacts caused by heart beats and breathing (moving diaphragm) still remain a major problem in MRI. ECG gating may overcome blurring artifacts to some extent but lengthens the time of examination. Continuous arrhythmia as well as claustrophobia are contraindications for MRI. Further help may come from rectangular changing of the read-out gradient, so that artifacts change their direction and no longer interfere with diagnostically important areas (Fig. 1a,b). T1-weighted images with ECG gating were best in delineating the outlines of the neoplasms. The signal intensities of fat layers in the mediastinum on T1-weighted images were helpful in differentiating between tumor and neighboring structures such as the aortic arch, the descending aorta, the left atrium, or the segmental bronchi. T2-weighted images suffered from a worse signal-to-noise ratio and from the fact that the signal of the tumor increases and therefore minimizes the contrast to the surrounding bright fat signal. Gradient-echo images (FFE) with a small flip angle (T2-weighted) produced mostly a bright signal in the aorta and in the left atrium, so that the tumor delineation from the fat was bad also (Fig. 1c)

Gadolinium-DTPA was administered to 11 patients and led to an increasing signal intensity of the tumor (T1-weighted), producing an image very similar to a T2-weighted one with the same disadvantages mentioned above. In one case, gadolinium demarcated in a sagittal plane a borderline between tumor and descending aorta, indicating noninvasion. In general, there was no need for gadolinium-DTPA.

The tumor length, which is no longer an aspect in modern TNM classification, is determined more precisely by MRI because of the direct imaging in coronal or sagittal planes than in CT, where the longitudinal extent must be calculated indirectly by adding the single slice thicknesses. Because of the extremely high soft tissue contrast in MRI, this modality is in individual cases superior to CT in estimation of infiltration of neighboring organs such as trachea, segmental bronchi, and descending aorta. This may provide important

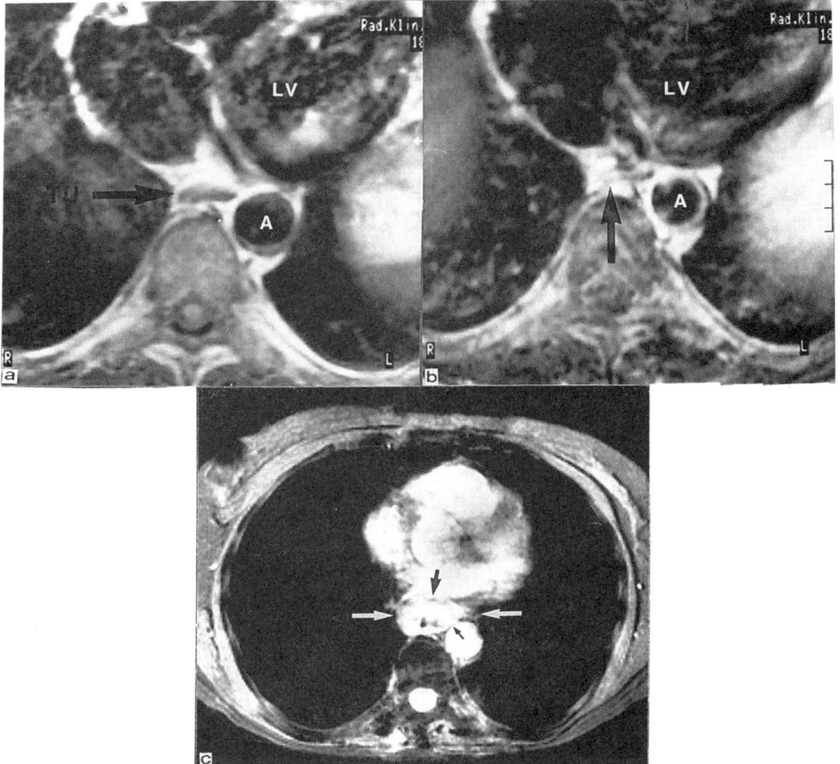

Figure 1: (a–c): The problem of blurring artifacts (sometimes even with ECG gating): the preparation direction in (a) is right to left and the esophagus is visible. In (b) the direction is anterior to posterior and no esophagus is detectable. In (c) the gradient echo sequence (FFE = fast-field echo) demonstrates a T2-weighted slice, which in general gives less information because of high signal intensity in heart and aorta and in the tumor itself. A = aorta, LV = left ventricle.

additional information, especially in those patients in whom tumor stenosis does not permit passage of an endoscope. This happens quite often if tumor penetration is more than 25 mm.

Based on both diagnostic and clinical information, only 10 patients out of the whole esophageal cancer group were operated upon. The diagnostic grading of these patients was compared using MRI, CT, and EUS. Data regarding the depth of tumor infiltration show a

Table I
Comparison of MRI, CT, and EUS with Histopathology and Intraoperative Findings Concerning Depth of Tumor Infiltration in 10 Patients

	Correct	*Overstaged*	*Understaged*	*Could Not Be Assessed*
MRI	4	4	1	1 (early cancer)
CT	4	3	2	1 (early cancer)
EUS	7	—	—	3 (stenoses)

tendency for overstaging by MRI and CT (Table I). Those tumors through which the endoscope could be passed were all classified correctly by EUS. Three nearly complete stenoses hampered endoscopic assessment and EUS produced no results (30%). MRI overstaged depth of penetration in four patients, while CT overstaged depth in three. Overall, EUS established a correct diagnosis of tumor infiltration in 70%, while MRI and CT were less accurate at about 40%.

Table II illustrates the findings concerning the regional lymph nodes in the 10 operated patients (Fig. 2a,b), which also includes those situated close to the lesser curvature of the stomach. EUS was superior, achieving nine correct classifications, in contrast to CT (six correctly staged patients) and MRI (three correctly staged patients). CT and MRI had a tendency of understaging the regional lymph node involvement, meaning these diagnostic modalities missed those nodes. In the case of distant lymph nodes in the celiac region, MRI

Table II
Comparison of MRI, CT, and EUS with Histopathology and Intraoperative Findings Concerning Regional Lymph Nodes (N1) in 10 Patients

	Correct		*Overstaged*	*Understaged*	*Could*
	N0	*N1*	*False +*	*False −*	*Not Be Assessed*
MRI	2	1	—	7	—
CT	2	4	—	4	—
EUS	2	7	—	—	1

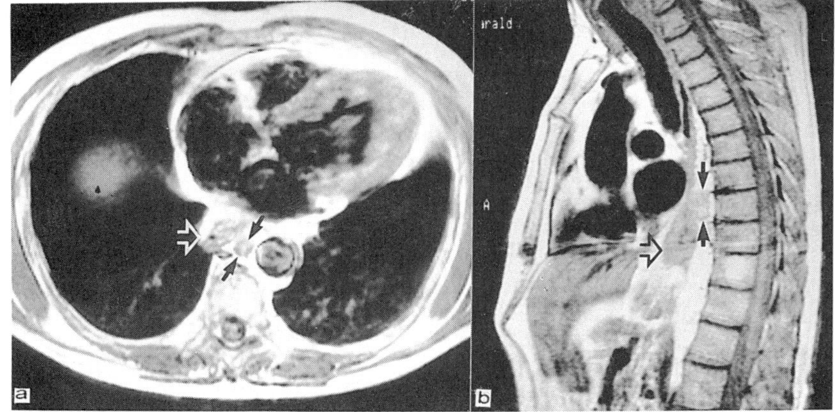

Figure 2: (a,b): The axial plane shows a lymph node (solid arrow) of about 10 (×) 15 mm between the esophageal tumor (open arrow) and the descending aorta. The lymph node is surrounded by fatty tissue. The sagittal plane confirms the node (closed arrow).

and CT were statistically superior to EUS, but missed the two patients with positive M1 lymph nodes that were seen by EUS (Table III).

Discussion

Increasing magnetic field strength and improvements in imaging data processing have produced an acceptable quality of MRI inves-

Table III
Comparisons of MRI, CT, and EUS with Histopathology and Intraoperative Findings Concerning Distant Lymph Nodes (M1) in 8 Patients*

	Correct		*Overstaged*	*Understaged*	*Could Not Be*
	M0	*M1*	*False +*	*False −*	*Assessed*
MRI	6	—	—	2	—
CT	6	—	—	2	—
EUS	3	2	—	—	3

* two patients could not be assessed histologically

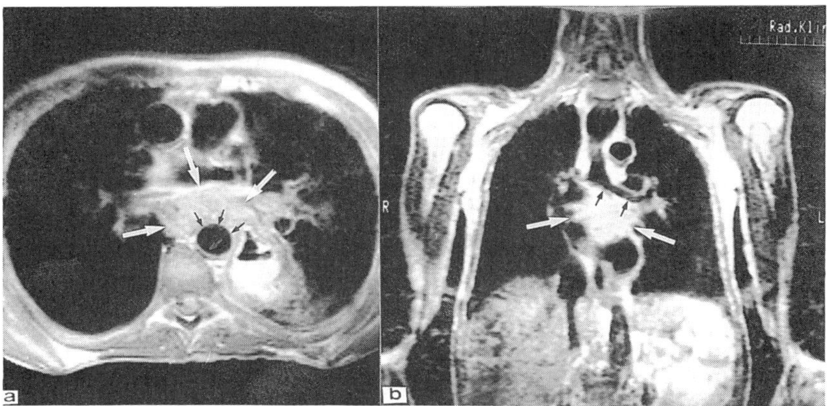

Figure 3: (a,b): Axial and coronal MRI of a T4 tumor. The tumor covers more than 90° of the aorta and no fat layer is seen (small solid arrow). The coronal plane demonstrates attachment to the left main bronchus over a long distance (small solid arrow). Invasion is possible but undetermined.

tigations in esophageal cancer. Imaging quality has particularly benefited from the introduction of ECG gating. One advantage of T1-weighted MR images is the signal loss in almost all vessels due to moving protons, offering a brilliant delineation between tumor and aorta (Fig. 3a). For the same reasons, excellent contrast can also be observed between soft tissue and the air-filled signal-free lumen of the trachea and the segmental bronchi. Furthermore, the high magnetic field strength of 1.5 T, which on the other hand makes ECG gating necessary, offers better spatial resolution compared to a low field MRI system.

The capability of MRI to demonstrate the tumor in sagittal and coronal planes allows a more precise estimation of the tumor size in the craniocaudal direction than by CT, although this superiority has no proven clinical importance. The coronal planes seem to give additional information concerning the involvement of bronchi or trachea (Fig. 3b). A broad attachment of the neoplasm over more than 3 or 5 cm makes tumor invasion likely, even if bulging of the tumor into the tracheal or bronchial lumen is not visible. The way to answer this question is by performing a transthoracic operative approach with inspection of the mediastinum, and separate histologic evaluation of the neighboring structures, a problem which is also involved in the judgment of lymph node enlargement. Transhiatal esophagectomy

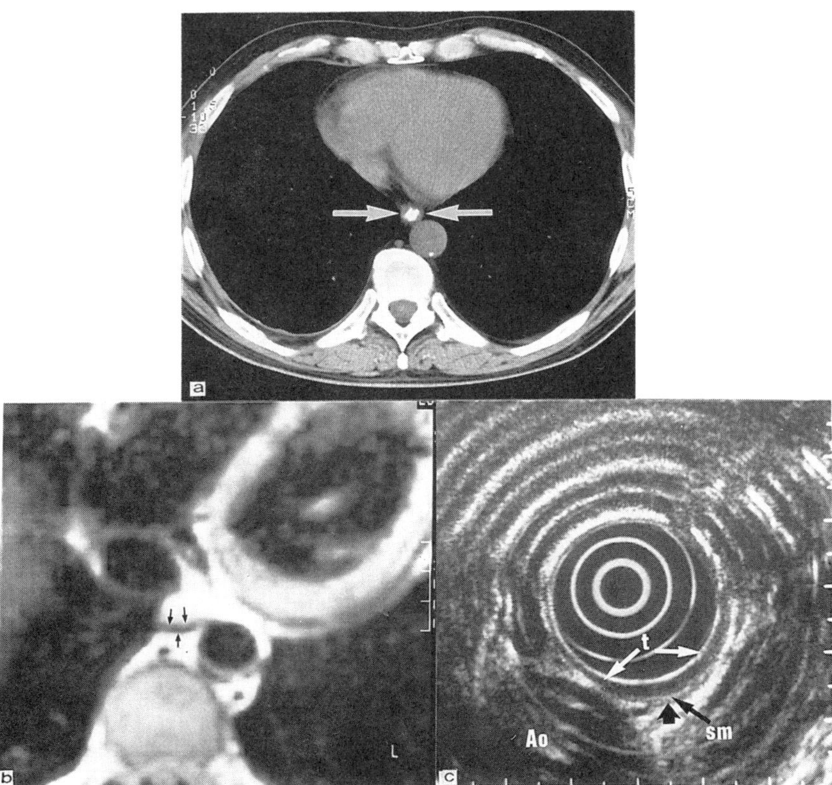

Figure 4: (a–c): In a T1 cancer, CT with oral contrast agent shows an irregular esophageal wall (medium solid arrow). The MRI cannot demonstrate the tumor reliably (small solid arrow). Endosonography (EUS) shows an echo-poor infiltration (medium solid arrow) limited to the submucosa. The muscularis propria (large solid arrow pointing up) is not involved. Ao = aorta, t = tumor, sm = submucosa.

in this situation is not acceptable as a means for assessing accuracy of clinical staging tests.

Early esophageal cancer that is restricted to the mucosa or submucosa (T1 stage) is normally not detectable by MRI or CT. Because these tumors do not even show severe clinical symptoms and an endoscope can always pass through the involved segment of the esophagus, EUS promises to be the method of choice for evaluating such patients (Fig. 4a,b,c). The TNM classification of larger tumors

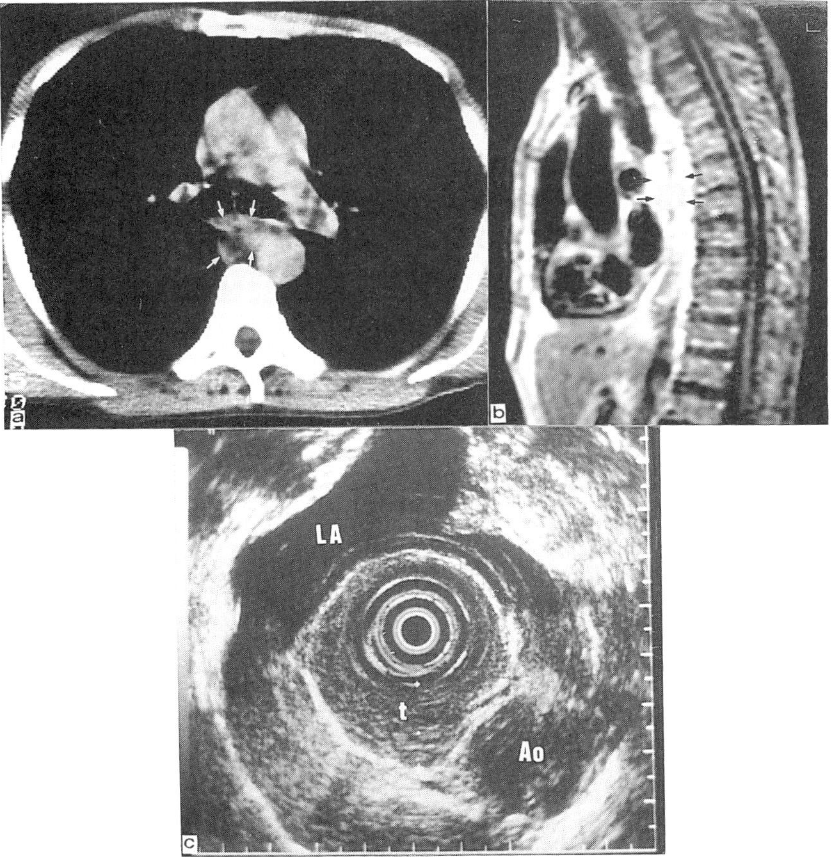

Figure 5: (a–c): A tumor staged as T2 by CT and MRI corresponded to stage T3 by EUS and postsurgical histopathology. The sagittal MRI plane shows a thin fat layer around the tumor (small solid arrow). EUS shows a circular growing advanced tumor with infiltration of all layers involving the periesophageal tissue. Ao = aorta, LA = left atrium, t = tumor.

is based on whether infiltration of adjacent tissues is present. In CT or MRI, the existence of a surrounding fat layer is a diagnostic hint of noninvolvement of mediastinal structures like the aorta or heart (indicating a T2 stage), whereas by EUS, the same patient may have infiltration of this fat layer seen by a disruption of the esophageal adventitia (indicating a T3 stage). The adventitia itself cannot be diagnosed by CT or MRI because of poorer spatial resolution (Fig. 5a,b,c).

MRI and CT seemed to overstage tumors according to the depth of infiltration, but appeared to understage the regional lymph nodes. Both modalities were insufficient for distinguishing a closely attached lymph node from the tumor itself. Although the spatial resolution of MRI was less than CT, MRI has more potential because of its higher soft-tissue contrast and the ability to image the tumor in multiple planes. The diagnostic value of MRI and CT was nearly equal in 80% of the cases. In about 10–20%, additional information was obtained by coronal and sagittal planes, especially concerning the infiltration of heart and aorta. The paramagnetic contrast agent gadolinium-DTPA was of limited value because the higher signal intensity of the perfused tumor eliminated the contrast to the fat layer.

Endosonography (EUS) seemed to be the method of choice for staging investigations because of its ability to detect T1 tumors. The advantage of EUS over CT and MRI was its ability to differentiate the layers of the esophageal wall and to estimate the involvement of the regional lymph nodes. Distant metastases in other organs could not be properly diagnosed by EUS. A further limitation was total or subtotal tumor stenosis present in 20–30% of the cases.

References

1. Ross J, O'Donovan P, Novoa R, et al: Magnetic resonance of the chest: Initial experience with imaging and in vivo T1 and T2 calculations. Radiology 152:95, 1984.
2. Mark A, Winkler M, Peltzer M, et al: Gated acquisition of MR images of the thorax: Advantages for the study of the hila and mediastinum. Magn Res Imaging 5:57, 1987.
3. Epstein D, Kressel H, Gefter W, et al: MR imaging of the mediastinum: A retrospective comparison with computed tomography. J Comput Assist Tomogr 8:670, 1984.
4. Von Schulthess G, McMurdo K, Tscholakoff D, et al: Mediastinal masses: MR imaging. Radiology 158:289, 1986.
5. Glazer G, Orringer M, Chenevert T, et al: Mediastinal lymph nodes: Relaxation time/pathologic correlation and implications in staging of lung cancer with MR imaging. Radiology 168:429, 1988.
6. Quint L, Glazer G, Orringer M: Esophageal imaging by MR and CT: Study of normal anatomy and neoplasms. Radiology 156:727, 1985.
7. Krestin G, Steinbrich W, Friedmann G, et al: Magnetic resonance tomography in carcinoma of the esophagus. Fortschr Roentgenstr 145:437, 1986 (in German).

8. Picus D, Balfe D, Koehler R, et al: Computed tomography in the staging of esophageal carcinoma. Radiology 146:433, 1983.
9. Quint L, Glazer G, Orringer M, et al: Esophageal carcinoma. CT findings. Radiology 155:171, 1985.
10. Halvorson R, Magruder-Habib K, Foster W, et al: Esophageal cancer staging by CT: Long-term follow-up study. Radiology 161:147, 1986.
11. Murata Y, Muroi M, Yoshida M, et al: Endoscopic ultrasonography in the diagnosis of esophageal carcinoma. Surg Endosc 1:11, 1987.
12. Tio T, Cohen P, Coene P, et al: Endosonography and computed tomography of esophageal carcinoma: Preoperative classification compared to the new (1987) TNM system. Gastroenterology 96:1478, 1989.

III.

Surgical Therapy: Editors' Overview

Surgical resection continues to be the primary mode of therapy for local control and possible cure of esophageal cancer. In recent years, controversy has developed over the appropriate extent of resection, particularly focusing on regional lymph nodes. Popular operations range from a strictly palliative transhiatal approach, which provides no significant nodal removal, to extended en bloc radical resection, promoted as a means to both decrease local recurrence and improve long-term survival. In this section on surgical therapy for esophageal cancer, it is apparent that many surgical groups have attempted to extend the scope of surgical resection, having become dissatisfied with results of more conventional operations. The section also includes chapters that focus on other facets of surgical techniques, including those used in esophageal reconstruction.

The section begins with a discussion of so-called superficial squamous cell carcinoma of the esophagus. As Gayet and his coauthors illustrate in Chapter 18, this term is a misnomer, since the primary lesion, thought to have a good prognosis because it is confined to the mucosa and submucosa, is often accompanied by regional nodal involvement. Their data support the contention that these cancers should be managed, under most circumstances, in a manner similar to that for invasive esophageal tumors.

In chapter 19, Endo and his colleagues describe their approach to cervical esophageal cancer based on a very large series of patients. The results illustrate the utility of exacting technique in resection of the primary tumor and regional nodes as well as in reconstruction. Their experience with jejunal autografts requiring microvascular anastomoses is among the best ever reported.

Chapters 20–23 focus on efforts, largely on the part of the Japanese, to improve long-term survival by means of more extensive nodal dissection. Their efforts illustrate several important points. First, nodal involvement, particularly in the cervical region, becomes more apparent as dissection becomes more radical. This underscores our inability to accurately stage patients clinically. Second, the data suggest that there may be a survival advantage provided by a more extensive nodal dissection. These studies are not based on randomization techniques, and all results are necessarily subject to criticisms stemming from this. The results, therefore, suggest the need for future controlled, randomized trials of routine versus extended nodal dissection in management of esophagael cancer.

The perceived enthusiasm for more radical surgical procedures for esophageal cancer present in prior chapters is tempered somewhat by data presented in Chapters 24 and 25. Huang and his co-workers support the utility of radical resection in patients with limited disease, but caution that extensive nodal involvement, when present, is a poor prognostic factor regardless of the extent of resection. They encourage exploration of multimodality therapy in this latter group of patients. These beliefs are echoed by Bardini et al. who similarly demonstrate the dependence of survival on nodal status regardless of the completeness of resection.

Appropriate therapy for Barrett's adenocarcinoma is addressed by Altorki and coauthors in Chapter 26. Their results illustrate several important points. The overall prognosis in patients with Barrett's adenocarcinoma is as poor as for patients with squamous cell cancer. Individual prognosis correlates well with pathological stage. Resection is possible in most patients and offers good palliation with a low rate of local occurrence when performed in a complete manner. Finally, the data show that surveillance, using endoscopy and cytology, provides the best means for early diagnosis and cure in this group of patients.

Chapters 27–30 address controversial methods for timing and techniques of reconstruction following esophagectomy for cancer. Chasseray et al. report a prospective randomized study comparing cervical versus intrathoracic esophagogastric anastomoses, demonstrating a significantly higher rate of anastomotic leaks in the neck than in the thorax. These findings may well be related to the surgical techniques used as well as to factors influencing gastric blood supply. Surprisingly, the long-term clinical outcome seems little affected by the choice of anastomotic site. A decrease in gastric blood flow during stomach transposition is reported by Nabeya and his co-workers.

They feel that by delaying the cervical esophagogastrostomy by several weeks, the likelihood of anastomotic leak is decreased, secondary to an improvement in gastric circulation, and the risk of aspiration pneumonia is also reduced. In contrast, Siewert et al. report that a brief delay of 2 to 3 days between esophagectomy and anastomosis offers no therapeutic benefit compared to immediate reconstruction. Perhaps with a longer delay they might observe improvements similar to those outlined above. Finally, Chapter 30 details results of a prospective study comparing stomach to colon as organs for esophageal substitution. Ando and his coauthors report a moderate advantage in using the colon, as transit time is faster and long-term weight gain is better than when the stomach is used.

18

Superficial Squamous Cell Carcinoma of the Esophagus: An Early Lesion of Good Prognosis? A Report of 58 Patients Resected

Brice Gayet, Corinne Vons, G. Molas,
Jacques Belghiti, François Fékété

The poor prognosis for squamous cell carcinoma of the esophagus has been attributed to its advanced stage when diagnosed.[1] Recent reports from China[2–5] and Japan[6–9] have described improved survival in "early" esophageal cancer with the 5-year survival rate ranging from 65% to 90%. Superficial squamous cell carcinoma (SSC) of the esophagus is a lesion with tissue invasion limited to the mucosa, or to the mucosa and submucosa, regardless of the presence of lymph node metastasis. So-called early esophageal carcinoma is a superficial cancer without metastasis. Confusion occurs between so-called early esophageal cancer, based on the preoperative presumptive diagnosis and SSC.[10–12]

In Western literature, recognition of SSC has been limited to single case reports or small series.[10,12–16] The only multicenter European study indicated a survival rate of 49% at 2.5 years.[17] In the present study we describe and analyze the pathological features and results of surgical resection of 58 cases of SSC seen between 1979 and 1987

Ferguson MK, Little AG, Skinner DB: Diseases of the Esophagus, Vol. I: Malignant Diseases. Futura Publishing Company, Inc., Mount Kisco, NY, © 1990.

Table I
Previous and Concomitant Disease in 29 Patients Operated on for Superficial Squamous Cell Carcinoma of the Esophagus

Previous and Concomitant Disease	*Number*
Carcinoma with	
Previous radiotherapy and chemotherapy	6
Total or partial gastric resection	2
Pulmonary resection	4
Hepatic cirrhosis	9
Cardiac insufficiency	6
Respiratory insufficiency	5
Alcoholic hepatitis	1
Esophageal tumor perforation	1
Total	34*

* Some patients had two previous or concomitant diseases.

in our institute. Data are compared to those obtained during the same period in 354 patients undergoing surgery for advanced squamous cell carcinoma (ASC) of the esophagus with tissue invasion extending to the muscular layer.

Patients and Methods

The case reports of 58 patients with squamous cell carcinoma of the esophagus in which tumor invasion was limited to the mucosa and submucosa (SSC), with or without lymph node metastasis, were retrospectively reviewed. There were 53 men and 5 women, aged between 32 and 75 years (mean 56 years). Thirty-four previous or concomitant disorders were present in 29 patients (50%) and are listed in Table I. Respiratory insufficiency was defined as a forced expiratory volume in 1 second (FEV_1) of less than 1 liter. Six patients (10%) were over 70 years of age. One patient, initially excluded from surgery, underwent an emergency operation because of an iatrogenic perforation of the tumor during endoscopic intubation. Esophagectomy, with complete posterior mediastinectomy and removal of lymph nodes of the celiac axis, was performed in all patients.[18] There were 40 intrathoracic anastomoses for tumors situated at the aortic (n = 1) and subaortic (n = 39) level and 18 cervical anastomoses for 2 cervical, 8 supra-aortic, and 8 subaortic tumors. Cervical esophagogastrostomy was performed without thoracotomy in 8 patients: 2 patients with cervical tumor, 5 patients with significant pulmonary insufficiency, and 1 patient with a tumor localized at the thoracic outlet that was considered and treated by the surgeon as a cervical tumor. One patient had a coloplasty.

The pathology reports and histologic slides were reviewed to determine the microscopic characteristics of the resected specimens. Sections were taken from (1) the suspicious zones; (2) adjacent and distant areas; (3) the margins of resection; (4) all lymph nodes. Patients were divided into two groups: mucosa (M) tumor group (patients with a tumor confined to the mucosa) and submucosa (SM) tumor group (patients with a tumor penetrating the submucosa). In SM tumor group patients, care was taken to detect "extensive carcinoma," defined as a carcinoma penetrating the submucosa with associated intramucosal portions of continuous malignant changes extending 20 mm or more from the penetrating lesion.[19,20] On the basis of the wall penetration, the lymph node involvement, and the presence or absence of metastases, the patients were also divided into five stages (Japanese classification).

Follow-up data were obtained for all patients. Survival rates were calculated for the whole group of patients, for the patients surviving the curative resection, in M and SM tumor groups, and with respect to lymph node involvement. Survival was defined with regard to death due to esophageal carcinoma only. Disease-free actuarial rates were also calculated in M and SM tumor groups.

Student's *t*-test was used to compare quantitative data and Fisher's exact test to compare qualitative data. Survival rates were calculated using the Kaplan-Meier method and the Log Rank test was used to compare actuarial survival curves.

Results

There were 16 patients in the M tumor group: 6 intraepithelial (IE), 10 muscularis mucosa (MM) tumors, and 42 patients in the SM tumor group. During the same period, an advanced squamous cell carcinoma was identified in 354 patients (Table II).

Lymph nodes were assessed in all cases. Lymph node involvement was present in 13 patients with SSC (22.4%), all of whom had an SM tumor. There was no lymph node involvement in patients in the M tumor group. Vascular invasion was present in 14 patients: 2

Table II
Vascular Invasion and Involvement of Lymph Nodes and Surgical Margin of Resection in 58 Patients with SSC and 354 Patients with ASC of the Esophagus

	Number	*Lymph Node Involvement*	*Vascular Invasion*	*Involvement of Surgical Margin of Resection*
SSC	58	13 (22.4%)	14 (24%)	5 (9%)
IE	6	0	0	1
MM	10	0	2	2
SM	42	13	12	2
ASC	354	(69%)	(40%)	(10%)

SSC = superficial squamous cell carcinoma of the esophagus, IE = intraepithelial, MM = muscularis mucosa, SM = submucosa, ASC = advanced squamous cell carcinoma of the esophagus.

patients with an MM tumor and 12 patients with an SM tumor. According to the Japanese classification, there were 45 stage 0, 5 stage II, 5 stage III, and 3 stage IV patients. Five patients had involvement of the surgical margin of resection. Three of them had postoperative radiotherapy and one had a resection of the anastomosis, but no residual tumor was found. Fifteen patients presented with multicentric lesions (25.9%). Seven of these patients had an M tumor (44%) and 9 had an SM tumor (19%). Twenty-five patients with an SM tumor

Table III
Characteristics of 58 SSC and 354 ASC of the Esophagus

	Multicentric Lesion	*Extensive Lesion*	*Association with Another Synchronous or Metachronous Carcinoma*
SSC	15 (25.9%)	25* (43%)	21 (36%)
IE	3 (50%)		5 (83%)
MM	4 (40%)		4 (40%)
SM	8 (19%)	25 (59.5%)	12 (28.6%)
ASC	15 (4.2%)	96 (27%)	37 (10.6%)

* Only patients in SM tumor group are considered.
SSC = superficial squamous cell carcinoma of the esophagus, ASC = advanced squamous cell carcinoma of the esophagus, IE = intraepithelial, MM = muscularis mucosa, SM = submucosa.

Table IV
Causes of Operative Deaths in 58 Patients Operated on for SSC of the Esophagus

Cause	*Number*
Complications of cirrhosis	
Variceal bleeding	1
Mesenteric infarction	1
Anastomotic leak	1
Pulmonary embolism	2
Respiratory failure	1
Cardiac infarction	1
Total	7*

* One other patient, initially rejected for surgery, was operated on for perforation and died of sepsis with fistula.
SSC = superficial squamous cell carcinoma of the esophagus.

had an extensive carcinoma (59.5%). An association of superficial esophageal cell squamous and another synchronous or metachronous carcinoma was found in 21 cases (36%), of which a squamous cell carcinoma was present in 13 patients (Table III).

All these data were compared to those obtained in patients with an ASC (Tables II and III). The differences between patients with SSC and those with ASC were all highly significant, except for the involvement of surgical margins of resection.

There were eight hospital deaths (13.8%). One patient, who was initially excluded from surgery, had an emergency operation after an iatrogenic perforation of the esophagus during endoscopic intubation and died postoperatively of sepsis. The causes of hospital deaths are listed in Table IV. Four patients had hepatic cirrhosis, one had alcoholic hepatitis at the time of surgery, one had preoperative major respiratory insufficiency, and one had been treated for previous gastric and testicular carcinoma with surgery, chemotherapy, and radiotherapy. During the same period, the hospital death rate in patients with ASC of the esophagus who underwent curative surgery was 5.5%.

The 5-year actuarial survival rate was 19% for all patients, with a mean survival time 27 ± 20 months. The 5-year disease-free rate (actuarial) was 55%. For patients surviving curative resection, the 5-year survival rate was 38%. The 5-year survival rate was 40% for IE and MM tumors, and 12.7% for SM tumors. The 5-year survival

Table V
Causes of Late Deaths in 19 Patients Out of 50 Patients Surviving Surgery, According to Depth of Wall Penetration of the SSC

Wall Penetration	*Recurrence*	*Another Carcinoma*	*Another Cause (alcohol related)*
Mucosa	1*	2	1
Submucosa	11	2	2
Total (50)	12	4	3

* Patient with involvement of surgical margin of resection.
SSC = superficial squamous cell carcinoma of the esophagus.

rate in patients with lymph node involvement was 11.7%, while in patients without lymph node involvement, it was 23.6%. This difference was not statistically significant. The 5-year disease-specific survival rate was 60%. Disease-free actuarial rates were 80% in group M and 43.6% in group SM, respectively (difference not statistically significant).

There were 19 late deaths. Twelve deaths were related to recurrence, of which 10 were local or regional (in three patients, the margin of resection was involved by the tumor) and two were metastatic recurrences. The relationship between the extent of invasion of the carcinoma and cause of late deaths is shown in Table V. There was no recurrence in the M tumor group, except in one patient with involvement of the surgical margin of resection. Deaths were related to another synchronous or metachronous carcinoma in four cases. Two patients are alive with recurrence. Thirty-five patients did not have any recurrence (70%) but nine developed another carcinoma (20%).

Discussion

This is a large series of SSC of the esophagus treated by resection. Our results suggest several points: (1) SSC should not be considered as an early cancer; (2) the optimism regarding survival after therapy of SSC of the esophagus is not completely justified; (3) SSC of the esophagus, except in cases where a distinction between mucosal and submucosal invasion can be made preoperatively, necessitates major radical surgical resection.

Clinical and histologic data suggest that SSC is not just an early ASC. The incidence of multicentric lesions observed in SSC and of extensive carcinoma observed in SM tumor group patients was significantly higher than in ASC (Table III). SSC seems rather to be a pathological entity with a specific pattern of development. Its frequent association with another synchronous or metachronous carcinoma, especially squamous cell carcinoma (Table III), is also an argument for this concept. The term "early cancer" employed in the literature has no histologic basis.

The hospital mortality rate of 13.8%, 12.2% for "operable" patients, and the 5-year actuarial survival rate of 19% are disappointing and compare unfavorably with those reported from China and Japan.[2,3,8,9] Hospital mortality was higher in this group of patients than the rate observed during the same period in patients with ASC after curative resection (5.5%). The main reason may be the high rate of previous or concomitant disease in this series (50%), including cirrhosis (15.5% versus 6.8% for ASC) and carcinoma (20.7% versus 8% in ASC) treated by radiotherapy or surgery, including simultaneous pulmonary or gastric resection. Indications for surgical resection were liberal in this group of patients due to their presumed good prognosis. Prognosis was not as good as expected on the basis of Asian literature, but agreed with results reported in Western literature. The presence of lymph node involvement in SM tumor group patients and associated synchronous and metachronous cancer in both groups account for this discrepancy. Regional and metastatic recurrences were more closely correlated with wall penetration than with lymph node involvement (Table V). Deaths were also related to the development of another carcinoma, which was particularly frequent in SSC.

The absence of lymph node involvement or recurrence in the IE-MM tumor group (except for one patient with involvement of surgical margin of resection) suggests that these patients could be given local treatment if they can be identified preoperatively. Progress in echoendoscopic examination may make this possible. In the absence of preoperative identification of the patients presenting with a tumor limited to the mucosa, the same surgical indications must be applied to patients with superficial cancer as to those with an invasive cancer. In this case, extensive surgical resection is necessary to ensure resection of all multifocal lesions and lymph node metastases.[21] Total esophagectomy with cervical anastomosis should be guided by vital staining for mucosal spread[9,13,22,23] and endosonography for submucosal spread. Patients in both groups should undergo frequent checkups to detect and treat the possible development of another carcinoma.

The term "early esophageal cancer" has no histologic or developmental basis. SSC is not always an early cancer, but seems to be a specific entity. Progress must be made in order to identify M tumor and SM tumor patients preoperatively in order to administer suitable therapy.

References

1. Earlam R, Cunha-Melo JR: Esophageal squamous cell carcinoma. A critical review of surgery. Br J Surg 67:381, 1980.
2. Guanrei Y, He H, Sungliang M, et al: Endoscopic diagnosis of 115 cases of early esophageal carcinoma. Endoscopy 14:157, 1982.
3. Guo-Quing W: Endoscopic diagnosis of 115 early esophageal carcinoma. J R Soc Med 74:502, 1981.
4. Huang GJ, Zhang DW, Wang GQ, et al: Dépistage précoce et résultats du traitement chirurgical du carcinome d'oesophage en Chine. Méd Hyg 39:2929, 1981.
5. Li MH, Li P, Li PJ: Recent progress in research on esophageal cancer in China. Adv Cancer Res 33:173, 1980.
6. Endo M, Ide H, Yoshino K, et al: Diagnosis and treatment of early esophageal cancer. In: Diseases of the Esophagus, Siewert JR, Hölscher AH (eds), Berlin, Springer-Verlag, 1988, p 375.
7. Nabeya K: Markers of cancer risk in the esophagus and surveillance of high-risk group. In: Precancerous Lesions of the Gastrointestinal Tract, Sherlock P, Morson BC, Barbara L (eds), New York, Raven Press, 1983, p 71.
8. Shimazu H, Kobori O, Shoji M, et al: Superficial carcinoma of the esophagus. Gastroenteral Jpn 18:409, 1983.
9. Yamada A, Hanyu F, Ide H, et al: Superficial esophageal cancer with special reference to x-ray diagnosis. In: Diseases of the Esophagus, Siewert JR, Hölscher AH (eds), Berlin, Springer-Verlag, 1988, p 126.
10. Benasco C, Combalia N, Pou JM, et al: Superficial esophageal carcinoma: A report of 12 cases. Gastrointest Endosc 31:64, 1985.
11. Monnier P: Le diagnostic au stade "précoce" du carcinome epidermoïde de l'oesophage. Méd Hyg 39:2937, 1981.
12. Schmidt LW, Dean PJ, Wilson RT: Superficially invasive squamous cell carcinoma of the esophagus: A study of seven cases in Memphis Tennessee. Gastroenterology 91:1456, 1986.
13. Barge J, Molas G, Maillard JN, et al: Superficial esophageal carcinoma: An esophageal counterpart of early gastric cancer. Histopathology 5:499, 1981.
14. Burke EL, Sturm J, Williamson D: The diagnosis of microscopic carcinoma of the esophagus. Am J Dig Dis 23:148, 1978.

15. Sotus PC, Majmudar B, Symbas PN: Carcinoma in situ of the esophagus. JAMA 239:335, 1978.
16. Winkler MJ, Miller DM, Ferlic RM: Superficial esophageal carcinoma diagnosed solely by endoscopy. Nebr Med J 63:184, 1978.
17. Froelicher P, Miller G: The European experience with esophageal cancer limited to the mucosa and submucosa. Gastrointest Endosc 32:88, 1986.
18. Fékété F, Gayet B, Place S, et al: 380 esophageal anastomoses with stapler. In: International Trends in General Thoracic Surgery, Delarue NC, Wilkins EW, Wong J (eds), Esophageal Cancer, Philadelphia, WB Saunders, 1986, p 63.
19. Kusielewicz H, Conte-Marti J, Parc R, et al: Cancer epidermoïde, superficiel et etendu en nappe de l'oesophage. Gastroenterol Clin Biol 8:33, 1984.
20. Bogomoletz WV, Molas G, Gayet B, et al: Superficial squamous cell carcinoma of the esophagus: A report of 76 cases and review of the literature. Am J Surg Pathol 13:535, 1989.
21. Mitomi T, Makuuchi H, Ogoshi K, et al: Treatment of so-called early esophageal carcinoma. In: Diseases of the Esophagus, Siewert JR, Hölscher AH (eds), Berlin, Springer-Verlag, 1988, p 381.
22. Mandard AM, Tourneux J, Gignoux M, et al: In situ carcinoma of the esophagus: Macroscopic study with particular reference to the Lugol test. Endoscopy 12:51, 1980.
23. Hix WR, Wilson WR: Detection of occult carcinoma of the esophagus by toluidine blue staining in high-risk patients. In: Diseases of the Esophagus, Siewert JR, Hölscher JH (eds), Berlin, Springer-Verlag, 1988, p 118.

19

Surgical Procedures for Cervical Esophageal Cancer

Mitsuo Endo, Kunihide Yoshino, Toru Takiguchi, Sigeru Yamazaki

Operative procedures for cancer of the cervical esophagus are selected from among three types according to tumor site and macroscopic findings of the lesions. If the lesion appears limited to the hypopharynx and cervical esophagus with no accessory lesions in the thoracic esophagus, pharyngolaryngo-cervical esophagectomy is performed and free jejunal autotransplantation is indicated. If there appears to be invasion of the thoracic esophagus, pharyngolaryngo-esophagectomy without thoracotomy is carried out and pharyngogastrostomy should be performed. If the cancer is located at the border between the cervical and the thoracic esophagus, pharyngoesophagectomy with thoracotomy is carried out and pharyngogastrostomy or pharyngocolostomy is performed. Systematic lymph node dissection in the upper and lower mediastinum and in the abdominal cavity must be performed.

Patients and Methods

In 72 cases, a pharyngoesophagectomy and reconstruction surgery were performed. In all of these cases, digestive tract reconstruction was carried out simultaneously. Autotransplantation of the je-

Ferguson MK, Little AG, Skinner DB: Diseases of the Esophagus, Vol. I: Malignant Diseases. Futura Publishing Company, Inc., Mount Kisco, NY, © 1990.

Table I
Operative Methods for Cervical Esophageal Cancer, 1965–1989

Pharyngolaryngocervical esophagectomy	
Autojejunal transplantation	31 (2)
Pharyngogastrostomy	5
Pharyngocolostomy	3
Pharyngolaryngoesophagectomy without thoracotomy	
Pharyngogastrostomy	22 (1)
Pharyngoesophagectomy and pharyngolaryngoesophagectomy with thoracotomy	
Pharyngogastrostomy	10
Pharyngocolostomy	1
Total	72 (3)

(Operative death)

junum was performed in 31 cases, while an esophagoplasty with the stomach or the colon based on a vascular pedicle was employed in eight cases. Pharyngolaryngectomy and blunt dissection of the whole esophagus followed by pharyngogastrostomy was carried out in 22 cases. Pharyngoesophagectomy with thoracotomy and pharyngogastrostomy or pharyngocolostomy was performed in 11 cases (Table I). The operative mortality rate was 4.2%.

Results

Lymph node metastases in the neck were mostly found in the deep cervical lymph nodes (52%) and in the supraclavicular lymph nodes (42%). However, the incidence of metastases to the thoracic paratracheal lymph nodes and the upper thoracic paraesophageal lymph nodes was relatively high, 21% and 15%, respectively (Table II). Therefore, a lymph node dissection should be carried out to include nodes within the upper mediastinum. Laryngectomy was performed in almost all cases except those involving a localized lesion at the junction of the cervical and thoracic esophagus. Thyroidectomy and combined resection of the large vessels were carried out in the infiltrative cases.

Nakayama's instrument for small vessel anastomosis was employed in 14 of 31 cases of autotransplantation of a free jejunal graft.[1–3] However, postoperative necrosis of the transplanted intestine was observed in three cases because of arterial sclerosis. In the

Table II
Incidence of Lymph Node Metastases in Cervical Esophageal Cancer

Location of Lymph Nodes	*Incidence of Metastases %*
Superficial cervical nodes	6
Cervical paraesophageal nodes	27
Deep cervical nodes	52
Retropharyngeal nodes	3
Supraclavicular nodes	42
Upper thoracic paraesophageal nodes	15
Thoracic paratracheal nodes	21
Perigastric nodes	3
Celiac nodes	3
Retropancreatic and hepatoduodenal nodes	3
Incidence of Lymph Node Metastasis	61

remaining 17 cases, jejunal free graft with microvascular surgery was transplanted successfully. Donor vessels included the lingual artery, the transverse cervical artery, and the superior thyroid artery, while the external jugular and the anterior jugular vessels were used as recipient veins. Anastomosis of the alimentary tract was performed either before or after vascular reconstruction. The pharyngojejunal anastomosis was end-to-end. In this procedure, it is very important that the jejunum interposed between the pharynx and esophagus should be as straight as possible (Fig. 1). In some cases, a loop of jejunum was interposed between the pharynx and esophagus. When the skin defect was large or the skin was not sutured because of undue tension, a myocutaneous (deltopectoral) flap was applied to cover the skin defect[4] (Fig 2).

Multiple cancer lesions were observed in the thoracic esophagus in 26% of cases of cervical esophageal cancer in which whole esophagectomy was performed. Most of them were superficial cancers (mucosal or submucosal lesions). Careful preoperative endoscopic examination of the thoracic esophagus was necessary to decide upon an operative technique. When the stricture was severe and the endoscope could not be passed through the tumor, endoscopy was performed during the operation when the thoracic esophagus was intended to be preserved.

In cases in which the thoracic esophagus was involved by tumor or when multiple superficial lesions in the thoracic esophagus were

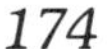

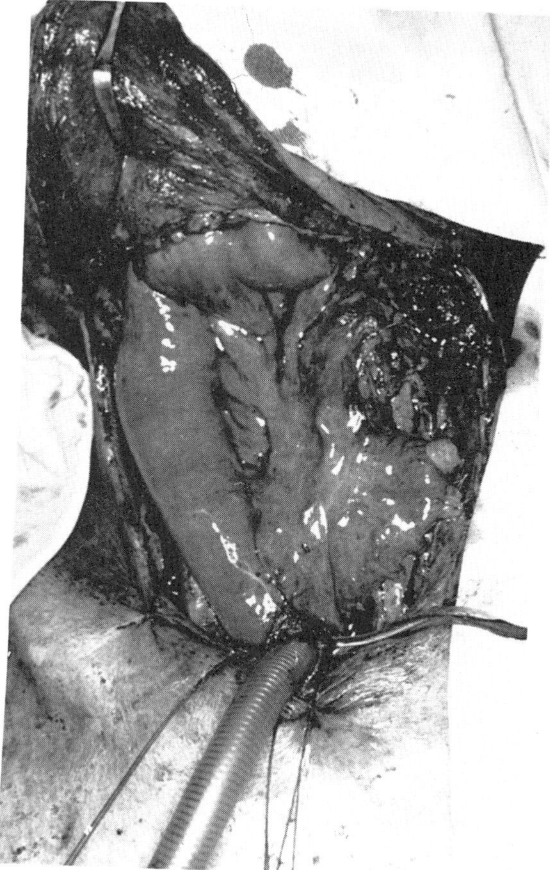

Figure 1: Cervical esophagoplasty by free jejunal autotransplantation.

suspected, blunt dissection of a whole esophagus was carried out and the stomach was pulled up to the pharynx through the mediastinum.[5,6] Anastomosis between the pharynx and the fundus of the stomach was performed in two layers.

When cancer was seen at the cervicothoracic border, or when mediastinal metastases were suspected by CT examination, pharyngectomy and total esophagectomy with thoracotomy was performed with pharyngogastrostomy or pharyngocolostomy. The lymph node dissection was performed along the whole esophagus,

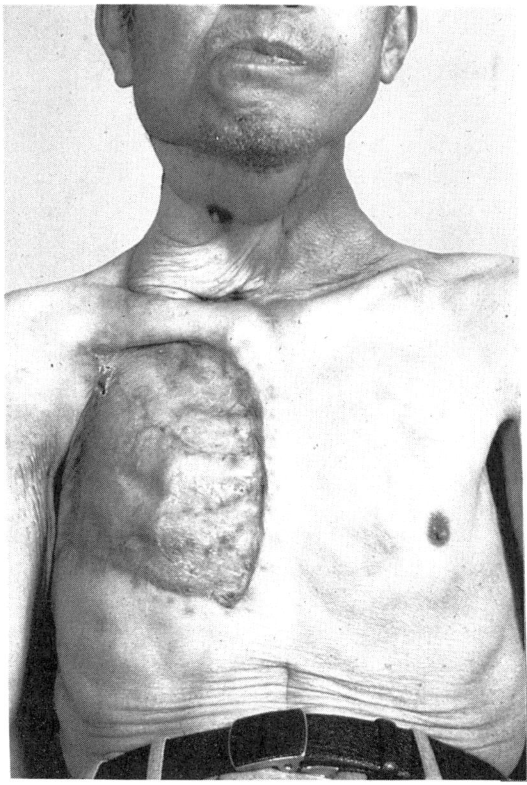

Figure 2: A skin defect was covered with pectoralis major myocutaneous flap.

accompanied by dissection of the cervical lymph nodes. The incidence of metastases in the upper paraesophageal and the thoracic paratracheal lymph nodes was high, while the incidence of metastasis in the lower mediastinum was relatively low.

The overall operative mortality rate was 4.2%. Mortality for the free jejunal autotransplantation and pharyngoesophagectomy without thoracotomy were 6.5% and 4.5%, respectively. The 5-year survival rate for the pharyngolaryngo-esophagectomy cases without thoracotomy was 33%, while that for the esophagectomy cases with thoracotomy was 14% and that for the pharyngolaryngo-cervical esophagectomy cases was 3%.

Discussion

Surgical treatment for cancer of the hypopharyngo-cervical esophagus involves resection, lymph node dissection, and esophageal reconstruction. Lymph node dissection is as extensive as possible, with removal of the regional lymph nodes, deep cervical lymph nodes, supraclavicular lymph nodes, and upper mediastinal lymph nodes. The method of reconstruction selected depends on the location occupied by the lesion. In cases in which the tumor is limited to the hypopharynx and cervical esophagus without recognizable multiple lesions, reconstruction by free bowel autotransplantation is employed. When the cervical esophageal cancer shows invasive features or when multiple lesions are suspected in the thoracic esophagus, pharyngolaryngo-esophagectomy by blunt dissection without thoracotomy is performed with a pharyngogastrostomy done through the posterior mediastinum. In cases in which the tumor is located at the cervicothoracic border or in which mediastinal metastases are suspected by CT examination, pharyngolaryngo-esophagectomy and lymph node dissection are performed via a thoracotomy.

References

1. Seidenberg B, et al: Immediate reconstruction of the esophagus by a revascularized isolated jejunal segment. Ann Surg 149:162, 1959.
2. Roberts RE, et al: Replacement of the cervical esophagus and hypopharynx by a revascularized free jejunal autograft. N Engl J Med 264:342, 1961.
3. Nakayama K, Tamiya T, Yamamoto K, et al: A simple new apparatus for small vessel anastomosis. Surgery 52:918, 1962.
4. Ariyan S: Further experiences with the pectoralis major myocutaneous flap for the immediate repair of defects from excisions of head and neck cancer. Plast Reconstr Surg 64:605, 1979.
5. Ong GB, et al: Pharyngogastric anastomosis after esophago-pharyngectomy for carcinoma of the hypopharynx and cervical esophagus. Br J Surg 48:193, 1960.
6. Akiyama H, Hiyama M, Miyazono H: Total esophageal reconstruction after extraction of the esophagus. Ann Surg 182:547, 1975.

20

Extended Dissection for Thoracic Esophageal Cancer Based on Preoperative Staging

Hiroko Ide, Fujio Hanyu, Yoko Murata,
Ataru Kobayashi, Akiyoshi Yamada,
Seiichiro Kobayashi

Introduction

Metastatic lymph nodes of thoracic esophageal cancer are mostly found in the mediastinum, abdomen, and sometimes in the cervical region. Since 1985, we have been resecting esophageal cancer with lymph node dissection based on preoperative staging by ultrasound, endoscopic ultrasonography, and computed tomography. In this chapter, we report the clinical effectiveness of extended dissection of three regions, particularly bilateral cervical dissection, among cases of total thoracic esophagectomy.

Materials and Methods

From January 1985 to September 1988, 203 of 258 cases of thoracic esophageal cancer were resected using a right thoracotomy based on preoperative staging. For preoperative lymph node detection, we used mainly conventional ultrasonography (US) and endoscopic ultraso-

Ferguson MK, Little AG, Skinner DB: Diseases of the Esophagus, Vol. I: Malignant Diseases. Futura Publishing Company, Inc., Mount Kisco, NY, © 1990.

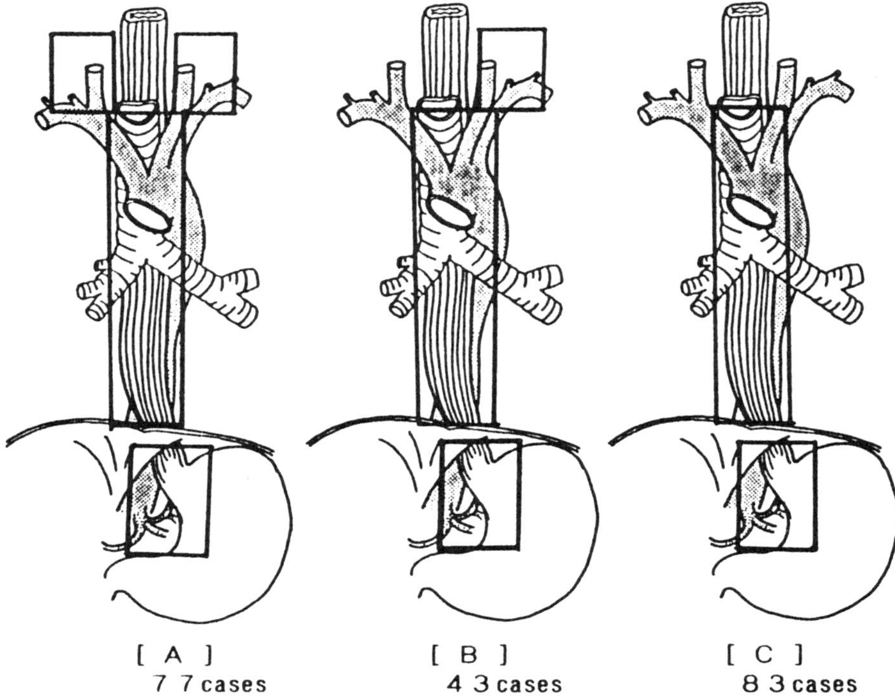

Figure 1: Type of dissection in the operation of thoracic esophageal cancer: 203 cases of right thoracotomy.

nography (EUS) with a diagnostic accuracy of 88–95%. Our indications for bilateral cervical dissection were (1) cases of upper thoracic cancer, (2) cases in which cervical lymph node enlargement was detected by EUS, and (3) cases of positive metastatic lymph nodes in the upper mediastinum detected by US or intraoperative findings. If the patient did not meet these criteria or had other factors indicating a palliative procedure was better, the dissection of cervical lymph nodes was omitted.

Using the type of lymph node dissection performed based on preoperative staging, 203 cases with right thoracotomy were divided into three groups: group A (extended dissection – 77 cases with mediastinal, abdominal, and bilateral cervical lymph node dissection); group B (standard approach plus some further degree of dissection – 43 cases with mediastinal, abdominal, and only left cervical lymph

Table I
Background Factors for Resected Esophageal Cancers with Right Thoracotomy Based on Preoperative Staging

Type of Nodal Dissection	*[A] Extended Dissection*	*[B] Standard + α Dissection*	*[C] Standard Dissection*
Number of Cases	77	43	83
Age (mean)	36–76 years (58 years)	35–76 years (58 years)	37–82 years (63 years)
Location of Tumor			
Upper	17 (22%)	2 (5%)	3 (4%)
Middle	51 (66%)	29 (67%)	59 (71%)
Lower	9 (12%)	12 (28%)	21 (25%)
pT of TNM			
pTis			2 (2%)
pT1	9 (12%)	5 (12%)	17 (20%)
pT2	10 (13%)	6 (14%)	14 (17%)
pT3	45 (58%)	27 (62%)	38 (46%)
pT4	13 (17%)	5 (12%)	13 (16%)
Stage			
O			2 (2%)
I	6 (8%)	4 (9%)	14 (17%)
IIA	6 (8%)	11 (26%)	20 (24%)
IIB	8 (10%)	3 (7%)	10 (12%)
III	28 (36%)	16 (37%)	34 (40%)
IV	29 (37%)	9 (21%)	5 (6%)

α = dissection of left cervical nodes
pT = pathological T status

node dissection); and group C (standard dissection – 83 cases with mediastinal and abdominal lymph node dissection only) (Fig. 1).

Group A showed a tendency towards more upper third cancers and stage IV disease, largely because bilateral cervical dissection was carried out. Compared with group A, group C contained more early stage cases, more elderly patients (the average age was 63, higher than the other two groups), and a greater number of high-risk cases (Table I).

Results

Table II shows the metastatic rate in each dissection group. The rate of lymph node metastases was 83% in the extended dissection

Table II
Lymph Node Dissection of Thoracic Esophageal Cancer Based on Preoperative Staging

Type of Nodal Dissection	*[A] Extended Dissection 77 cases*	*[B] Standard + α Dissection 43 cases*	*[C] Standard Dissection 83 cases*
Rate of Node Metastases			
Total	83%	63%	54%
Mediastinal Nodes	69%	35%	45%
Abdominal Nodes	48%	44%	42%
Cervical Nodes	31%	14%	—
Total Number of Positive Nodes	387	109	181
(Average)	5.0	2.5	2.1

α = dissection of left cervical nodes

group (A), 63% in group B, and 54% in the standard dissection group (C). The metastatic rate was higher in group A, which had the highest rate of mediastinal and cervical lymph node metastases, 69% and 31%, respectively. The average number of metastatic lymph nodes was 5.0 in group A, more than double the number in group C.

Table III
Incidence of Cervical Lymph Node Metastases in Groups A and B

	Cervical Region Dissected Cases	*Incidence of Cervical Metastasis (%)*
No. of Cases	120	30 (25%) right (11), left (16), bilateral (3)
Location of Tumor		
Upper	19	9 (47%)
Middle	80	18 (23%)
Lower	19	3 (16%)
pT of TNM		
pT1	14	1 (7%)
pT2	16	2 (13%)
pT3	69	21 (30%)
pT4	18	6 (33%)

Table IV
Operative Results of Esophageal Cancer According to the Type of Dissection

	[A]	[B]	[C]
Average Time of Operation	365 min (±80 min)	354 min (±73 min)	305 min (±90 min)
Intraoperative Bleeding	1047 ml (±555 ml)	1061 ml (±497 ml)	985 ml (±820 ml)
Mortality Rate	7.8%	0%	2.4%
Rate of Hospital Death (>1 month)	5.1%	4.6%	3.6%

Table III shows the incidence of cervical lymph node metastases in patients in whom cervical dissection was performed. The cervical metastatic rate was 47% in upper third cases, 22% in middle third cases, and 16% in lower third cases. The cervical metastases were on the right side in 11 patients, on the left side in 16 patients, and were bilateral in three patients. This shows that the rate of involvement of cervical lymph nodes on the right side is the same as on the left side. According to the TNM classification, we found that about one third of patients with T3 or T4 tumors had cervical node metastases, although even though one submucosal cancer (T1) had cervical metastasis.

Table IV shows the operative results for each type of dissection. The average time of operation was 365 minutes in group A, 345 minutes in group B, and 305 minutes in group C. This indicates that the operation takes slightly longer if we add a cervical lymph node dissection. There was no difference in the average blood loss in each group.

The operative mortality rate was 7.8% in group A, 0% in group B, 2.4% in group C. The operative mortality rate of group A is slightly higher than that of other groups, but there was not a significant difference in the hospital death rate.

Table V describes the postoperative morbidity in each group. Intensive care requiring mechanical ventilation more than 2 days was necessary in 25% of patients in the extended dissection group (A) followed by 22% in group C which included many elderly and high-risk cases. The rate of tracheotomy was 32% in group A, 26% in group C, and 14% in group B, showing a slightly higher rate in group A.

Table V
Postoperative Care and Complications by Type of Dissection

	[A]	[B]	[C]
Mechanical Ventilation over 48 Hours	25%	14%	20%
Tracheostomy	31%	14%	24%
Postoperative Complications	52%	33%	42%
Pneumonia	23%	5%	22%
Anastomotic leak	12%	12%	13%
Paralysis of Recurrent Nerve	16%	2%	4%
Insufficient Circulation	8%	2%	4%

The postoperative complication rate was higher in group A followed in order by group C and group B.

Recurrent nerve paralysis was significantly higher in the extended dissection group (A) but the occurrence of anastomotic leakage showed no difference among the three groups. Among the cases of moderate or severe recurrent nerve paralysis, almost all were cases of left or bilateral paralysis. In group A, recurrent nerve paralysis was particularly frequent in cases of upper mediastinal lymph node metastases. It was concluded that the paralysis was due to the upper mediastinal dissection rather than to the cervical dissection.

Concerning operative mortality, many of the group A and C cases were elderly patients (over 70 years old), and many palliatively resected cases developed pneumonia. In cases of hospital death, there were many pulmonary complications requiring long-term admission. However, cases of hospital death were mostly due to recurrent cancer treated with palliative resection.

Figure 2 shows the cumulative survival rate of each group for curatively resected cases. Among the three groups, there was no significant difference in survival rate. The extended dissection group (A), which included many advanced cases with a high metastatic rate, yielded the same survival curve as the standard dissection group (C), which included many cases with a low clinical metastatic rate. We believe that extended dissection of three regions, including the bilateral cervical region, is effective in improving the long-term survival rate.

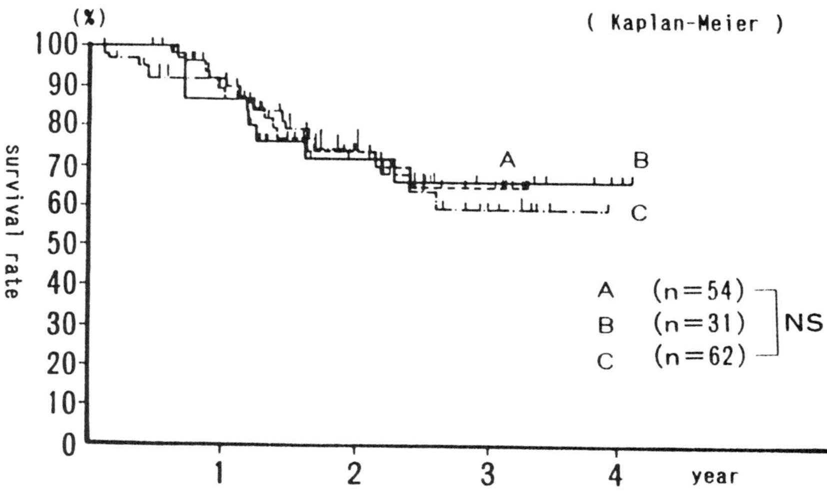

Figure 2: Survival curves of curatively resected esophageal cancer based on preoperative staging: cases of right thoracotomy (TWMC, June 1989).

Figure 3 shows the cumulative survival rates of node-negative cases treated by standard curative resection with right thoracotomy from 1980 to 1984 and node-negative cases of curative resection based on preoperative staging from January 1985 to September 1988. There is no difference in the 1 to 2-year survival rate, but at 3 years and beyond the survival rate of cases dissected based on preoperative staging is significantly greater ($p<0.05$).

Figure 4 shows the cumulative survival curve of curatively resected node positive cases. Improvement in the 1 to 2-year survival rate was obtained by dissection based on preoperative staging in the period after 1985 ($p<0.05$–0.01).

Table VI shows the recurrence pattern for each group. Group A, which included many cases with a high rate of lymph node metastases, showed a tendency to lymphatic nodal recurrence (80%) and disseminated recurrence (20%). However, in group C, which included many cases of low-grade metastases, lymphatic recurrence was seen in 53%. This was lower than the 80% of group A or the 68% of the standard dissection group without cervical region dissection treated by right thoracotomy before 1984. Organ metastases were seen in about 50% of each group, and local recurrence was approximately

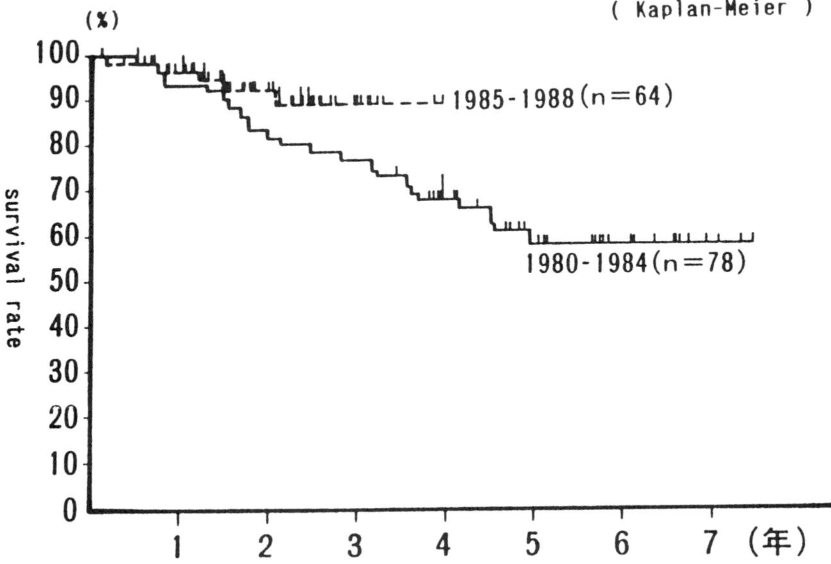

Figure 3: Survival curves of curatively resected esophageal cancer without lymph node metastases: cases of right thoracotomy (TWMC, June 1989).

10% in each. There was no difference related to whether or not the cervical node dissection was performed.

Discussion

In esophageal cancer, lymph node status is as important a factor for prognosis as is local extent of the tumor. Since 1972, we have been trying approaches in which we dissect two regions (mediastinum and abdomen) and give postoperative T-shaped irradiation to prevent cervical and upper mediastinal recurrence.[1] However, the 5-year survival rate of resected cases in our institute and our country is only about 22–23%.[2,3] Therefore, we are now trying several combination therapeutic strategies to increase the survival rate.[4] Extended dissection of the three regions including the upper mediastinal paratracheal and bilateral cervical area has been performed in a multicenter study for several years in Japan.[5,6]

Since 1985, we have selected the approach for and type of dissection for thoracic esophageal cancer resection based on preoperative

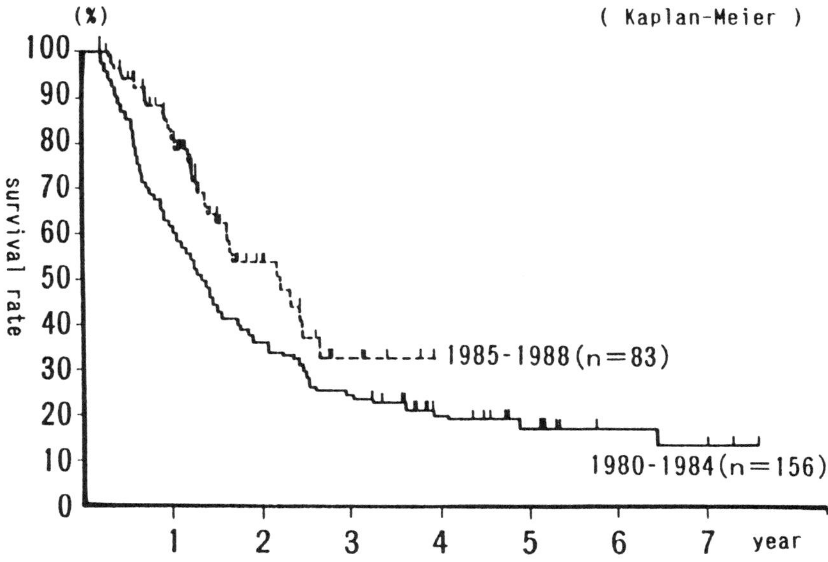

Figure 4: Survival curves of curatively resected esophageal cancer with lymph node metastases: cases of right thoracotomy (TWMC, June 1989).

Table VI
Recurrence Patterns of Thoracic Esophageal Cancer

	[A] Extended Dissection 13 Cases	*[C] Standard Dissection 20 Cases*	*1980–1984 Standard Dissection 92 Cases*
Lymphatic Recurrence	80%	53%	68%
Cervical Nodes	(46%)	(30%)	(29%)
Mediastinal Nodes	(40%)	(30%)	(51%)
Abdominal Nodes	(13%)	(8%)	(22%)
Local Recurrence	20%	15%	17%
Organ Metastasis	53%	53%	50%
Dissemination	20%		3%
Anastomotic Recurrence	7%		4%

staging by EUS, US, and CT scanning. In our institute, the preoperative detection of lymph node enlargement is performed by US for the cervical and abdominal regions and by EUS for the mediastinum. These ultrasonographic examinations for detection of lymph nodes are very useful compared to CT scanning because they can detect 3–5 mm diameter lymph nodes and yield greater than 90% diagnostic accuracy.[7]

Extended dissection with dissection of the bilateral cervical area based on preoperative staging produced an increase in the long-term survival rate, even though the rate of metastases to lymph nodes in the extended dissection group (A) was as high as 83% overall and 31% in the cervical region. These data demonstrate the efficacy of extended dissection based on preoperative staging. However, this more extensive operation does result in a slightly longer operative time and more frequent occurrence of moderate and severe recurrent nerve paralysis.

Since complications and operative death were particularly common in palliative resections of advanced cancers in the elderly, cases recognized as such will not be considered for such an operation in the future.

References

1. Endo M, Ide H, et al: Postoperative irradiation in the prevention of recurrence in patients with cancer of the thoracic esophagus. J Clin Oncol 11:247, 1981.
2. Ide H, Hanyu F, et al: Operative results of thoracic esophageal carcinoma. Jpn Geka-Tiryo 60:671, 1989.
3. Japanese Society for Esophageal Diseases: The annual reports of registered esophageal cancer cases in Japan. 1985.
4. Ide H, Hanyu F, et al: Multidisciplinary treatment of thoracic esophageal carcinoma. Jpn J Cancer Chemother 15:589, 1988.
5. Iizuka T, Ide H, Kakegawa T, et al: Preoperative radioactive therapy for esophageal carcinoma. Chest 93:1054, 1988.
6. Akiyama H: Cardinals in the regional lymph node dissection in surgery of thoracic esophageal cancer. In: Disease of the Esophagus, Siewert JR, Hölscher AH (eds), Berlin, Springer-Verlag, 1988, pp 416–420.
7. Murata Y, Okushima N, et al: The value of ultrasonography for preoperative staging of esophageal carcinoma. In: Disease of the Esophagus, Siewert JR, Hölscher AH (eds), Berlin, Springer-Verlag, 1988, pp 154–158.

21

Cervical-Thoracic-Abdominal Lymph Node Dissection for Intrathoracic Esophageal Carcinoma

Masahiko Tsurumaru, Hiroshi Akiyama,
Harushi Udagawa, Yoshimasa Ono,
Masatoshi Suzuki, Goro Watanabe

Introduction

It is a well-recognized fact that intrathoracic esophageal carcinoma tends to have widespread lymph node metastases to the mediastinum, abdomen, and the neck. Until several years ago, a cervical lymph node metastasis was regarded as clinical evidence of advanced tumor and unresectability. However, we have two patients who developed cervical lymph node metastases after the initial operation and survived more than 5 years after subsequent neck dissection or radiotherapy. These experiences suggested that a more extensive lymph node dissection of the superior mediastinum as well as bilateral neck dissection might improve the prognosis. We started doing bilateral neck dissection simultaneous with mediastinal and abdominal lymphadenectomy 5 years ago. We call this procedure "cervical-thoracic-abdominal (CTA) lymph node dissection." In this chapter, the results

Ferguson MK, Little AG, Skinner DB: Diseases of the Esophagus, Vol. I: Malignant Diseases. Futura Publishing Company, Inc., Mount Kisco, NY, © 1990.

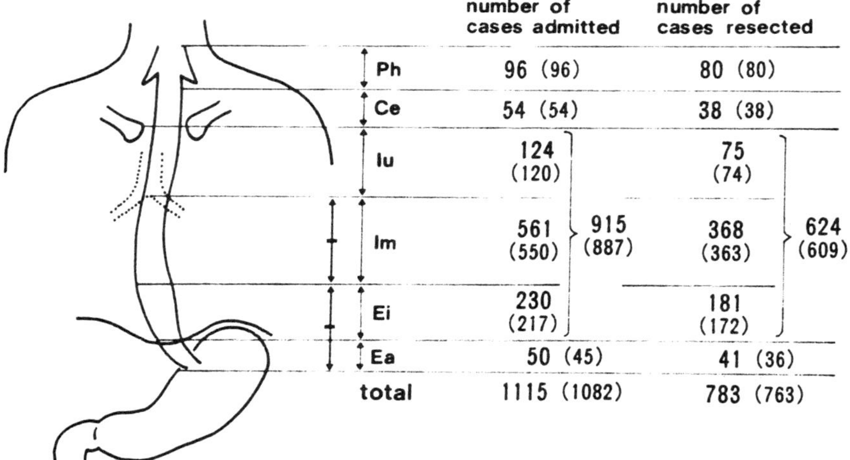

	number of cases admitted		number of cases resected	
Ph	96 (96)		80 (80)	
Ce	54 (54)		38 (38)	
Iu	124 (120)	915 (887)	75 (74)	624 (609)
Im	561 (550)		368 (363)	
Ei	230 (217)		181 (172)	
Ea	50 (45)		41 (36)	
total	1115 (1082)		783 (763)	

Figure 1: Incidence of tumors in each region of the esophagus. Ph = pharyngeal, Ce = cervical, Iu = upper thoracic, Im = middle thoracic, Ei = lower thoracic, Ea = abdominal esophagus.

of CTA dissection with regard to patterns of lymph node metastasis and survival are reviewed.

Materials and Methods

In the past 5 years, 1,115 cases of esophageal carcinoma were admitted to Toranomon Hospital (Fig. 1). Of the 915 cases of intrathoracic esophageal carcinomas, 887 cases were squamous cell carcinomas. Among the 609 resected cases, 310 patients underwent the conventional thoraco-abdominal (TA) lymph node dissection while 182 cases underwent CTA lymph node dissection. These 182 cases were reviewed to analyze the pattern of lymph node metastasis and outcome of cervical-thoracic-abdominal lymph node dissection.

Initially, CTA dissection was carried out only in the patients with clinically evident cervical lymph node metastases confirmed by ultrasonography and in patients with carcinoma of the upper esophagus. This initial series of 17 patients and the latest 37 patients were excluded in evaluation of prognosis.

Results

The frequency of lymph node metastasis is shown in Figure 2 a and b. Most (74.2%) of the patients who underwent CTA dissection had metastatic lymph nodes, including 34.1% for cervical lynph node metastases, 59.9% for mediastinal lymph node metastases and 50.0% for abdominal lymph node metastases.

Carcinoma of the upper third of the esophagus showed 43.3% with positive lymph nodes in the neck, 53.3% in the superior mediastinum, 20.0% in the middle mediastinum, 6.7% in the lower mediastinum, and 20.0% in the superior gastric area. Carcinoma of the middle third of the esophagus showed 33.0% with positive lymph node metastases, 38.0% in the superior mediastinum, 37.0% in the middle mediastinum, 22.0% in the lower mediastinum, and 44.0% in the superior gastric area. Carcincma of the lower third of the esophagus showed 29.2% with positive lymph node metastasis in the neck, 33.0% in the superior mediastinum, 52.1% in the middle mediastinum, 33.3% in the lower mediastinum, and 64.6% in the superior gastric area. A high incidence of metastatic nodes to the neck was noted even for the tumors located in the lower esophagus.

The distribution of the positive lymph nodes in the neck is illustrated in Figure 3. The most common site of cervical lymph node metastases was to the lymph node group along the right recurrent laryngeal nerve (17.3%). About 90% of the positive nodes were confined within the triangle which was bounded by the omohyoid muscle, clavicle, and esophagus. Lymph node metastases did develop on both sides of the neck. The relative frequency of positive lymph nodes was 24.2% on the right side and was 18.1% on the left. Bilateral cervical lymph node metastases developed at a rate of 8.2%.

Figure 4 shows the relative frequency of positive lymph nodes in the three regions (mediastinum, abdomen, neck). Mediastinal lymph node metastases developed in 109 patients (59.9%), cervical lymph node metastases in 62 cases (34.1%), and abdominal lymph node metastases in 91 cases (50.0%). Thirty-nine (21.4%) out of the 182 patients who had a CTA dissection had lymph node metastases to three regions simultaneously. This accounted for 62.9% of the 62 cases with cervical lymph node metastases, and may indicate the degree of malignancy of such tumors. Cervical lymph node metastases without any node metastasis elsewhere occurred in four patients. Cervical and abdominal lymph node metastases without mediastinal lymph node metastasis developed in five patients.

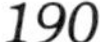

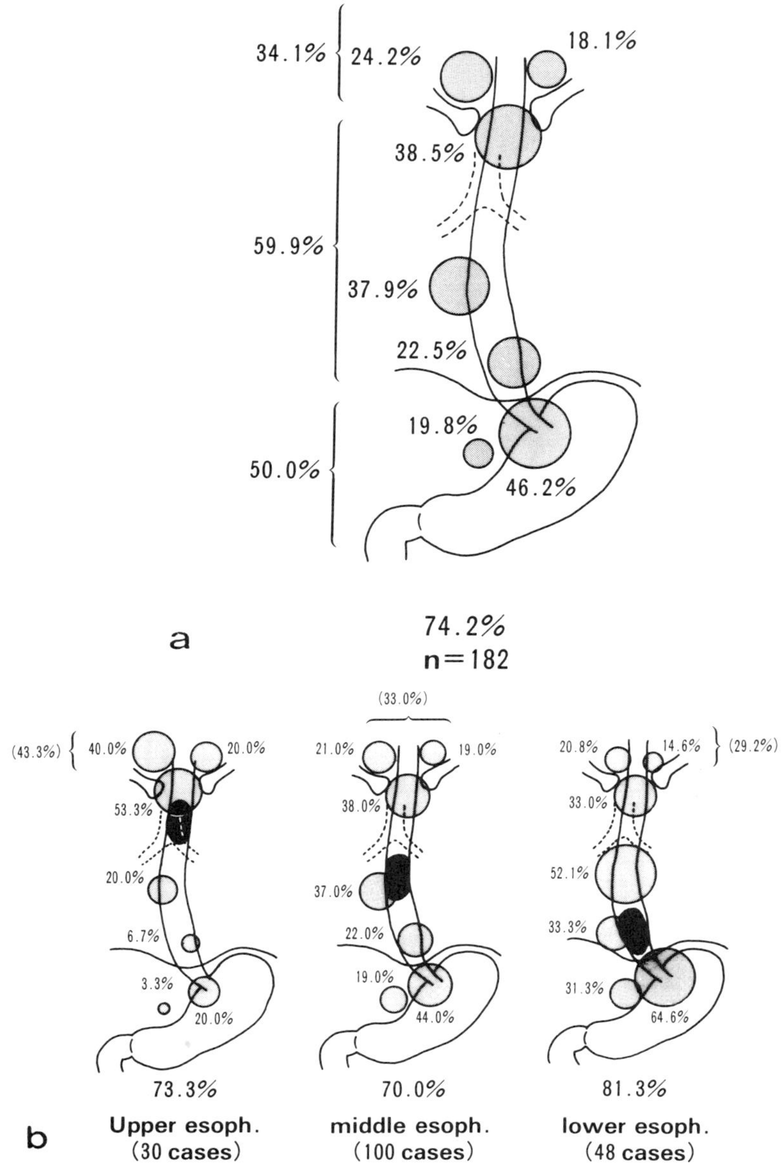

Figure 2: Frequency of lymph node metastases among patients undergoing cervical-thoracic-abdominal dissection. (a) Overall incidence. (b) Incidence by location of the primary tumor.

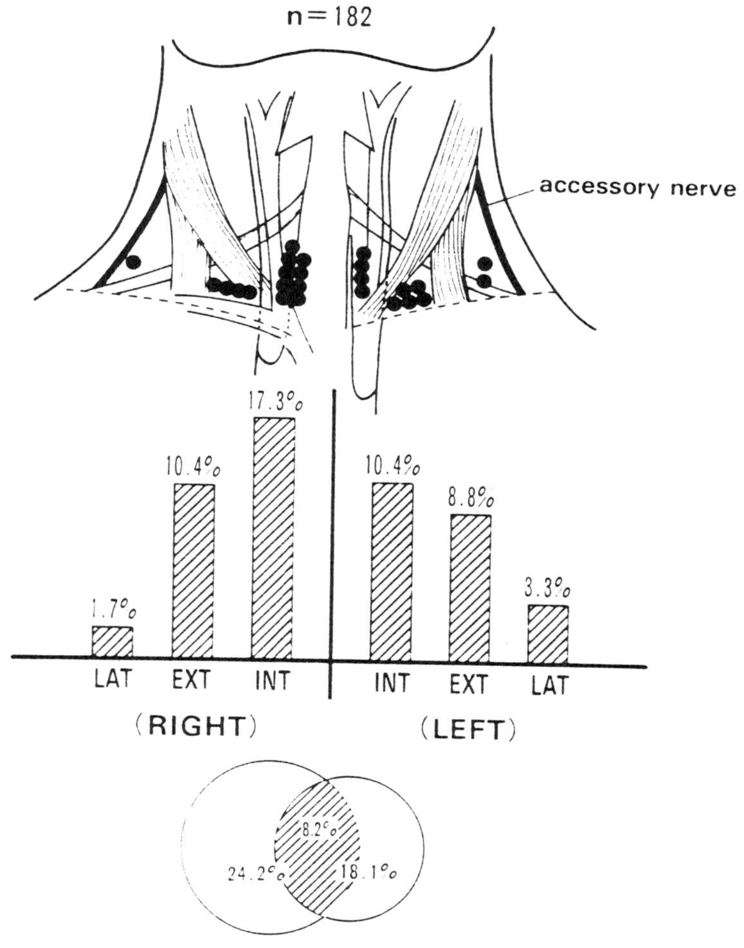

Figure 3: Distribution of positive cervical lymph nodes (LN).

Survival curves for 182 patients treated with CTA dissection were compared to conventional TA dissection (Fig. 5a). Survival rates after CTA dissection are 83.0% for 1 year, 63.3% for 2 years, 57.5% for 3 years, and 47.5% for 4 years. However, there is no statistically significant difference between the survival rates of the CTA dissection and TA dissection groups. Some subgroups were analyzed to further

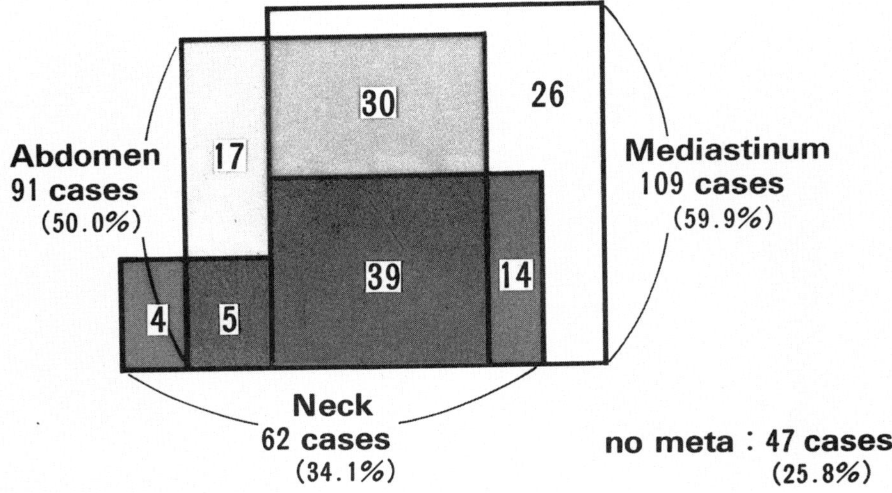

Figure 4: Regional distribution of lymph node metastases (182 patients).

evaluate the influence of CTA dissection pertaining to the prognosis. The 182 patients who underwent CTA dissection were divided into four subgroups according to the status of the mediastinal and the abdominal lymph nodes (Fig. 5b–e). A statistically significant difference was obtained for the subgroup of patients with positive mediastinal nodes and positive abdominal nodes [M(+)A(+)]. For the subgroup of patients with positive mediastinal nodes and negative abdominal nodes [M(+)A(-)], no significant difference was observed. This was also true for the subgroup of patients with negative mediastinal nodes and positive abdominal nodes [M(-)A(+)]. For the subgroup of patients with negative mediastinal nodes and negative abdominal nodes [M(-)A(-)], no difference could be seen by a generalized Wilcoxon test, however, a significant difference by Z test was observed at 2 years and 3 years. Statistical significance was also obtained for the subgroup of the patients without metastatic nodes in the superior mediastinum (Fig. 5f).

Discussion

We analyzed the modes of recurrence after esophagectomy with lymph nodes in the mediastinum and the abdomen. The recurrences

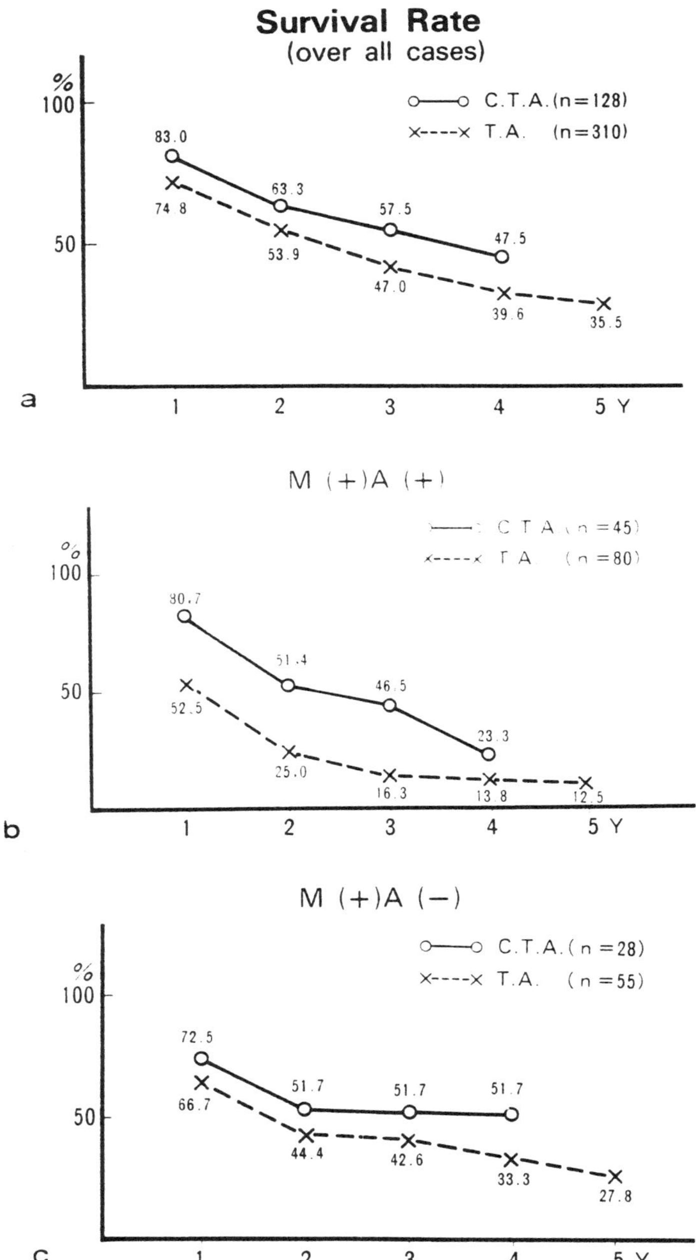

Figure 5: Survival rates for resected patients. (a) Overall rates. (b) Patients with involved mediastinal and abdominal nodes. (c) Patients with involved mediastinal but negative abdominal nodes. Continued.

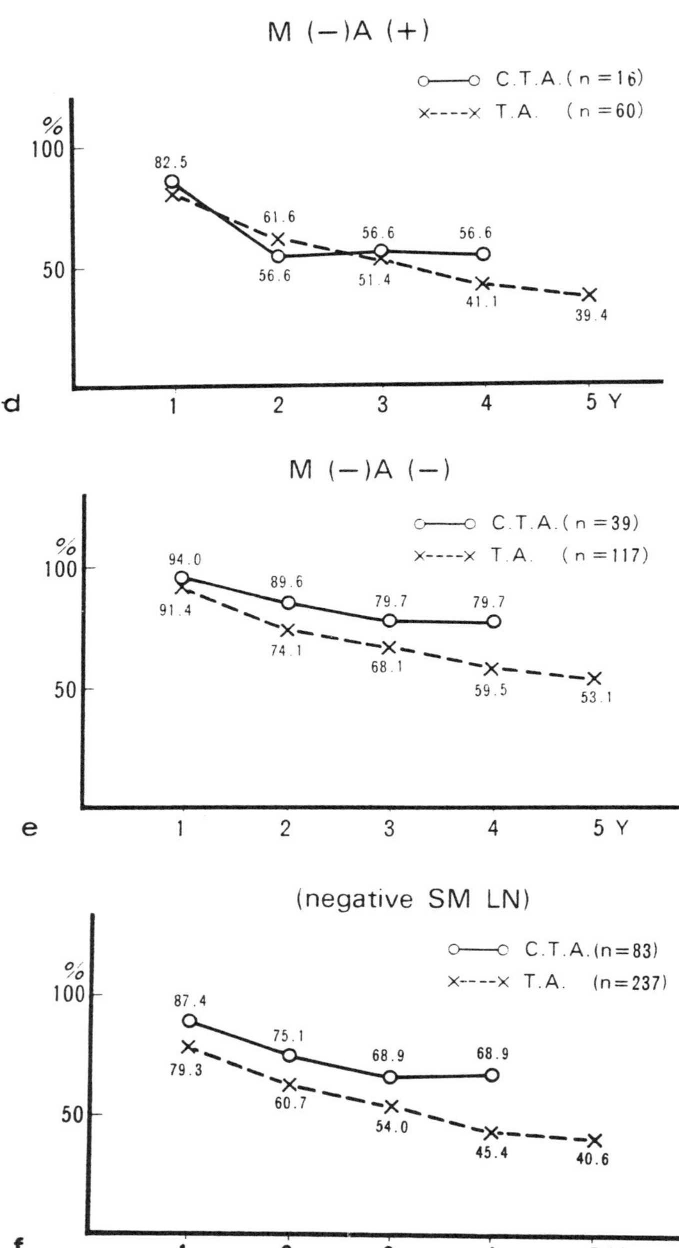

Figure 5: Survival rates for resected patients. (d) Patients with negative mediastinal but positive abdominal nodes. (e) Patients with negative mediastinal and abdominal nodes. (f) Patients with negative superior mediastinal nodes.

Table I
Modes of Recurrence According to the Location of Tumor

	LN Metastases					
	Cervical	*Mediastinal*	*Abdominal*	*Blood-borne*	*Local*	*Others*
Upper esophagus 15 cases	5 (33.3%)	3 (20.0%)	0	5 (33.3%)	2 (13.3%)	2
Middle esophagus 65 cases	15 (23.1%)	16 (24.6%)	3 (4.6%)	30 (46.2%)	1 (1.5%)	13
Lower esophagus 32 cases	6 (18.6%)	1 (3.1%)	4 (12.5%)	23 (71.9%)	0	7
Total 112 cases	26 (23.2%)	20 (17.9%)	7 (6.3%)	58 (51.8%)	3 (2.7%)	22

as shown in Table I were those initially recognized. Although blood-borne metastases occur most often, clinical recurrences at the cervical and superior mediastinal lymph nodes are also frequent. These data suggest that a more extensive lymph node dissection which includes a bilateral neck dissection may improve the prognosis. This is one of the underlying motives for starting the CTA dissection. CTA dissection provided us with more accurate information about the extent of lymph node metastases of squamous cell carcinoma of the intrathoracic esophagus. Close attention should be paid to the high incidence of metastatic lymph nodes in the neck and the superior mediastinum, especially in the cases of carcinoma of the upper esophagus. However, the possibility of cervical node metastases should not be ignored even among the cases of carcinoma of the lower esophagus. Although we expected CTA dissection to yield statistically significant differences in the survival curve for all cases, the prognosis remained the same. However, two subgroups showed statistically significant improvement in their survival curves. One of them is the subgroup with negative superior mediastinal lymph nodes. The group without lymph node metastasis might be composed of two subgroups, the true negative and the false negative (meaning those cases with micrometastasis) groups. This false negative group is thought to have a better survival rate. Therefore the patients who are assessed to have no lymph node metastasis by preoperative evaluation should be included as candidates for CTA dissection. Although CTA could not yield a significantly better survival rate, we have a couple of patients who have survived more than 4 years despite obvious lymph node metastatic spread to three regions at the initial operation. Therefore, CTA dissection can be justified as the radical operation for carcinoma which is located in the thoracic esophagus.

22

A Comparative Study Regarding Surgical Treatment for Thoracic Esophageal Cancer According to the Procedure of Lymph Node Dissection

Hiroshi Watanabe, Hoichi Kato, Hiroshi Tachimori

Introduction

At the National Cancer Center (Tokyo) from 1962 to 1982, surgical treatment with preoperative irradiation was the standard procedure for esophageal carcinoma. A cooperative, prospective, randomized study to evaluate the effectiveness of preoperative irradiation in curatively resected esophageal carcinoma was performed in 264 cases in eight institutions during 1982 and 1983, which was supported by a Grant-in-Aid for Cancer Research (56-SI) from the Ministry of Health and Welfare in Japan. Based on the survival curves in this study, postoperative irradiation alone was found to be superior to preoperative plus postoperative irradiation.[1] As a result, since 1983 we have not performed preoperative irradiation but have performed surgery first as a standard procedure. With this procedure, we have been able

Ferguson MK, Little AG, Skinner DB: Diseases of the Esophagus, Vol. I: Malignant Diseases. Futura Publishing Company, Inc., Mount Kisco, NY, © 1990.

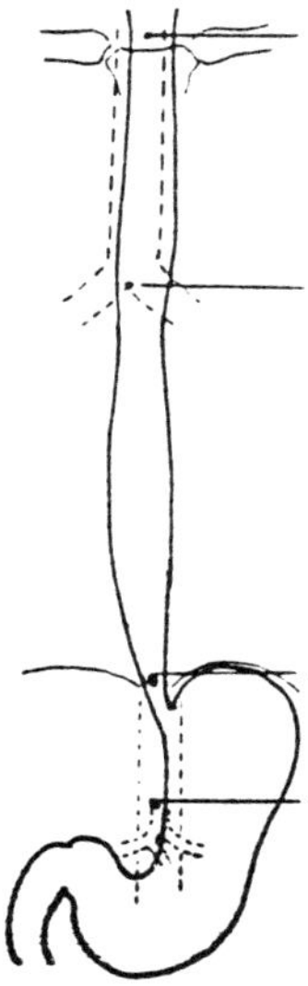

Group of lymph nodes	O group (n=105)	E group (n=71)
Upper mediastinal	40.9%	66.7%
Lower mediastinal	51.4	56.3
Superior gastric (Paracardiac & lesser curvature)	57.1	54.9
Left gastric & celiac	33.3	38.0

Figure 1: Rate of positive lymph nodes per number of cases with lymph node metastasis.

to perform an extensive lymph node dissection in the superior mediastinum.

Materials and Methods

In this comparative study, the first group was designated the O (ordinary) group, referring to 144 patients with preoperative irradiation followed by a lymph node dissection that was not extensive or complete. The second group was designated the E (extensive) group, referring to 82 patients without preoperative irradiation but followed by extensive and complete dissection of the lymph nodes.

Patients in both groups had squamous cell carcinoma limited to the thoracic esophagus, and underwent the same operative procedure, a subtotal esophagectomy with cervical esophagogastrostomy by the substernal route. In the O group, the preoperative irradiation total dose was 30–40 Gy. Both groups received a postoperative irradiation total dose of 50 Gy.

Table I
Background Factors Between O Group and E Group

Factor	*O Group*	*E Group*	X^2	*P Value*
Sex				
male	121	98	2.44	NS
female	23	10		
Age				
up to 59	71	44	2.20	NS
over 60	73	64		
Location of lesion				
upper	11	10	3.25	NS
middle	108	70		
lower	25	28		
Degree of lymph node metastasis*				
n_1	40	38	5.85	NS
n_2	50	35		
n_3	40	18		
n_4	14	16		
Histologic depth of invasion*				
a_0	32	41	7.52	$p < 0.05$
a_1–a_2	87	50		
a_3	21	17		

* Classification from guidelines for the clinical and pathological studies for carcinoma of the esophagus.[2]

Results

Background factors for the patients are noted in Table I, including sex, age, primary tumor location, and the degree of lymph node involvement.[2] There were no differences between the two groups. The incidence of invasion to the adventitia was significantly different between the groups ($p<0.05$ difference by the chi-square test using the FREQ procedure[3] of the SAS program software on a mainframe computer of the National Cancer Center, Tokyo). However, since the O group had preoperative irradiation, the difference was felt to be unimportant.

Considering both groups regarding the spread of cancer to the lymph nodes in the upper mediastinum (Fig. 1.), the O group reported a 40.9% incidence, while the E group reported a 66.2% incidence. This clearly shows that more cancer was removed from the

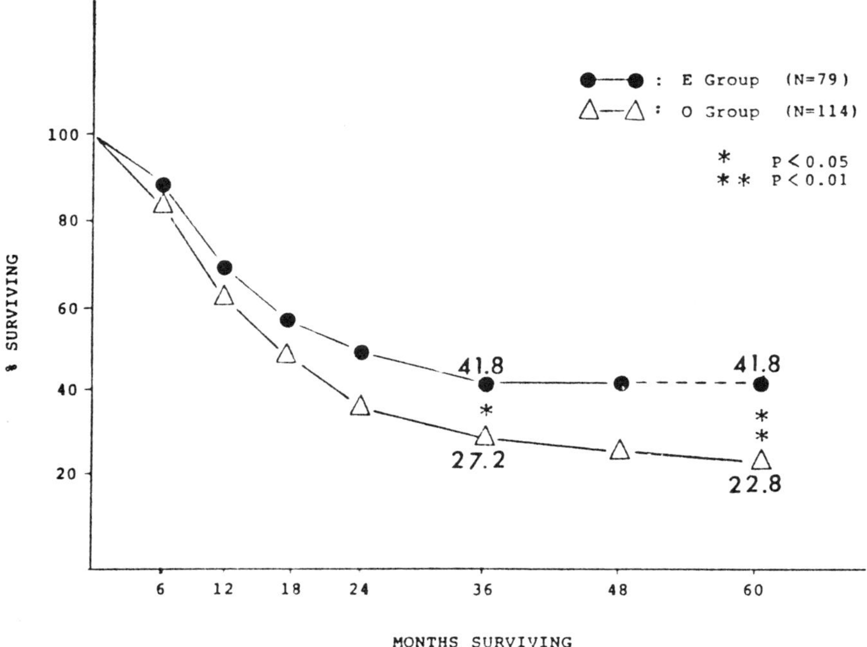

Figure 2: Comparison of survival after extensive versus ordinary lymph node dissection.

lymph nodes in the upper mediastinum of the E group compared to the O group. Below the carina, the lower mediastinal lymph nodes revealed metastases in 51.4% of the O group and 56.3% of the E group. The superior gastric lymph nodes (pericardiac, lesser curvature lymph nodes) were involved in 57.1% of the O group and in 54.9% of the E group. The lymph nodes in the region of the left gastric artery and the celiac artery showed a metastasic rate of 33.3% for the O group and 38.0% for the E group. There was very little difference in percentage of cancer metastasis in these lymph nodes between the two groups.

In the superior mediastinum, the upper right nodes (chiefly around the right recurrent laryngeal nerve), had a positive rate of 39 of 82 cases for the E group (47.6%), while in the upper left nodes (chiefly around the left recurrent laryngeal nerve), the rate of involvement was 17 of 82 (20.7%) (Table II). Consequently, it should

Table II
Rate of Positive Lymph Nodes in Upper Mediastinum for Patients (N = 82) Undergoing Extensive Node Dissection

		No. of Cases with Positive Lymph Nodes	*%*
Location of Lymph Nodes	Right Nodes (chiefly, around right recurrent laryngeal nerve)	39	47.6
	Left Nodes (chiefly, around left recurrent laryngeal nerve)	17	20.7

be emphasized that it is important to completely dissect the lymph nodes of the upper mediastinal group.

The survival curves (Kaplan-Meier method) of both groups is seen in Figure 2. Since the E group does not have a follow-up of 5 years, the 3-year survival rate was compared for both groups. The O

Table III
Results of Surgical Treatment* for Carcinoma of Thoracic Esophagus

	No. of Resected Cases	*Operative Death*** No. (%)*	*Hospital Death**** No. (%)*
Ordinary lymph node dissection (O Group)	144	8 (5.6)	9 (6.2)
Extensive lymph node dissection (E Group)	82	0 (0)	6 (7.3)

* Surgical procedure: Subtotal esophagectomy with cervical esophagogastrostomy by the substernal route
** Died within 30 days after operation
*** Died during the hospitalization, excluding operative death

group survival rate was 23.5% and the E group survival rate was 32.3% at 3 years after the operation, suggesting that the prognosis for the E group is better. The O group operation death rate was eight cases out of 144, or 5.6%, while the E group had no death at all (Table III). The hospital death rate for the O group was nine cases out of 144, or 6.2%, while the E group was six cases out of 82, or 7.3%. Overall early mortality for the E group and the O group was 7.3% and 11.8%, respectively.

Discussion

In many prior studies, the highest rate of lymph node involvement was found in the superior gastric region.[4,5] However, in our study, the highest incidence of nodal metastases was in the upper mediastinum. The distribution of nodal metastases in this region was influenced by operative technique and perioperative therapy, being higher in patients with more extensive dissections and lower in those who had preoperative radiotherapy.

Postoperative recurrences of thoracic esophageal carcinoma are observed mainly in the upper mediastinum or cervical region.[6] The cause of these recurrences may be an inadequate dissection of lymph nodes in the upper mediastinum. We believe a reasonable operation for thoracic esophageal carcinoma is total esophagectomy with complete lymphadenectomy. As the most commonly affected upper mediastinal node groups include those along the right and left recurrent laryngeal nerves, these regions should be included in the dissection to improve long-term survival.

References

1. Iizuka T, Ide H, Kakegawa T, et al: Preoperative radioactive therapy for esophageal carcinoma. Chest 93:1054, 1988.
2. Japanese Society for Esophageal Disease: Guidelines for the clinical and pathologic studies for the carcinoma of the esophagus. Jpn J Surg 6:69, 1976.
3. The FREQ procedure. SAS user's guide: Statistics, 5th edition. Cary, N.C., SAS Institute, 1985, p 403.
4. Akiyama H, Tsuramaru M, Kawamura T, et al: Principles of surgical treatment for carcinoma of the esophagus. Ann Surg 194:438, 1981.
5. Watanabe H: Late results of locally adjuvant chemotherapy with entubed

solidified bleomycin against abdominal lymph node metastasis after surgical treatment of esophageal cancer. In: Diseases of the Esophagus, Siewert JR, Holscher AH (eds), Berlin, Springer-Verlag, 1988, p 349.

6. Isono R, Onoda S, Ishikawa T, et al: Studies on the causes of deaths from esophageal carcinoma. Cancer 49:2173, 1982.

23

Evaluation of Lymphadenectomy of Intrathoracic Esophageal Cancer in Terms of Patient Survival

Kaichi Isono, Kazuaki Okuyama, Takenori Ochiai

Introduction

Postoperative survival rates for patients with esophageal cancer are poor. One of the reasons for that is the high recurrence rate of the cancer in the lymph nodes.[1,2] We have performed surgery for esophageal cancer for more than 20 years and have tried to improve the patient survival. Our efforts have been directed to dissection of potential metastatic lymph nodes as completely as possible. Recently we have introduced radical lymphadenectomy covering three fields: the neck, the mediastinum, and the abdomen. This chapter describes the incidence of metastatic lymph nodes and the effect of the lymphadenectomy on long-term patient survival in esophageal cancer.

Materials and Methods

A total of 560 patients with esophageal cancer underwent esophagectomy between 1965 and the end of 1988. Since 1983, 118 pa-

Ferguson MK, Little AG, Skinner DB: Diseases of the Esophagus, Vol. I: Malignant Diseases. Futura Publishing Company, Inc., Mount Kisco, NY, © 1990.

tients received a radical lymphadenectomy including three fields: the neck, the mediastinum, and the abdomen along with esophagectomy. The operative procedure for thoracic esophageal cancer consisted of total thoracic esophagectomy and reconstruction with a gastric tube through the substernal route. The lymph nodes of the neck and upper mediastinum were completely removed at the time of three-field lymphadenectomy. The lymph nodes dissected at the operation are illustrated in Figure 1. We classified the extent of the lymphadenectomy into four grades: grade 0 – lymphadenectomy was not performed, such as during a blunt dissection; grade 1 – dissection of adjacent lymph nodes which are defined as group 1 lymph nodes by the Guidelines of the Japanese Society for Esophageal Diseases;[3] grade 2 – dissection of group 2 lymph nodes of the classification of the Society; grade 3 – dissection of distant lymph nodes classified as group 3 or 4 by the Society's definition. Grade 3 lymphadenectomy is also referred to as a three-field (bilateral neck, mediastinum, and abdomen) lymphadenectomy.

Results

The overall postoperative mortality rate was 5.0% in 560 patients who underwent esophageal cancer surgery from 1965 until 1988. The mortality rate improved from 12.5% in the period between 1965 and 1969 to 2.0% between 1980 and 1988 (Table I).

Some distant lymph nodes that were not dissected during our early experience showed a high metastatic rate in the recent group of patients. Those are the lymph nodes located along the bilateral recurrent nerves, the bifurcation of the trachea, and bilateral supraclavicular fossae (Fig. 1). A total of 118 patients with intrathoracic esophageal cancer underwent lymphadenectomy of the three areas of the neck, mediastinum, and abdomen along with esophagectomy. As a result, 39 of the 118 patients (33.1%) showed lymph node metastases to the neck, 55 (46.6%) to the mediastinum and 53 (44.9%) to the abdominal nodes (Table II).

The extent of the lymphadenectomy was divided into four grades. The proportion of the patients receiving the different grade of the lymphadenectomy was compared between the six different periods from 1959 to 1988. The number of patients receiving the grade 2 lymphadenectomy increased gradually, and the grade 3 lymphadenectomy was performed only in the latest period from 1983 to 1988.

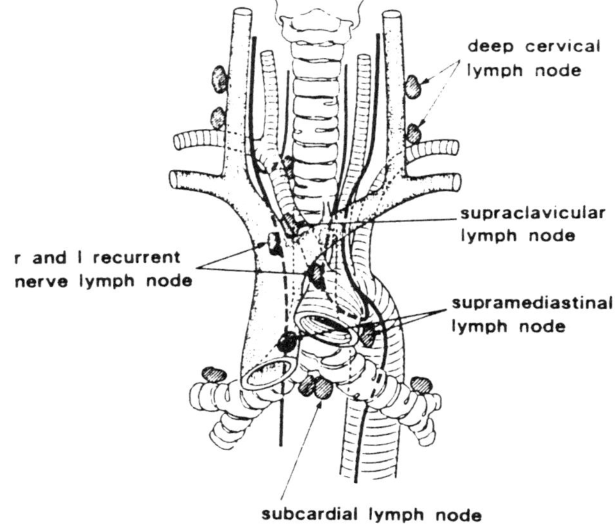

Figure 1: Dissected lymph nodes at grade 3 lymphadenectomy.

The 5-year survival rate of each period has gradually improved as shown in Figure 2. The 5-year survival rate was 30.5% in the latest period.

The survival rate is compared among the patients who had lymph node metastasis either to one, two, or three areas of the neck, mediastinum, and abdomen. The survival rate of the patients who had positive lymph nodes in one area was statistically better than that of

Table I
One-Month Mortality Rate after Surgery of Thoracic Esophageal Cancer

Period	*No. of Cases Resected*	*No. of Cases Dying Within 1 Month*	*Mortality Rate*
1965–69	112	14	12.5%
1970–74	83	4	4.8
1975–79	116	5	5.0
1980–88	249	5	2.0
Total	560	28	5.0

Table II
Lymph Node Metastatic Rate in the Neck, Mediastinum, and Abdomen in 118 Patients Receiving Three-Field Lymphadenectomy

Location of Lymph Node	*No. of Cases with Positive Nodes*	*Metastatic Rate*
Neck	39	33.1%
Mediastinum	55	46.6
Abdomen	53	44.9

the patients showing metastases in two or three areas (Fig. 3). The survival rate curves were compared between the patients receiving either grade 2 or grade 3 lymphadenectomy (Fig. 4). The survival rate was better in patients receiving three-field lymphadenectomy. The survival rate of the patients receiving three-field lymphadenectomy was much better in patients stage 0, I, II, and III; however, the difference was not evident in patients with stage IV disease (Fig. 5).

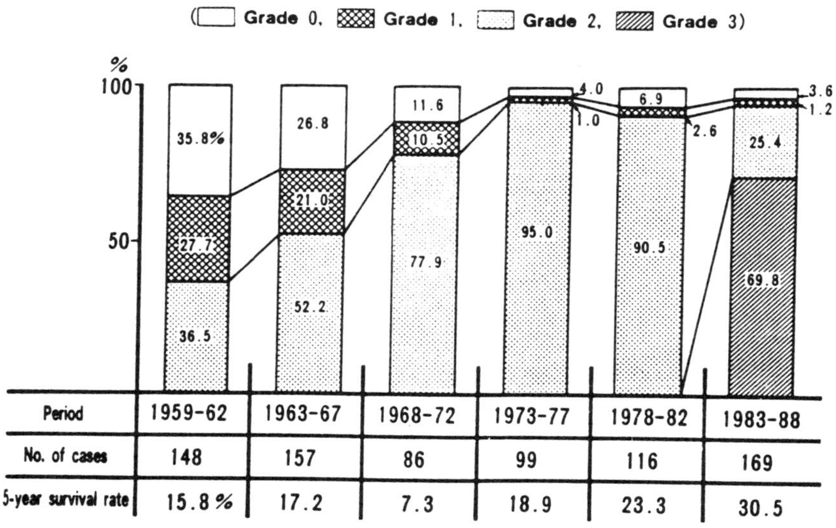

Figure 2: Grade of lymphadenectomy and five-year survival rate by periods.

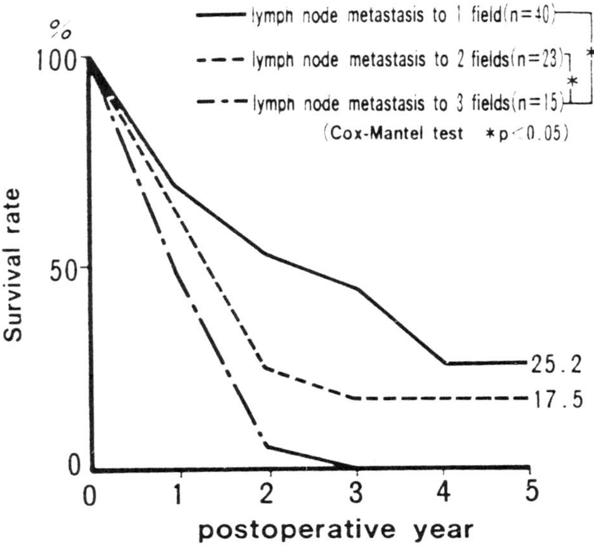

Figure 3: Survival rate curves of patients having lymph node metastasis either in 1, 2 or 3 fields.

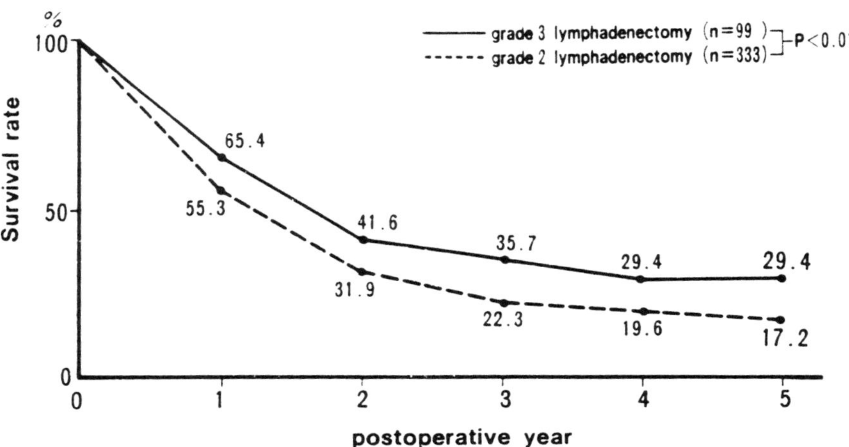

Figure 4: Survival rate curves of patients receiving either grade 2 or grade 3 lymphadenectomy.

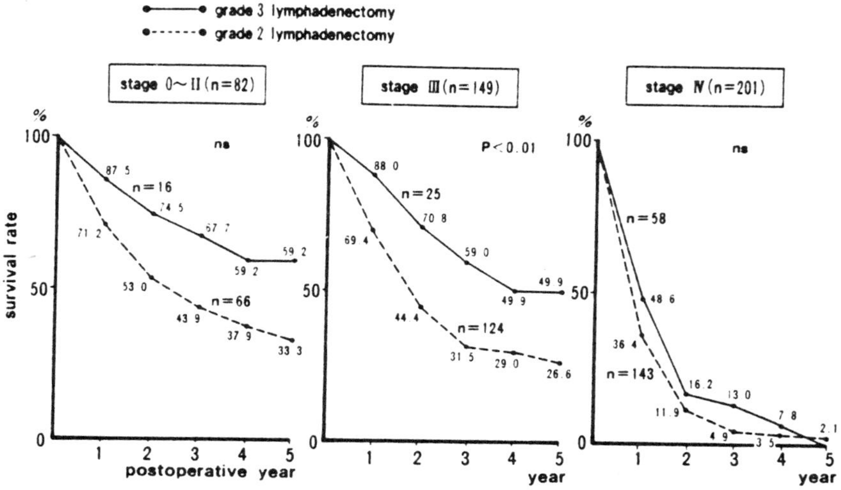

Figure 5: Survival rate curves according to the cancer stage.

Discussion

Long-term survival of esophageal cancer patients is not good. The main reason is that the esophageal cancer shows a high frequency of recurrence rate, especially in lymph nodes and distant organs. In an attempt to improve postoperative patient survival, we have introduced combined therapy with radiation, chemotherapy, and immunotherapy after operation with the lymph node dissection by group 2. These treatment regimens, however, were not satisfactory to cure the cancer. We have emphasized the high recurrence rate of the cancer in the lymph nodes of the upper mediastinum and para-aortic region.[4]

Recently we adopted the radical lymphadenectomy including regions of the neck, mediastinum, and abdomen.[5] We have performed the treatment of the three-field lymphadenectomy with combined therapy in 118 patients since 1983. This procedure is now a routine one in our institution. In order to determine whether the extensive lymphadenectomy is useful for improvement of patient survival, the present investigation was performed to determine the effect of three-field lymphadenectomy on the long-term patient survival.

The postoperative mortality rate improved from 12.5% during the period from 1965 to 1969 to 2.0% of that from 1980 to 1988, suggesting that extensive lymphadenectomy was safe to perform in patients under 70 years of age. The mortality rate of patients over 70 years old was as high as 11%, as compared to 1.1% for those under 70. Histologic studies showed that the metastatic rate to the neck is as high as 33.1%, similar to the metastatic rates of 46.6% and 44.9% in the mediastinal and abdominal nodes. This suggests that the lymphadenectomy of the neck is mandatory for a curative operation.

Three-field lymphadenectomy on patient survival was favorable in terms of the long-term patient survival, but this favorable effect was not seen in stage IV cancer. In conclusion, three-field lymphadenectomy is mandatory for esophageal cancer operation according to the indication based on the patient's condition, such as cancer stage or patient age.

References

1. Nishi M, Hiramatsu Y, Hioki K, et al: Risk factors in relation to postoperative complications in patients undergoing esophagectomy or gastrectomy for cancer. Ann Surg 207:148–154, 1988.
2. Pradihan GN, Eng J-B, Sabanathan S. Left thoracotomy approach for resection of carcinoma of the esophagus. Surg Gynecol Obstet 168:49–53, 1989.
3. Japanese Society for Esophageal Diseases: Guidelines for the clinical and pathologic studies on carcinoma of the esophagus. Jpn J Surg 6:69–78, 1976.
4. Sato H, Isono K: Antethoracic esophagogastrostomy through the right thoracic approach for esophageal cancer. Gastroenterol Surg 6:636–647, 1983 (in Japanese).
5. Isono K, Sato H, Koike Y, et al: Operative procedures of thoracic esophageal cancer using CUSA. Operation 35:1219–1227, 1981 (in Japanese).

24

Prognostic Significance of Lymph Node Metastasis in Surgical Resection of Esophageal Carcinoma

Guo Jun Huang, Ke Lin Sun

Introduction

Despite the high incidence of esophageal carcinoma in China, most patients are seen at relatively advanced stages of the disease. In a series of 1159 resections for nonirradiated esophageal carcinoma reported by Huang et al. in 1985, lymph node metastases were found in 593 of the cases, an incidence of 51.2%.[1] It is obvious that practically all of the nonresectable cases, which accounted for about 16% of our cases operated upon, showed lymph node metastases, although fixation of the primary tumor with severe invasion to the surrounding vital organs usually constituted the chief cause of nonresectability. Consequently, the actual incidence of lymph node metastasis of patients who had surgery was at least 67%.

The present study evaluates the prognostic significance of lymph node metastasis following surgical resection of esophageal carcinoma, based on a retrospective analysis of patients operated on over 5 years previously.

Ferguson MK, Little AG, Skinner DB: Diseases of the Esophagus, Vol. I: Malignant Diseases. Futura Publishing Company, Inc., Mount Kisco, NY, © 1990.

Materials and Methods

The present series consisted of 474 consecutive resections of non-irradiated intrathoracic squamous cell carcinoma of the esophagus carried out in a period of 4 years ending 1984.

Operation was done through a left posterolateral thoracotomy approach when the tumor was located in the middle or lower esophagus, and through a right approach when it was located in the upper thoracic segment or higher. The usual practice of resection was to eradicate as completely as feasible all the connective and tumor-bearing tissues around the esophagus, and the draining lymph nodes of the perigastric group up to the root of the left gastric artery, the paracardial, the paraesophageal and the mediastinal groups including the hilar, the paratracheal, and the subcarinal groups, along with the dissection and mobilization of the esophagus and the stomach, which was used in all cases as a substitute for the resected esophagus. No attempt was made to do overextensive lymph node dissection. Total esophagectomy was not a routine practice except in cases with high thoracic or cervical lesions.

Results

In 349 (73.6%) of the 474 resections, the operation was classified as curative with no evidence of residual tumor as evaluated by the surgeons and by pathological examination of the resected specimens, while in the remaining 125 cases (26.4%), it was classified as palliative because of incomplete excision of the primary tumor due to extra-esophageal invasion in 62 (49.6%), metastatic lymph nodes inaccessible to resection in 48 (38.4%), and organ metastases, residual tumor at surgical margins, or multiple primaries in 15 (12%) of the cases.

Of the 474 resections, positive lymph node metastases (LNM) were found in 211 patients for an incidence of 44.5%. In the entire series, the total number of lymph nodes removed and pathologically examined was 5,382, averaging 11.4 nodes per patient. There were 690 nodes found to be involved by tumor, an incidence of lymph node involvement of 12.8%.

The overall 5-year survival rate of the entire series was 30.6% (145/474). It was 44.9% (118/263) in patients without LNM and 12.8% (27/211) in those with LNM. In the curative resection group, it was 52.2% (107/205) in those without LNM and 17.4% (25/144) in those

Table I
Prognostic Factors Influencing 5-Year Survivals in 474 Resections for Nonirradiated Squamous Carcinoma of the Esophagus

Factors	% 5-Year Survival (cases)	p Value
Overall	30.6 (145/474)	
With LNM*	12.8 (27/211)	
Without LNM	44.9 (118/263)	0.0001
Curative resections	37.8 (132/349)	
With LNM	17.4 (25/144)	
Without LNM	52.2 (107/205)	0.0001
Palliative resections	10.4 (13/125)	
With LNM	3.0 (2/67)	
Without LNM	19.0 (11/58)	0.0035

* LNM = Lymph node metastasis

with LNM, while in the palliative resection group, it was 19.0% (11/58) in those without LNM and only 3.0% (2/67) in those with LNM. All of these differences were of high statistical significance (Table I).

In the group of 145 patients with positive LNM, when the metastatic lymph nodes were less than 5 in number, the 5-year survival rate was 14.7% (27/184); it was 19.4% (25/129) with a curative resection and 3.6% (2/55) with a palliative resection, a difference of statistical significance. However, when the metastatic lymph nodes were over 5 in number, there was no 5-year survivor with either a curative or a palliative resection (Table II). Similarly, when the metastatic lymph nodes were less than 50% of those removed, the 5-year survival rate

Table II
Five-Year Survivals in Relation to Number of Metastatic Lymph Nodes (MLN)

Number of MLN	% 5-Year Survival (cases)	p Value
Less than 5	14.7 (27/184)	
Curative resections	19.4 (25/129)	
Palliative resections	3.6 (2/55)	0.0057
Over 5	0 (0/27)	
Curative resections	0 (0/15)	
Palliative resections	0 (0/12)	

Table III
Five-Year Survivals in Relation to Percent of Metastatic Lymph Nodes (MLN) Removed

% MLN Removed	*% 5-Year Survival (cases)*	*p Value*
Less than 50	14.8 (26/176)	
Curative resections	19.8 (24/121)	
Palliative resections	3.6 (2/55)	0.0049
Over 50	2.9 (1/35)	
Curative resections	4.3 (1/23)	
Palliative	0 (0/12)	

was 14.8% (26/176); it was 19.8% (24/121) with a curative resection and 3.6% with a palliative resection, a difference of statistical significance. When the metastatic lymph nodes were over 50% of those removed, the 5-year survival rate was only 2.9% (1/35); it was 4.3% (1/23) with a curative resection and 0% (0/12) with a palliative resection (Table III).

Discussion

It is widely accepted that surgery remains the first choice of treatment for carcinoma of the esophagus, and that meticulous lymph node dissection is an important integral part of oncologic surgery. However, surgical resection, no matter how extensive, is a regional treatment ineffective to any cancer beyond its scope. Surgery is relatively ineffective in extirpating microscopic or subclinical tumor foci, and bears the potential risk of iatrogenic cancer cell dissemination due to surgical manipulation.

The present study showed that completeness of resection and lymph node status are two important prognostic factors that significantly influence long-term survival, and that they are closely interrelated. Our analysis showed that with a curative resection and absence of lymph node metastases, the prognosis was the best in this series with a 5-year survival rate of 52.2%. On the contrary, with a palliative resection and presence of lymph node metastases, the prognosis was the poorest with a 5-year survival rate of only 3.0%. Our analysis also showed that the more extensive the lymph node metastases, the less favorable was the prognosis even with a curative resection. All of these findings indicate that radical surgery is of great prognostic importance when the cancer process is relatively early and localized, but is of much less prognostic importance when the disease process is relatively advanced.

In an analysis of long-term results of surgical treatment in 1,647 patients with carcinoma of the esophagus reported by Huang et al.,[2] the 5-, 10-, 15- and 20-year survival rates were 29.6% (390/1317), 22.5% (210/933), 19.7% (122/620), and 11.0% (20/181), respectively. This analysis showed that recurrence and/or metastasis of the initial cancer were the main obstacles to long-term survival, as they constituted the causes of death in as many as 40.0% of patients who died over 5 years and 24.2% of those who died over 10 years after resection, even though in 85.1% of these patients, the initial resection was classified as curative. These findings indicate that in the majority of cases with relatively advanced carcinoma of the esophagus, surgery is of limited value in completely eradicating the cancer, even though the resection may appear to fulfill all the criteria of a curative operation.

It is the authors' belief that when the tumor with its metastatic process is relatively localized, there is a good chance of complete eradication of the tumor-bearing tissues by surgery, and in such cases extensive dissection of lymph nodes is of value in improving the survival. However, when the tumor is more advanced with relatively widespread lymph node and other metastases, the chance of completely eradicating all tumor-bearing tissues, even by extensive lymph node dissection, is small, and in so doing the chance of iatrogenic dissemination of cancer cells is great. Under such circumstances, it is advisable to resort to judicious use of combination therapy rather than to rely on overextending the scope of resection with the risk of increasing operative morbidity and mortality.

Summary

Surgery remains the first choice of treatment for carcinoma of the esophagus, and meticulous lymph node dissection is an important integral part of oncologic surgery. However, in relatively advanced cases of this disease, surgery is of limited value in complete eradication of cancer involvement, and further improvement in treatment results will depend on more judicious use of multimodality therapy rather than on overextending the scope of operation.

References

1. Huang GJ, Wang LJ, Liu JS, Cheng GY, Zhang DW, Wang GQ, Zhang RG: Surgery of esophageal carcinoma. Semin Surg Oncol 1:74, 1985.
2. Huang GJ, Wang LJ, Zhang DW, Zhang RG: Late results of surgical treatment for carcinoma of the esophagus. In: Siewert JR, Hoelscher AH (eds), Diseases of the Esophagus, Berlin, Springer-Verlag, p 641, 1988.

25

Prognostic Factors for Squamous Cell Carcinoma of the Thoracic Esophagus After Curative Resection

Romeo Bardini, Carlo Castoro, Paolo Sorrentino, Alberto Ruol, P. Borelli, Antonella Ruffatto, Carlo Tremolada, Alberto Peracchia

Introduction

Results of treatment for squamous cell carcinoma of the thoracic esophagus are unsatisfactory. The overall 5-year survival averages 15%.[1] Curative resection is the treatment of choice whenever possible, but most patients die of recurrence within 2 years after operation, and the 5-year survival after curative resection does not exceed 25% in large series.[1] Many different prognostic factors have been considered in the staging of esophageal carcinoma after curative resection.[2–4] In this chapter, we present a statistical analysis of prognostic factors in a homogeneous group of 262 patients who underwent curative resection for cancer of the thoracic esophagus to assess the predictive value of pathological factors.

Ferguson MK, Little AG, Skinner DB: Diseases of the Esophagus, Vol. I: Malignant Diseases. Futura Publishing Company, Inc., Mount Kisco, NY, © 1990.

Table I
Prognostic Factors Considered for the Univariate Analysis

Sex
Age
Tumor site
Tumor length
Macroscopic appearance
Histologic grading
Number of mitoses per microscopic field
Histologic pattern
pT according to the TNM staging
pN according to the TNM staging
Number of metastatic nodes
Degree of nodal involvement
Vascular invasion
Lymphocytic stromal reaction
Pattern of local spread
Multifocality of cancer

Materials and Methods

We selected a homogeneous group of patients with squamous cell carcinoma of the thoracic esophagus, without visceral metastases, who underwent curative resection through a right thoracotomy. This approach permits a total thoracic esophagectomy and mediastinal lymphadenectomy. Patients who had undergone preoperative chemotherapy or radiation therapy were excluded. All patients were followed until death or for a minimum period of 2 years. Using the above criteria, 262 patients were selected out of all patients with squamous cell carcinoma of the esophagus treated between 1980 and 1986. Mean age was 56.6 years (range 32–75) and male/female ratio was 4:1. The site of cancer was the upper thoracic esophagus in 44 (16.8%), the middle esophagus in 140 (53.4%), and the lower esophagus in 78 (29.7%) patients.

Survival estimation was performed with the product-limit Kaplan-Meier test. Univariate analysis was performed according to Mantel-Cox and Breslow tests (BMDP 1L) and the Cox model (BMPD 2L) was then used for multivariate analysis. Prognostic factors considered for the univariate analysis are shown in Table I. All were prospectively registered in a computerized clinical record that has been used for

Table II
Results of the Univariate Analysis

Parameter	Categories	p Value
Tumor site	Upper, middle, lower	0.01
Tumor length	<2, >2 <5, >5 cm	0.01
pT	1, 2, 3, 4, (4)	<0.0001
pN	1, 2	<0.0001
Number of involved nodes	0, 1, >1	<0.0001
Vascular invasion	yes/no	0.04

patients with esophageal cancer since 1980. The histologic parameters were reviewed to confirm the already stored data. For the multivariate analysis, only the factors showing a significant influence on survival on the basis of the univariate analysis were considered.

Results

Univariate Analysis

The univariate analysis showed the following factors had significant influence on survival: tumor site, tumor length, depth of wall penetration (pT), nodal involvement (pN), number of metastatic nodes, site of metastatic nodes, and vascular invasion. Table II shows the detailed "categories" of each parameter and the corresponding p value.

Regarding nodal involvement, we considered as N1 paraesophageal, mediastinal, pericardial nodes, and those along the lesser gastric curvature, while N2 nodes included distant abdominal nodes such as those of the celiac axis. The overall 5-year survival rate was 23.4% (Fig. 1). Figure 2 shows the survival curves for the pN pattern.

Multivariate Analysis

The estimated survival function, according to the Cox Model, confirmed a statistical significance only for pT, pN, both site and number of metastatic nodes, and tumor site. Tumor length and vascular invasion did not prove to be of significant prognostic value.

The multivariate analysis showed that the single most important

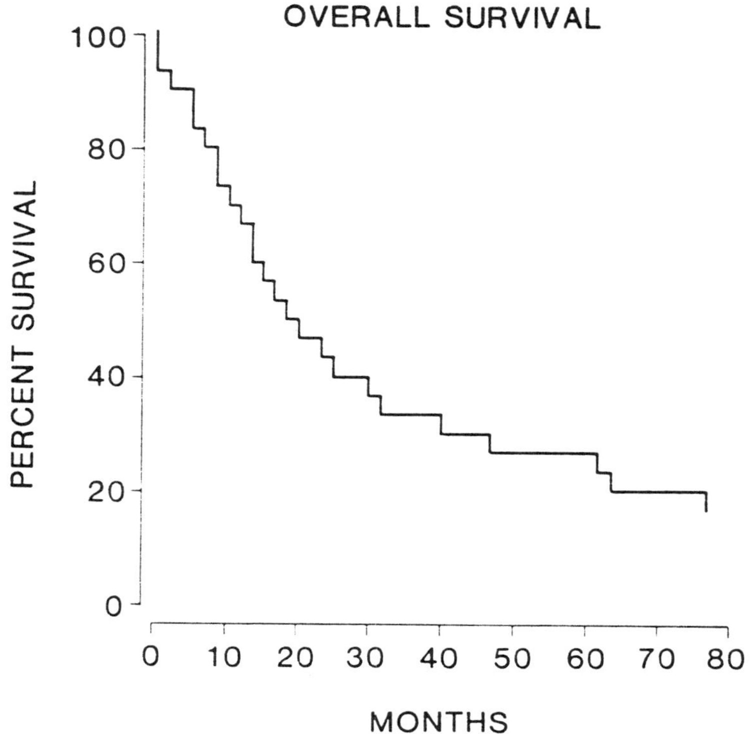

Figure 1: Overall survival curve.

prognostic factor was lymph node status and that the statistical relevance of the pT pattern was mainly dependent on the presence or absence of node metastases.

No statistical difference was found between pT1 and pT2, and pT3 patients with the same pN pattern. On the contrary, there was a significant difference in survival between pN0 and pN1 patients with the same pT pattern. Since the presence of lymph node metastasis was significantly dependent on the depth of wall penetration, pT and pN cannot be considered independent variables.

The best statistical predictive value was obtained classifying these patients as shown in Table III. This stage grouping was obtained by combining pT, pN, site and number of metastatic nodes. Figure 3 shows the corresponding estimated survival curves.

The multivariate analysis confirmed the statistical prognostic sig-

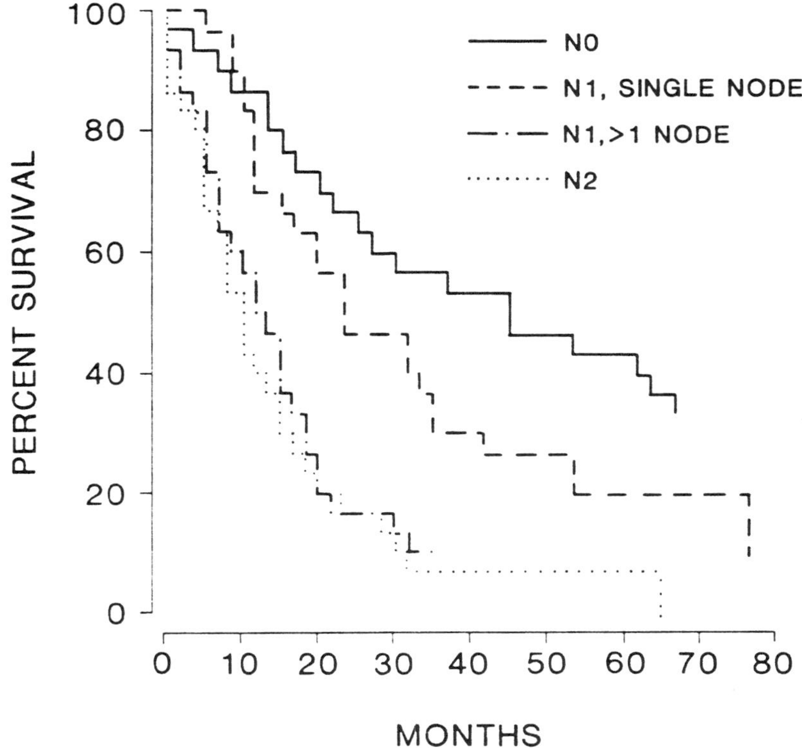

Figure 2: Lymph node status: survival curves for patients with different pN pattern.

Table III
Cox Model: Stage Grouping Obtained by Combining pT, pN, Site, and Number of Metastatic Nodes

Stage pTN1:	pT 1, 2, 3 without lymph node metastasis
Stage pTN2:	pT 1, 2, 3, 4 with one regional metastatic node and pT 4 without node metastasis
Stage pTN3:	pT 1, 2, 3, 4 with two or more regional metastatic nodes or with metastases to distant abdominal nodes (N2)

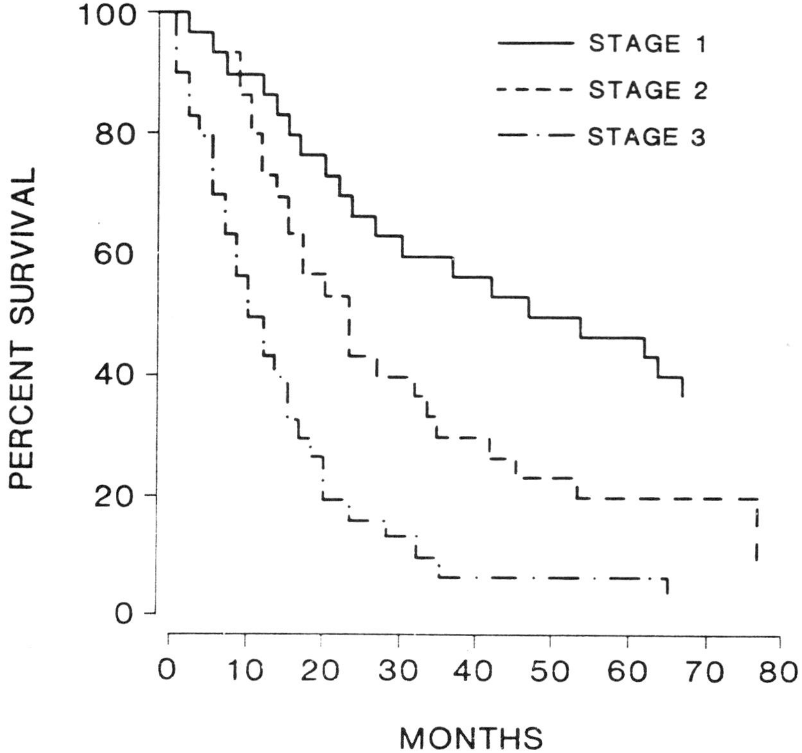

Figure 3: Stage: survival curves.

nificance of the site of the tumor. Figures 4–6 show the estimated survival function (Cox model) combining tumor state and tumor site. The result of this statistic model leads to nine numbers that are referred to as risk values, one for each subgroup of patients. These risk values can be applied to the overall survival curve of the population of this study to predict survival of patients belonging to each of the nine subgroups. The risk values are tabulated in Figures 4–6.

Discussion

Different studies have shown that the prognostic value of the pathological classifications currently used for esophageal cancer is

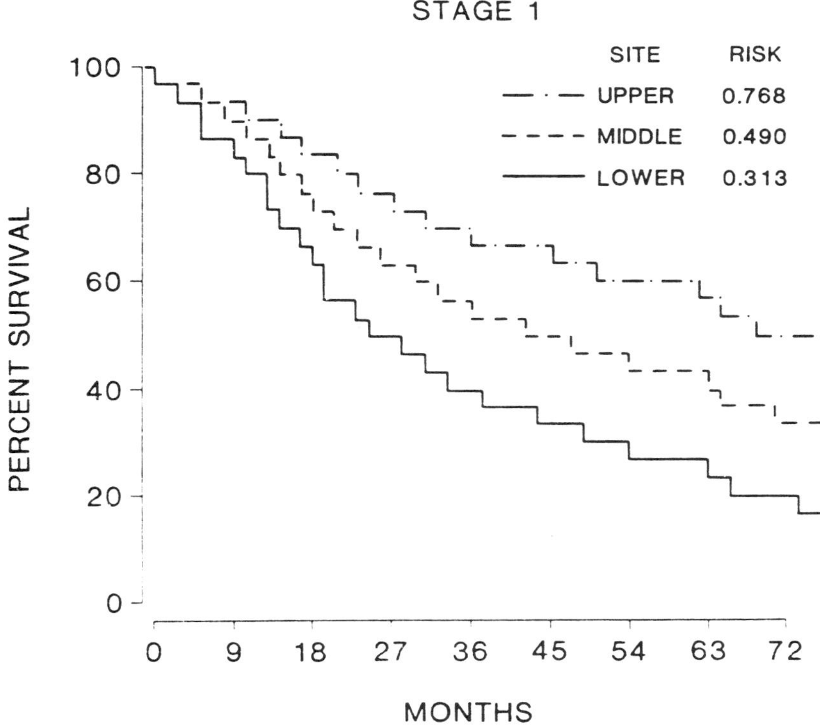

Figure 4: Cox model: survival curves for stage 1 patients.

only approximate. Pathological staging of esophageal cancer was an important topic of discussion during the Third World Congress of the ISDE in 1986 and, in 1988, a meeting on the TNM classification of esophageal carcinoma was held in Tokyo by the Research Committee of the ISDE. The modified TNM classification, which was published in 1987,[4] is an important contribution to the staging of esophageal cancer. Regarding postoperative staging, much more importance was given to the lymph nodal status.

In previous studies, we stressed the importance of lymph nodal status and site of cancer.[5] The present study was designed to further delineate the usefulness of these data. We tried to include macroscopic elements as well as more detailed histologic data. The multivariate analysis showed that depth of wall penetration (pT), nodal status (pN), and site of cancer are significant prognostic factors.

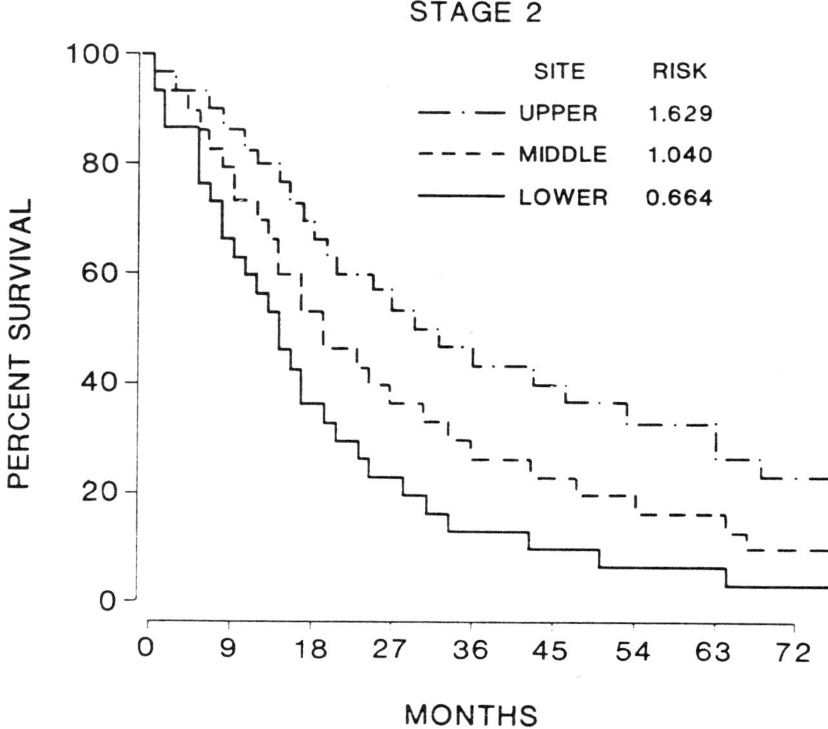

Figure 5: Cox model: survival curves for stage 2 patients.

Nodal status, including number and site of metastatic nodes, was the single most important prognostic factor. Our data suggest that the depth of wall penetration and nodal status are not independent prognostic factors, and that a better prognostic prediction can be obtained combining these two factors, referred to here as "pTN stage." Three pTN stages were obtained with a corresponding 5-year survival rate of 46% for stage 1, 18% for stage 2, and 5% for stage 3. The prognostic value of site of cancer has been stressed by the multivariate analysis; the Cox model obtained combining pTN stage and site of cancer together showed the best significant prognostic value in our patients. From this statistical model, a numeric value, which we called risk value, has been obtained for each subgroup of patients.

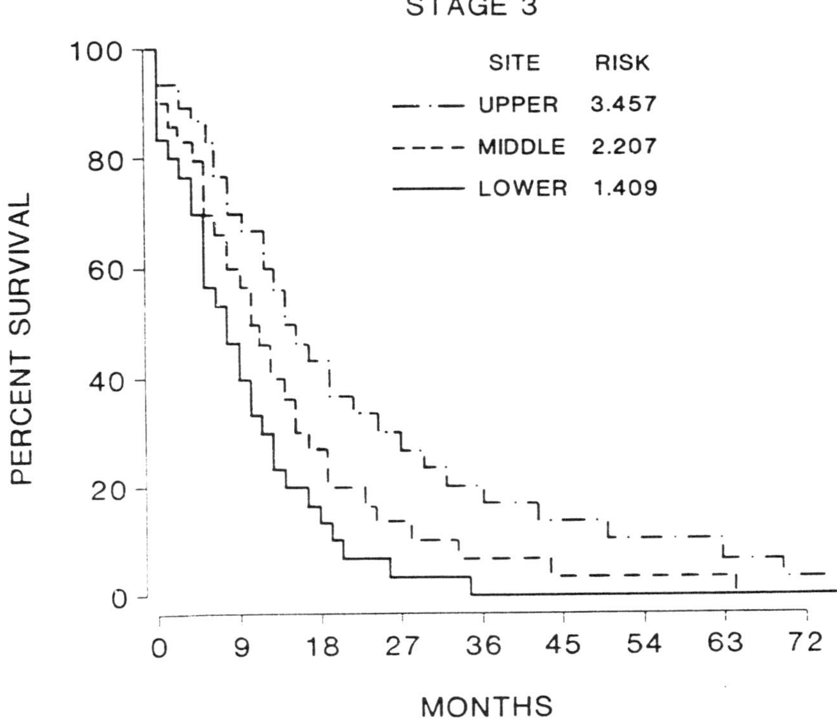

Figure 6: Cox model: survival curves for state 3 patients.

Conclusion

The present study shows that nodal status is the single most important prognostic factor for squamous cell carcinoma of the thoracic esophagus after curative resection. The prognostic value of wall penetration is dependent mainly on lymph node involvement. The site of cancer is a significant prognostic factor.

ACKNOWLEDGMENTS: This study was partially supported by a grant from the AIRC (Associazione Italiana per la Ricerca sul Cancro).

References

1. Richelme H, Baulieux J, eds: Le traitment des cancer de l'oesophage. Paris, Masson, 1986, pp 103–121.

2. Akiyama H, Tsurumaru M, Kawamura T, Ono Y: Principles of surgical treatment for carcinoma of the esophagus. Analysis of lymph node involvement. Ann Surg 194:438, 1981.
3. Skinner DB, Little AG, Ferguson MK, et al: Selection of operation for esophageal carcinoma based on staging. Ann Surg 204:391, 1986.
4. UICC: TNM Classification of Malignant Tumors, 4th edition, Berlin, Springer-Verlag, 1987.
5. Sorrentino P, Ruol A, Castoro C, et al: Prognostic significance of tumor stage and lymph node involvement in thoracic esophageal cancer. In: Diseases of the Esophagus, Siewert JR, Holscher AH (eds), Berlin, Springer-Verlag, 1988, pp 709–713.

26

Barrett's Adenocarcinoma: Long-Term Survival and Recurrence Patterns

Nasser K. Altorki, David B. Skinner, Mark K. Ferguson, Alex G. Little

Introduction

Since Barrett reported his initial observation of a columnar-lined esophagus, the topic remains subject to controversy. Barrett believed the condition to be congenital with an intrathoracic stomach and a congenitally short esophagus.[1] Allison and Johnstone later demonstrated that the columnar-lined structure was in fact esophagus and suggested an acquired etiology for it.[2] A flurry of investigations in the last decade confirmed the association of Barrett's esophagus with severe gastroesophageal reflux;[3] however, unequivocal proof of an acquired or congenital origin remains elusive. The controversy would be of little consequence were it not for the premalignant nature of the abnormal epithelium. Adenocarcinoma arising in ectopic gastric mucosa has been reported as early as 1953 in Europe[4] and 1955 in this country.[5] Adenocarcinoma of the esophagus is now reported with increasing frequency and some surgical series place its incidence at 20–40%.[6–8] This report reviews our experience with Barrett's adenocarcinoma over a 15-year interval.

The definition of Barrett's carcinoma is complicated by the ne-

Ferguson MK, Little AG, Skinner DB: Diseases of the Esophagus, Vol. I: Malignant Diseases. Futura Publishing Company, Inc., Mount Kisco, NY, © 1990.

Table I
Demographics

Number of Patients:	40
Male/female:	38/2
Race:	100% white
Age Range:	38–74
	56 (mean)
	58 (median)

cessity to distinguish it from the routine adenocarcinoma of the cardia. For the purpose of this report, the diagnosis was made when adenocarcinoma arose in association with a columnar-lined esophagus where remnants of the benign columnar epithelium are documented histologically.

Materials

Between 1974 and 1988, 42 patients were referred for the evaluation and treatment of adenocarcinoma arising in association with a columnar-lined esophagus. Two patients had tumors arising in heterotopic columnar epithelium in the cervical esophagus and are not included in this analysis.

There were 38 males and two females ranging in age between 38 and 74 years (mean 56). The median age of 58 years is lower than the median age for patients with squamous cell carcinoma seen in our institutions. All patients were white, in contrast to the overall racial mix for patients with esophageal carcinoma referred to us of whom two-thirds were black. Twenty-two patients were smokers and 23 gave a history of alcohol intake either socially or on a more regular basis. Overall, there were 14 patients (35%) who were both drinkers and smokers (Table I).

Dysphagia (mean duration 80 days) was the main presenting symptom in 34 patients. Six patients had no dysphagia at presentation, all of whom had early lesions, four of which were detected by a Barrett's surveillance program. Twenty-five patients (62%) had longstanding history of heartburn. Fourteen had hiatal hernias demonstrated by gastrointestinal barium studies. Endoscopy was performed in all patients. Endoscopically, tumors were located between 26 and 31 cm from the incisors in nine patients and at 31–34 cm in six. Twenty-

Table II
Treatment

Inoperable:	5
Esophagectomy:	35
En bloc	24
Standard	10
Transhiatal	1

five patients had their tumors located at 35–40 cm from the incisors. The diagnosis was established by endoscopic biopsy in all patients. Twenty-five patients underwent endoscopic direct brush cytology with three false-negative interpretations. Computed tomography (CT) of the chest and upper abdomen was utilized in clinical staging in the latter period of the study and was thus performed in 24 patients. Attempts at clinical staging were guided by the WNM staging system previously evaluated and published.[9] CT accurately predicted wall penetration in 75% of patients but was not sensitive in predicting nodal involvement, being accurate in only 57% of patients.

Results

Six patients had metastatic disease at time of presentation. One patient who had a palliative resection had an isolated metastatic lesion in his left adrenal gland and survived for 11 months postoperatively. A total of 35 patients underwent esophagectomy employing the en-bloc technique in 24, a standard transthoracic resection in 10, and a transhiatal approach in one. The operation was performed through a right thoracotomy in eight patients while a left thoracotomy was employed in 26 (Table II).

There were four hospital deaths for an operative mortality of 11% (Table III). Two patients died from a perioperative myocardial infarction, one from pneumonia and one from a pulmonary embolus. All hospital deaths occurred during the first phase of the study between 1974 and 1981. With advances in intraoperative and postoperative monitoring techniques there have been no hospital deaths in 20 patients operated on since 1982.

Complications occurred in 17 patients for a 48% morbidity incidence (Table IV). Cardiopulmonary complications were seen in six

Table III
Hospital Mortality
4/35 (11%)

Myocardial infarction	2
Pneumonia	1
Pulmonary embolus	1
A. 1974–1981	4/15
B. 1982–1988	0/20

patients. Lobar collapse occurred in one patient, while delayed pulmonary embolus occurred following discharge in another. Atrial fibrillation requiring treatment was seen in two patients, congestive heart failure in one, and a nonfatal subendocardial infarction in one. Anastomotic leaks occurred in two patients (6%). One leak occurred following intrathoracic esophagocolostomy and the other occurred after cervical esophagogastrostomy. Both healed uneventfully with drainage and nutritional support. Necrosis of the tip of the gastric tube occurred in two patients in both of whom barium studies demonstrated an intact anastomosis with contrast extravasation at the tip of the gastric tube. Both healed with drainage. Prolonged chest tube drainage was required in five patients. Chylothorax developed in one patient after transhiatal esophagectomy and required insertion of a pleuroperitoneal shunt.

Final staging was based on pathological examination of the resected specimen for extent of wall penetration (W), as well as nodal involvement by malignant disease (N) (Table V).[9] The degree of wall penetration was classified into three categories: W0 for tumors con-

Table IV
Morbidity
17/35 (48%)

Cardiopulmonary		*Other*	
Lobar collapse	1	Anastomotic leaks	2
Delayed PE	1	Gastric tip necrosis	2
Atrial fibrillation	2	Wound infection	1
CHF	1	Prolonged CT drainage	5
Nonfatal MI	1	Chylothorax	1

Table V
Pathological Staging

WNM	*TNM*	*N*
W0N0	T1N0	4
W1N0	T2N0	2
W1N1	T2N1	1
W2N0	T3N0	3
W2N1	T3N1	9
W1–W2/N2	T2N1/T3N1	16
M1	—	5
TOTAL		40

fined to the mucosa or submucosa, W1 for tumors with less than full wall penetration, and W2 for tumors extending through the full thickness of the muscularis propria. The degree of nodal involvement was also classified into three categories: NO for no nodal involvement, N1 where there were four or fewer nodes involved with tumor, and N2 for involvement in five or more nodes. The final staging for all patients is shown in Table III as well as their corresponding stage by the modified current TNM system.[10]

Survival

Among 31 patients surviving esophagectomy, nine (25%) are alive, of whom seven have no evidence of disease with a mean and median follow-up of 3.5 and 3 years, respectively. One patient died 6 years postoperatively from unrelated causes. Two are alive with known recurrence 1 and 3 years following esophagectomy. Of the remaining 26 patients, 23 died with metastatic disease including five unresected patients, two died from chemotherapy-related complications, and the last patient died from massive gastrointestinal hemorrhage 2 months postoperatively (Table VI). Predictably, staging was the most important determinant of survival (Table VII). Among seven patients alive with no evident disease (NED), four had early lesions confined to the mucosa or submucosa, or partially penetrating the wall of the esophagus with negative nodes. All were patients who had their tumors detected by a Barrett's surveillance program. One patient with WINI is alive with no evidence of disease 1 year post-

Table VI
Overall Survival

Alive NED to date	7
Alive with disease	2
Dead NED at 6 years	1
Operative mortality	4
Chemotherapy-related death	2
Sudden death at 2 mos	1
Death with metastatic disease	23
TOTAL	40

NED = no evidence of disease

operatively and one with W2N0 had no recurrent disease at 2 years. For all unresected patients, the mean survival was only 3 months.

Recurrence

Recurrence patterns among 20 patients surviving esophagectomy are shown in Table VIII. Distant metastases occurred in 19 patients with no predilection for a specific site. Among 31 patients surviving esophagectomy, three had anastomotic or mediastinal recurrences. One patient developed a mediastinal recurrence 3 years following standard transthoracic esophagectomy. Two other patients developed both local and distant recurrences. Anastomotic recurrence occurred in one patient while recurrence occurred in the mediastinum in the other. The mean and median time to recurrence were 6 and 8 months, respectively.

Table VII
Survival

WNM	*TNM*	*Alive NED*	*Total*
W0/N0	I	3	4
W1N0	IIA	1	2
W1N1	IIB	1	3
W2N1	III	1	9

Four detected by Barrett's surveillance regimen.
NED = no evidence of disease

Table VIII
Recurrence Patterns

Local (mediastinal/anastomotic)			3
Distant metastases			19
Neck nodes	4	Skin	2
Bone	4	Liver	2
Lungs	3	Pericardium	1
Abdominal nodes	2	Unspecified	1
Brain	1		

Time to recurrence: Mean = 6 months
Median = 6 months

Discussion

The controversies surrounding the columnar-lined esophagus are no less today than when the condition was initially observed more than 30 years ago. Circumstantial evidence abounds on either side of the etiological fence to suggest an acquired or congenital origin. Regardless of its pathogenesis, columnar epithelium lining the tubular esophagus is now widely regarded as premalignant. Among the various recognized types of columnar lining identified in the esophagus, the specialized intestinal type has been most frequently associated with carcinoma.[11]

The prevalence of carcinoma arising in this metaplastic (or congenital) lining has ranged between 8% and 46% in various reports,[11–13] perhaps reflecting the nature of referral patterns rather than true prevalence. Figures reflecting actual incidence have been recently put forth by several investigators. Cameron and colleagues found an incidence of one in 400 patient years of follow-up[14] while Spechler et al. reported an incidence of one in 175 patient years of follow-up.[15] These studies may underestimate the true incidence as the mean follow-up of 3 to 3.5 years in these studies is a relatively short time in the biological life cycle of neoplasia. Nevertheless, the incidence based on these data is about 30–40-fold higher than the incidence of esophageal carcinoma in the general population. Translated into number of new cases per 100,000, it calculates to 500 new cases per year. The actual incidence of Barrett's adenocarcinoma therefore remains an unanswered question. Confounding the matter even further is the belief by at least some that most adenocarcinomas of the esophagus, including those arising in the sphincter region, may represent Barrett's adenocarcinoma in which all remnants of the Barrett's columnar lining has been replaced by tumor. Among cases referred to us for esophageal carcinoma, the incidence of Barrett's adenocarcinoma has remained a steady 20–25% over the last decade.

In this chapter, we reviewed our experience with these tumors in which remnants of the columnar lining could be identified either postresection or endoscopically in the case of unresected cases. The demographic features of these patients have been pointed out previously. The lower mean age in comparison to squamous cell tumors of the esophagus, the marked male predominance, and the exclusive occurrence in white patients is striking and intriguing. A long-standing history of heartburn was present in two-thirds of patients and is in keeping with previously published observations.[11] The role of smoking and alcohol ingestion as potential promoters of carcinogenesis is again suggested by the fact that one-third of the entire group were both drinkers and smokers.

Among the 40 patients reviewed, 37 were explored and 35 were successfully resected. The resectability rate of 95% for those explored and 88% for the whole group is among the highest reported.[6] Obviously, in evaluating these results, a certain degree of pre-referral selection bias cannot be excluded. Patients were not considered candidates for resection in the presence of documented metastatic disease and this is supported by the short mean survival of that group. Interestingly enough, one patient with an isolated adrenal metastasis underwent a palliative resection and survived for 11 months postoperatively.

The hospital mortality of 11% for the entire group was related to postoperative cardiopulmonary complications. The strides achieved in critical care over the last decade have had a tremendous impact on the hospital mortality for esophagectomy. We are gratified by the fact that there were no deaths among 20 resected patients operated on since 1982. However, esophagectomy continues to be an operation associated with a significant morbidity. Eleven patients (31%) developed major complications, the majority of which were cardiopulmonary. Minor complications occurred in another six patients.

The compelling influence of staging on survival is evident. Among five patients with W1-W0/N0 surviving the operation, four are long-term survivors with no recurrences and the fifth died of unrelated causes 6 years postoperatively. On the contrary, among 16 patients with five or more nodes involved with carcinoma, only one is alive. The salutary effect of surgery is difficult to evaluate in this small group of patients. However, an interesting observation is the disease-free interval observed in each stage following esophagectomy. While the mean disease-free interval for W2N1 was 465 days, recurrences occurred after a mean of 125 days in patients with N2 disease. In most patients, recurrence occurred at distant sites. There appears to be no particular predilection for a specific organ site with metastases occurring randomly in all sites.

Of nine operative survivors, seven are free of disease at a mean follow-up period of 3.5 years and a median interval of 3 years. Four of those patients were detected by a Barrett's surveillance program and offer a strong argument for the use of endoscopic or cytologic surveillance of all patients with Barrett's esophagus.

Among 18 patients operated on more than 5 years ago by the en-bloc technique, three survived 5 years with no evidence of disease for an absolute survival, a figure similar to that reported by Logan in 1963 among 250 patients operated on by the same technique for cancer of the cardia. The adoption of Logan's operation at that time was precluded by a high operative mortality.

Summary

Barrett's adenocarcinoma is being recognized with increasing frequency and generally has a poor prognosis. About 50% of patients in our study had unfavorable disease in the form of distant metastases or extensive nodal involvement (N2) at time of diagnosis. However, palliation could be achieved in the great majority of patients (95%) by esophagectomy. The procedure can now be performed with a reasonable mortality and acceptable morbidity. The hope for cure lies foremost in early detection of tumors at which point a truly curative resection could be done. A small group of patients with more advanced loco-regional disease could still be salvaged by en-bloc resection.

References

1. Barrett NR: Chronic peptic ulcer of the oesophagus and gastroesophagitis. Br J Surg 38:175, 1950.
2. Allison PR, Johnstone AS: The oesophagus lined with gastric mucous membrane. Thorax 8:87, 1953.

3. Iascone C, DeMeester TR, Little AG, Skinner DB: Barrett's esophagus. Arch Surg 118:543, 1983.
4. Morson BC, Belcher JR: Adenocarcinoma of the esophagus and ectopic gastric mucosa. Br J Cancer 6:127, 1953.
5. McCorkle RG, Blades B: Adenocarcinoma of the esophagus arising in aberrant gastric mucosa. Am J Surg 21:781, 1955.
6. Ellis FH, Gibb SP, Watkins E: Esophagogastrectomy: A safe, widely applicable, and expeditious form of palliation for patients with carcinoma of the esophagus and cardia. Ann Surg 198:531, 1983.
7. Skinner DB: En bloc resection for neoplasms of the esophagus and cardia. J Thorac Cardiovasc Surg 85:59, 1983.
8. Galanduik S, Hermann RE, Gassman JJ, Cosgrove DM: Cancer of the esophagus: The Cleveland Clinic experience. Ann Surg 203:101, 1986.
9. Skinner DB, Dowlatshahi KD, DeMeester TR: Potentially curable cancer of the esophagus. Cancer 50:2571, 1982.
10. Hermanek P, Sobin (eds): TNM Classification of Malignant Tumors, New York, Springer-Verlag, 1987 pp 40–42.
11. Skinner DB, Walther BC, Riddell RH, Schmidt H, et al: Barrett's esophagus: Comparison of benign and malignant cases. Ann Surg 198:554, 1983.
12. Naef AP, Savary M, Ozzello L, Pearson FG: Columnar-lined lower esophagus. Surgery 70:826, 1975.
13. Radigan LR, Glover JL, Shipley FE, Shoemaker RE: Barrett's esophagus. Arch Surg 112:486, 1977.
14. Cameron AJ, Ott BJ, Payne WS: The incidence of adenocarcinoma in columnar-lined (Barrett's) esophagus. N Engl J Med 313:857, 1985.
15. Spechler SJ, Robbins AH, Rubins HB et al: Adenocarcinoma and Barrett's esophagus: An overrated risk? Gastroenterology 87:927, 1984.

27

Esophagectomy for Carcinoma:
Cervical or Thoracic Anastomosis

Vincent Chasseray, G.K. Kiroff, J.L. Buard, Bernard Launois

Introduction

Carcinoma of the esophagus remains a surgical challenge with esophagectomy having high morbidity and mortality. A previous review of the results from our digestive surgical unit in Rennes has confirmed that much of this mortality is caused by leakage from intrathoracic anastomoses. In contrast, in our early experience with the Akiyama operation, we had only one death for 27 patients treated. These two factors, combined with the theoretical advantage of improved tumor clearance following cervical anastomosis, encouraged us to compare cervical and thoracic anastomoses for squamous cell carcinoma of the lower two-thirds of the esophagus. We were especially interested in three factors: (1) the incidence of anastomotic dehiscence; (2) operative mortality; and (3) long-term survival for the two groups.

Methods

Over a 4-year period (May 1982–December 1986), all patients who presented with squamous cell carcinoma of the middle or lower third

Ferguson MK, Little AG, Skinner DB: Diseases of the Esophagus, Vol. I: Malignant Diseases. Futura Publishing Company, Inc., Mount Kisco, NY, © 1990.

Table I
Preoperative Characteristics

	Cervical Anastomosis	*Thoracic Anastomosis*	
Smokes	42 (98%)	42 (86%)	(ns)
Pack Years	30 (0–98%)	19 (0–60%)	(ns)
Bronchitis	12 (29%)	11 (22%)	(ns)
Alcohol Use	42 (98%)	43 (88%)	(ns)
Weight Loss (%)	5.6% (0–20%)	3.9% (0–21%)	(ns)
Albumin (mg %)	43.3 (33–48.1%)	43.3 (33–47.1%)	(ns)
Vital Capacity	+8% (−48% to +53%)	+8% (−28% to +62%)	(ns)
FEV1	+7% (−57% to +80%)	+5% (−42% to +54%)	(ns)
Age	59 (41–73)	59 (47–75)	(ns)

Weight loss is expressed as a percentage of the pre-morbid weight. Vital capacity and forced expiratory volume, 1 second (FEV1) are expressed as a percentage of normal (+ or −) age and weight corrected.

of the esophagus and who where considered operable on clinical grounds were randomized to receive either cervical or thoracic anastomosis. Cervical anastomoses were performed either by MacKeown's technique resulting in an orthotopic gastroplasty or by Akiyama's method with retrosternal gastroplasty. Thoracic anastomoses were carried out by a midline laparotomy and right thoracotomy with an anastomosis at the apex of the right thorax. We preferred stapled anastomoses in both groups.

Thirty-one patients were subsequently excluded either because of the patient's medical condition, nonresectability of the tumor, or because macroscopic disease was left behind in the posterior mediastinum in one patient allocated to the thoracic anastomosis group. The remaining 92 patients had a median age of 59 years. Forty-nine were randomized to thoracic and 43 to cervical anastomoses. Of these, eight were performed by Akiyama's method and 35 by a modified MacKeown's technique.

The two patient groups were comparable with respect to major preoperative risks factors. Thus, smoking, pre-existing lung disease, pulmonary function, alcohol consumption, weight loss, nutrition, and age were similar in the two groups (Table I). Tumor level was also similar, with the median superior tumor margin at 30 cm for the thoracic anastomosis group and 28.5 cm for the cervical anastomosis group. All patients underwent the same routine preoperative assessment including hematology, biochemistry, chest radiology, pulmonary function testing, endoscopy and biopsy of the tumor, and bronchoscopy.

The operative technique was standardized as far as gastroplasty and gastric mobilization were concerned. The stomach was completely mobilized outside of the gastroepiploic arcade, the left gastric artery was divided close to its origin, and the duodenum was extensively mobilized. We routinely fashioned a tubed gastroplasty by serial application of GIA™ staples (USSC) parallel to the greater curvature and we then oversewed this staple line; the important lymph node-bearing area related to the cardia and lesser curvature was removed (Fig. 1).

Results

The two groups were similar with respect to the extent of disease. Thus, 43% of patients receiving thoracic anastomoses had lymph node metastases, of which four were mediastinal only, while the remaining 17 were intra-abdominal. Nearly 49% of the cervical anastomosis patients had involved nodes, seven were mediastinal only, while the remaining 14 were intra-abdominal. The resected specimens were all examined by an independent pathologist for measurement of the tumor-free superior margin. These measurements were performed on the fresh specimen and did not include the 2 or 3 cm of esophagus lost by our technique of performing a stapled anastomosis without a pursestring suture. Nevertheless, the patients receiving cervical anastomoses had a significantly greater superior tumor clearance (Fig. 2).

One of the most serious complications following esophagectomy is leakage from the anastomosis. Anastomotic fistula was significantly more common following cervical anastomoses. Although respiratory complications were more common following intrathoracic anastomosis, this difference was not significant. Other complications occurred with a similar frequency (Table II.) Mortality at 30 days for the two groups was similar: seven thoracic anastomosis patients died compared to four cervical anastomosis patients. It should be noted that two of these cervical anastomosis deaths were the result of mediastinitis following a leak from the anastomosis.

Complete follow-up is available on these 92 patients for a median of 30 months. There has been no recurrent dysphagia due to malignancy. However, 15% of the thoracic anastomosis and 23% of the

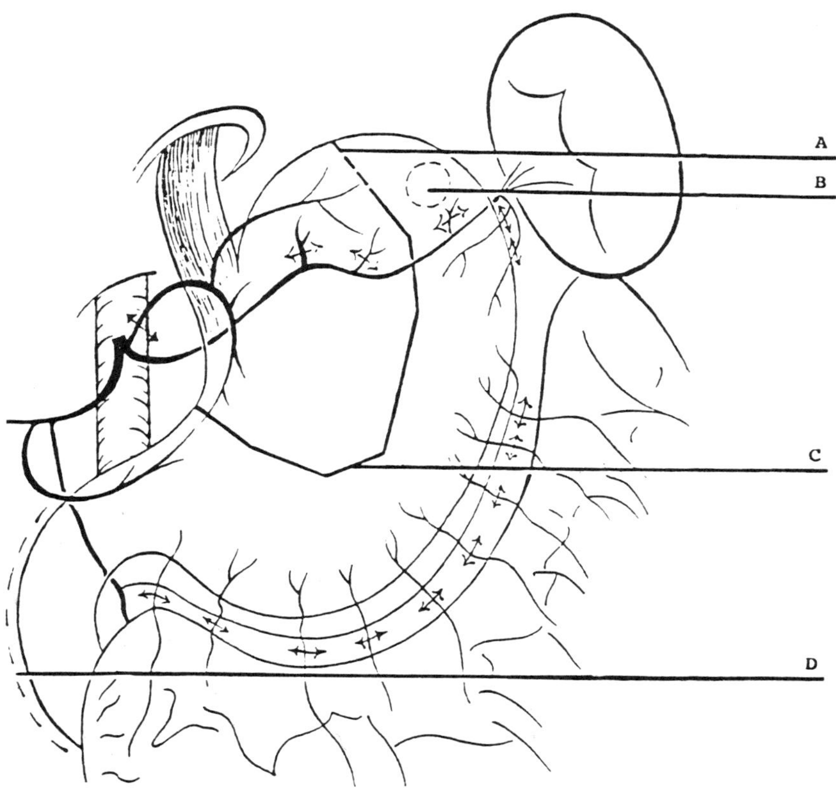

Figure 1: A standardized gastroplasty was used to replace the esophagus. A = line of eventual section with TA 55[R] (USSC), B = site of stapled anastomosis on the posterior wall, C = line of section with GIA ™ (USSC), D = mobilization of the duodenum.

cervical anastomosis patients had some degree of benign stricture requiring at least one dilation. The overall median survival for all patients combined is 22 months, with a 2-year survival rate of 46.6% and 30% at 40 months. The median survival time was similar for the two groups. For the cervical anastomosis group, the median survival time was 23 months (range 1–52 months), and for the thoracic anastomotic group, it was 20 months (range 1–48 months). The similar survival patterns are illustrated in Figure 3. Despite the superior

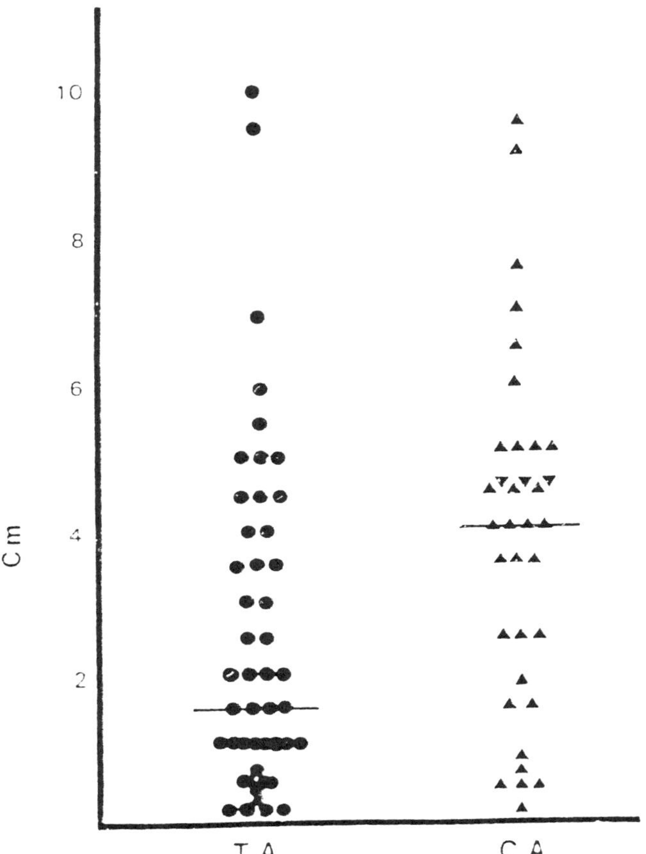

Figure 2: Length of esophagus macroscopically free of tumor above the upper limit of the lesion. TA = group treated with thoracic anastomosis, CA = group treated with cervical anastomosis.

tumor clearance achieved by cervical anastomosis, long-term results are the same.

Instead, survival is highly dependent on the stage of the disease. If patients from both groups were combined, those with carcinomas confined to the mucosa and submucosa (11 patients) had a 24-month survival rate of 90%; those with penetration of the esophageal wall without invasion of a neighboring structure or involvement of lymph nodes (28 patients) had a lower 24-month survival rate of 60%. In-

Table II
Significant Complications

	Cervical Anastomosis	*Thoracic Anastomosis*	
Anastomotic Leak	11 (26%)	2 (4%)	($p < 0.02$)
Respiratory	8 (16%)	14 (29%)	(ns)
Chylothorax	2 (5%)	4 (8%)	(ns)
Other	6 (14%)	6 (12%)	(ns)

Overall 41 patients (44%) sustained one or more serious complications.

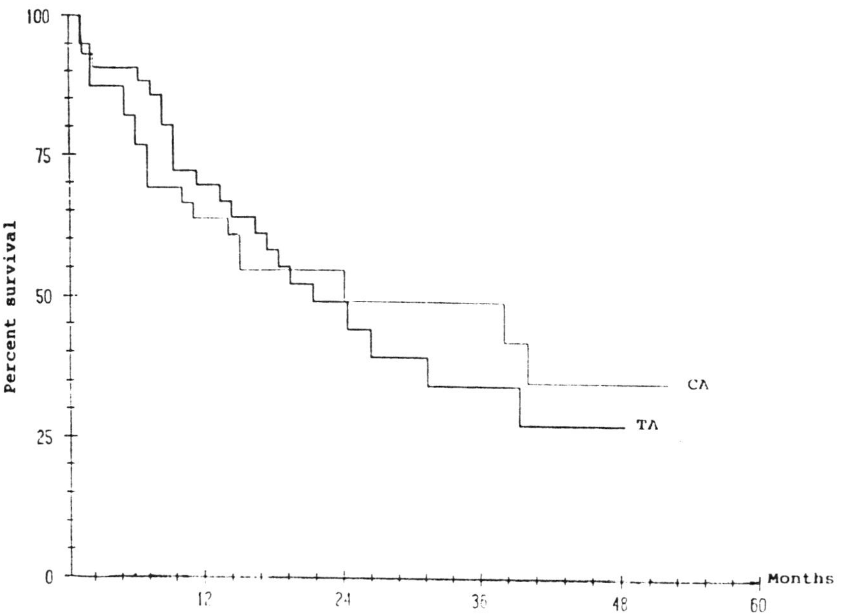

Figure 3: There was no significant difference in the length of survival time between patients treated by laparotomy and right thoracotomy (TA) and those treated by laparotomy, right thoracotomy, and cervicotomy (CA).

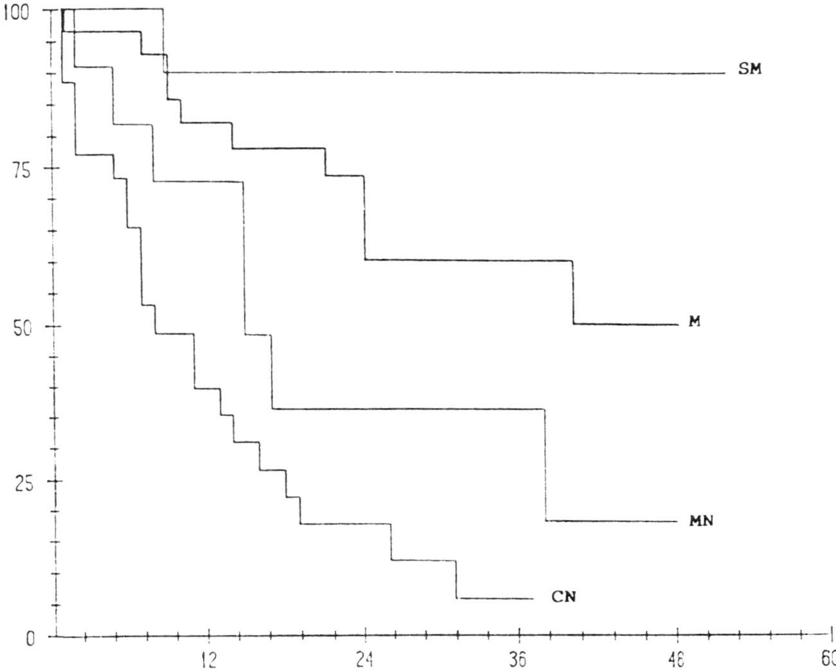

Figure 4: Survival rate is related to the extent of the disease. SM = tumor confined to the mucosa and submucosa only, M = tumor involving the muscularis but without lymph node involvement or extension to adjacent structure, MN = involvement of mediastinal nodes only, CN = involvement of intra-abdominal nodes.

volvement of mediastinal nodes (11 patients) was associated with a 24-month survival rate of 37%, whereas invasion of the celiac or lesser curvature nodes (26 patients) resulted in a lower rate of 18%, as illustrated in Figure 4.

Summary

Anastomic leak is significantly more common following cervical anastomosis. The incidence of other complications is similar and there is no significant difference in the early mortality. In this series, we observed no recurrent dysphagia due to malignancy in either group, although benign stricture is common regardless of the anastomotic site chosen. Survival was independent of the level of the anastomosis despite the increased length of esophagus resected with a cervical anastomosis, but was highly dependent on the extent of the disease. We conclude that there is no advantage in a cervical anastomosis for the majority of squamous cell carcinoma of the inferior two-thirds of the esophagus; in fact, there may be a disadvantage because of the high incidence of cervical fistula.

28

Two-Stage Esophagogastrostomy for Esophageal Reconstruction

Kin-ichi Nabeya, Tateo Hanaoka, Kimio Onozawa, Tetsuya Nyumura, Osamu Kimura, Chou-o Kaku

Introduction

In recent years, with improvements in nutritional control,[1] esophageal cancer operations have become much safer than in the past years. However, with the rising trend of elderly and poor risk cases, patient selection and postoperative management are still of great consequence.[2,3] In this study, the Doppler blood flow meter[4] was utilized to measure the hemodynamic state of the reconstructive gastric tube, and anastomotic leaks and pulmonary complications were compared in patients undergoing one-stage and two-stage anastomoses.

Materials and Methods

One hundred six patients underwent resection for esophageal cancer, in whom a one-stage anastomosis was made in 52 cases and a two-stage anastomosis was made in 54 cases. A two-stage anastomosis is a method in which the first stage of the procedure consists

Ferguson MK, Little AG, Skinner DB: Diseases of the Esophagus, Vol. I: Malignant Diseases. Futura Publishing Company, Inc., Mount Kisco, NY, © 1990.

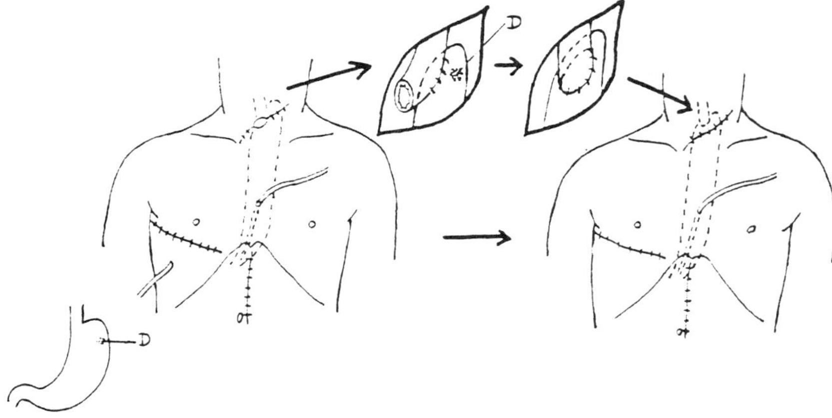

Figure 1: Two-stage esophagogastrostomy. D = anastomotic point blood flow measured by Doppler method.

of a right thoracotomy and esophagectomy. A gastric tube is made and raised to the neck by an antethoracic or retrosternal route and is fixed only to the esophageal posterior wall with four stitches. After approximately 3 weeks, as a second-stage procedure, the remnant of the esophageal stump is resected and the anastomosis is completed (Fig. 1). During this procedure, the Doppler blood flow meter was used to measure blood flow of the estimated anastomotic point in the reconstructive gastric tube. The Doppler blood flow meter consists of the MUV2100 and pencil-type probe of Nippon Koden Co., Ltd. and the recorder of San-ei Surgical Monitor Type 123. The postoperative complications, leakages, and pulmonary complications were compared in the one-stage and two-stage anastomosis groups. Statistical analysis was performed using the chi-squared and Student's *t*-tests.

Results

In 52 cases of one-stage anastomosis, the rate of blood flow at the estimated anastomotic point in the gastric tube was measured. The blood flow at the time of laparotomy was 360 ± 60 Hz with the Doppler blood flow meter. Assuming this as standard, the blood flow at the time of completion of the gastric tube dropped 29%, and at the time of anastomosis completion, this decreased by a total of 38%.

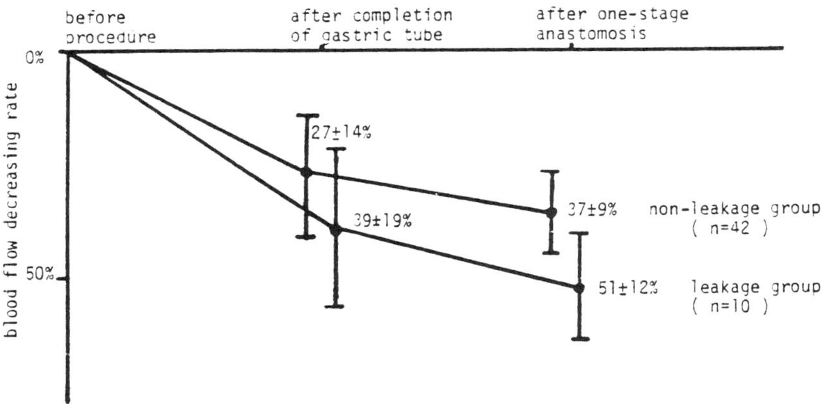

Figure 2: Changes of blood flow at anastomotic point of gastric tube (comparative study on leakage and nonleakage groups).

The 52 cases were divided into nonleakage and leakage groups, 42 cases and 10 cases, respectively, and comparisons were made. After completion of the gastric tube, the rate of blood flow in the nonleakage group dropped 37% ± 14%, while after anastomosis, it decreased by a total of 27% ± 9%. However, in the leakage group, the rate of blood flow after completion of the gastric tube decreased by 39% ± 19%, while after anastomosis the total decrease was 51% ± 12% ($p<0.05$) (Fig. 2). In tubes made from the entire stomach, blood flow dropped 29% ± 18%; in gastric tubes formed from the greater curvature, flow decreased by 33% ± 18% (no difference). Placing the reconstruction tube through an antesternal route resulted in a flow decrease of 15% ± 11% while through the retrosternal route this decrease was 12% ± 8% (no difference).

A comparison of blood flow in the gastric tube was made between the first operation and the second operation for 12 patients who had the two-stage operation. In comparison with the blood flow at completion of the first operation, the blood flow during the second operation, esophagogastrostomy, increased an average of 54% ± 25% (Fig. 3).

The 52 cases of one-stage anastomosis and 54 cases of two-stage anastomosis were compared for incidence of major leaks, those necessitating resuture or tube insertion, and minor leaks that healed spontaneously. The rate of anastomotic leakage in the one-stage an-

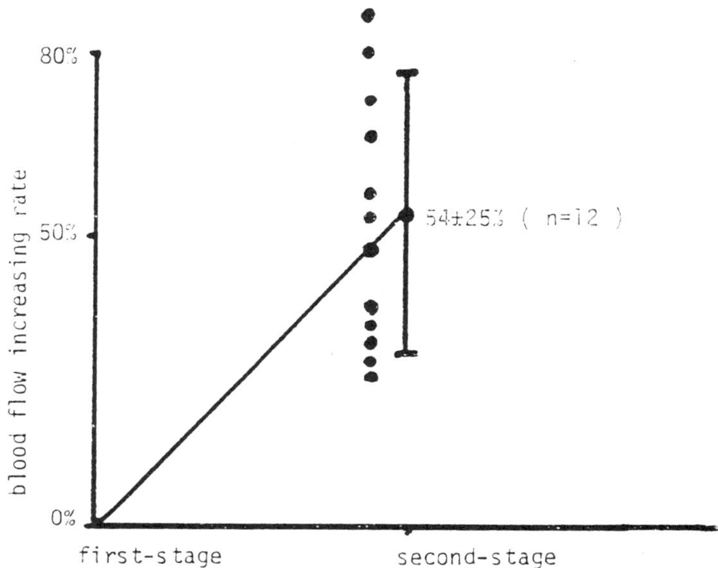

Figure 3: Increasing rate of blood flow at anastomotic point of gastric tube in two-stage esophagogastrostomy. Duration interval was 22 ± 5 days.

astomosis group was 19.2% versus 9.2% in the two-stage anastomosis group (Table I).

Pulmonary complications requiring tracheotomy and long-term respiratory control were classified as major. In the one-stage anastomosis group the incidence was 32.6%, while in the two-stage an-

Table I
Anastomotic Leakages in One-Stage and Two-Stage Esophagogastrostomy at the Neck

		Leakage		
	Cases	*Major*	*Minor*	*Total*
One-stage anastomosis	52	6 (3)	4	10 19.2%
Two-stage anastomosis	54	2 (1)	3	5 9.2%

( ) = operative death

Table II
Postoperative Pulmonary Complications in One-Stage and Two-Stage Esophagogastrostomy at the Neck

		Pulmonary Complications		
	Cases	*Major*	*Minor*	*Total*
One-stage anastomosis	52	8 (3)	6	14 (32.6%)
Two-stage anastomosis	54	3 (1)	5	8 (14.8%)

( ) = operative death

astomosis group this was 14.8% (Table II). Operative deaths numbered three cases in the one-stage group and one in the two-stage group.

Discussion

Generally, management of anastomotic leakages[5] and pulmonary complications[6] is the most difficult part of esophageal cancer surgery. Of all causes of anastomotic leakage, decreased blood flow of the reconstructed organ is the most serious. There are many methods[7] for measuring blood flow in these organs and among them, the Doppler method stands out as a safe and simple one.[4]

With this Doppler blood flow meter, measurements of blood flow of reconstructed gastric tubes after esophagectomy were made. Blood flow at the anastomotic point of the gastric tube decreased considerably with completion of the gastric tube, pulling-up of the gastric tube, and again with the anastomotic procedures. In the one-stage anastomosis, comparisons of nonleakage and leakage groups revealed that the blood flow in the leakage group decreased significantly ($p<0.05$). We believe that anastomotic leakage is more likely to occur in cases in which the blood flow decreased over 50%. On account of these leakages, the two-stage anastomosis was adopted. After a 3-week interval between the one-stage and two-stage procedure, a 54% blood flow increase at the anastomotic point was observed. Further, the gastric tube healed to the surrounding tissues, so adequate anastomotic orifice could be constructed, making stenoses rare.

The occurrence rate of leakage and pulmonary complications in 52 cases of one-stage and 54 cases of two-stage anastomosis were compared. The two-stage anastomosis was much safer than the one-stage anastomosis. Operative deaths amounted to three in the one-stage group and one in the two-stage group. All cases were advanced cancer and two were palliative resection cases. The main mortality factor was pulmonary complications developing into multiple organ failure.[8]

To solve these difficulties the two-stage anastomosis is recommended as this has merits in operative safety as follows: (1) anastomotic leakage is decreased at the cervical wound which would otherwise develop into a serious complication, (2) reflux of digestive juices is cut off immediately after the operation and aspiration pneumonia is prevented, (3) saliva accumulation is decreased and the oral cavity is kept clean.

The two-stage anastomosis does have the drawbacks of prolonging resumption of oral intake of food and the duration of hospitalization. However, when its advantages are taken into consideration, particularly for the poor risk elderly patients with pulmonary disorders and with diabetes, this two-stage anastomosis is highly indicated.

References

1. Daly JM, Masson E, Ciacco C, et al: Parenteral nutrition in esophageal cancer patients. Ann Surg 196:203, 1982.
2. Sugimachi K, Inokuchi K, Ueno H, et al: Surgical treatment for carcinoma of the esophagus in the elderly patient. Surg Gynecol Obstet 160:317, 1985.
3. Peracchia A, Bardini R, Ruol A, et al: Carcinoma of the esophagus in the elderly (70 years of age or older), indications and results of surgery. Dis Esophagus 1:147, 1988.
4. Wright CB, Hobson RW: Prediction of intestinal viability using Doppler ultrasound technics. Am J Surg 129:642, 1975.
5. Peracchia A, Bardini R, Ruol A, et al: Esophagovisceral anastomotic leak. A prospective statistical study of predisposing factors. J Thorac Cardiovasc Surg 95:685, 1988.
6. Sugimachi K, Ueno H, Natsuda Y, et al: Cough dynamics in esophageal cancer: Prevention of postoperative pulmonary complications. Br J Surg 69:734, 1982.
7. Zarins CK, Skinner DB, Rhodes BA, et al: Prediction of the viability of revascularized intestine with radioactive microspheres. Surg Gynecol Obstet 138:576, 1974.
8. Eiseman B, Beart R, Norton L: Multiple organ failure. Surg Gynecol Obstet 144:323, 1977.

29

En Bloc Esophagectomy: When to Reconstruct the Food Passage?

Jörg Rüdiger Siewert, Holger Bartels, Jochen Lange, Jürgen D. Roder, Arnulf H. Hölscher

Introduction

Postoperative mortality after esophagectomy still is an essential factor contributing to the bad prognosis of esophageal cancer. Attempts to reduce this mortality have included limited transmediastinal surgery, preoperative parenteral nutrition, or standardization of reconstruction. Our own efforts in this context have included a two-staged operation, meaning a temporal interruption between esophageal resection and reconstruction of the upper GI tract (48–72 hours). This concept is based on an analysis of postoperative respiratory function following esophagectomy.[1] As the results of a pilot study were promising, we performed a prospective randomized controlled study to investigate this therapeutic concept.

Patients and Methods

The study was performed between October 1, 1986 and December 31, 1988. Criteria for transthoracic esophagectomy[2] included tumor localization (intrathoracic esophagus) or tumor type (all intrathoracic squamous cell carcinomas; adenocarcinoma in the middle third of the esophagus). Patients who had preoperative radio- and/or chemo-

Ferguson MK, Little AG, Skinner DB: Diseases of the Esophagus, Vol. I: Malignant Diseases. Futura Publishing Company, Inc., Mount Kisco, NY, © 1990.

therapy were excluded. The indications for preoperative radio-chemotherapy were tumors above the tracheal bifurcation which seemed not completely resectable (R_0) on the basis of preoperative staging or esophageal carcinomas below the bifurcation with distant metastases (M_+ according to UICC 1987).[3] Patients with an indication for transmediastinal esophagectomy because of tumor type and tumor localization (all adenocarcinomas of the distal esophagus, small very distally localized squamous cell carcinomas) were not included in the study. However, this group (group III) was prospectively documented and evaluated in comparison to the other study patients.

After the patients gave their informed consent, they were preoperatively randomized to one of the two therapeutic procedures: direct reconstruction (group I) or reconstruction with delayed urgency after 48–72 hours (group II).

In all cases, a so-called en bloc resection of the esophagus was performed; together with the esophagus, all the mediastinal lymph and fatty tissue including the azygos vein and the thoracic duct were resected.[2] The reconstruction was usually done by an interposition of a gastric tube formed from the greater curvature.[4,5] In selected cases, the transverse colon together with the splenic flexure vascularized by the left colic artery was interposed. After achievement of a complete tumor resection (so-called R_0-resection), the reconstruction was performed in the posterior mediastinum, whereas in advanced tumors or when there was a suspicion of incomplete local resectability (R_1- or R_2-resection), a retrosternal route in the anterior mediastinum was used. Transmediastinal esophagectomy was done from the cervical region and through the hiatus using a technique described elsewhere.[6] In these cases the reconstruction was done according to the same principles as after transthoracic esophagectomy.

The criteria for the evaluation of the different procedures' postoperative course (respiratory function, complications, and postoperative mortality) were recorded prospectively and analyzed after finishing the study.

Results

Between October 1, 1986 and December 31, 1988, 137 patients underwent esophagectomy. Group I (en bloc esophagectomy with direct reconstruction) included 26 patients. Group II (transthoracic en bloc resection + reconstruction with delayed urgency after 48–72

Table I
Personal Data, Risk Estimation and Tumor Stages of the 95 Patients Esophagectomized During the Time Period of the Study

	Transthoracic Esophagectomy		*Transmediastinal Esophagectomy*	
	Direct Reconstruction (Group I)	*Reconstruction After 48–72 Hrs. (Group II)*	*Direct Reconstruction (Group III)*	*Patients Total*
Patients (n)	26	24	45	95
Age ($\bar{x}$) years	54.7	55.5	58.9	56.4
Weight (kg)	64.8	64.3	68.4	65.8
Height (cm)	168	170	167	168
ASA I + II	13 (50%)	11 (46%)	24 (53%)	48 (50.5%)
ASA > II	13 (50%)	13 (54%)	21 (47%)	47 (49.5%)
T_{1-2} N_{0-1} M_0	11 (42%)	8 (33%)	20 (44%)	39 (41%)
T_{3-4} N_+ M_0	15 (58%)	16 (67%)	25 (56%)	56 (59%)

ASA = American Society of Anesthesiologists class

hours) included 24 patients. During the same period, another 45 patients had a transmediastinal esophagectomy. Age, distribution of sexes, tumor stages, and risk factors were comparable for both groups as well as for group III (transmediastinal esophagectomy + direct reconstruction) with the exception of tumor type (Table I).

Besides groups I–III, another 42 patients were esophagectomized during the same time period. These patients had preoperative radio-chemotherapy because of their tumor localization and tumor stages. They are not included in this evaluation because they are the subject of another study (preoperative radio-chemotherapy in non-R_0 resectable esophageal carcinomas). The intra- and postoperative data of all groups are listed in Table II. Postoperative complications (bleeding, anastomotic leakage, sepsis, respiratory, cardiac, and liver disorders) and especially the most important parameters of 30-day mortality, or hospital mortality, respectively, are listed in Table III.

Discussion

Reduction of postoperative mortality following esophagectomy is of central importance to the improvement of the prognosis of esophageal carcinoma. As a consequence, the efforts of many surgical teams

Table II
Intra- and Postoperative Data of the 95 Patients Esophagectomized During the Time Period of the Study

	Transthoracic Esophagectomy		*Transmediastinal Esophagectomy*	
	Direct Reconstruction (Group I)	*Reconstruction After 48–72 Hrs. (Group II)*	*Direct Reconstruction (Group III)*	*Patients Total*
Duration of anesthesia (hrs.)	6.9	8.4	5.5	6.6
Units of packed RBC	3.1	2.9	2.5	2.75
Reconstruction procedure				
stomach	21 (81%)	21 (87%)	38 (84%)	80 (84%)
colon	5 (19%)	3 (13%)	7 (16%)	15 (16%)
Artificial ventilation postoperatively (hrs.)	34.7	72	38	45.7
ICU treatment (days)	9.2	12.9	9.6	10.3

RBC = red blood cells

concentrate on this aim. During the last years, however, little progress has been made through new or improved surgical methods (e.g., transmediastinal esophagectomy) or new therapeutic concepts (e.g., preoperative parenteral nutrition). More progress has occurred through the combination of many small refinements, including preoperative evaluation of risk factors, standardization of esophagectomy and reconstruction, and postoperative intensive care with improved techniques of artificial respiration. Another contribution to this progress has been the concentration of esophageal surgery at a limited number of centers with extensive experience.

Our own efforts to reduce the risk of esophagectomy by staged resection should also be considered in this context. The analysis of postoperative lung function in our patients has shown that in the immediate period after esophagectomy, a deterioration of gas exchange occurs due to a relatively high right-to-left shunt (more than 20%). Therefore, this situation is a sequela of esophagectomy. The consequences are a perfusion/ventilation mismatch caused by

Table III
Local and General Complications in the Postoperative Course as Well as Mortality of the 95 Patients Esophagectomized During the Time Period of the Study

	Transthoracic Esophagectomy		*Transmediastinal Esophagectomy*	
	Direct Reconstruction (Group I)	*Reconstruction After 48–72 Hrs. (Group II)*	*Direct Reconstruction (Group III)*	*Patients Total*
Local complications				
hemorrhage	2 (7.7)	1 (4.1%)	2 (4.4%)	5 (5.3%)
anastomotic leakage	4 (15%)	5 (20%)	7 (15.0%)	16 (16.8%)
sepsis	1 (3.8%)	1 (4.1%)	1 (2.2%)	3 (3.2%)
total	7 (26.9%)	7 (29.1%)	10 (22.2%)	24 (25.3%)
General complications				
respiratory	1 (3.8%)	2 (8.3%)	2 (4.4%)	5 (5.3%)
cardiac	1 (3.8%)	1 (4.1%)	3 (6.6%)	5 (5.3%)
hepatic	2 (7.6%)	1 (4.1%)	—	
total	4 (15.3%)	4 (16.6%)	5 (11.1%)	13 (13.7%)
Mortality				
30 days	—	1 (4.1%)	1 (2.1%)	2 (2.1%)
hospital	1 (3.2%)	1 (4.1%)	2 (4.2%)	4 (4.2%)

compression atelectasis which can be reduced by prophylactic postoperative ventilation with positive end-expiratory pressure (PEEP). These data led to the concept of routine postoperative artificial respiration after esophagectomy.[7] By application of this management, shunt volume, respiratory function, and respiratory index usually normalized within 48 hours.[8] Consequently, a delay of 48 hours seemed appropriate prior to performing reconstruction of the food passage. The results of a pilot study[9,10] proved this concept. Therefore, we started a prospective controlled study on October 1, 1986, to evaluate the value of reconstruction with delayed urgency by objective criteria.

This study was comprised of 95 patients with esophageal cancer (Table I). Another 42 patients who had been operated during the same time period were excluded from the study because of preoperative radio-chemotherapy. The distribution of the groups shows that in nearly half of the cases in our patients a transmediastinal esophagectomy was indicated because of tumor localization and tumor type. The other patients were reconstructed in a randomized order either directly or with delayed urgency (after 48–72 hours postoperatively). These three groups do not show differences concerning the patients' characteristics. In addition, an analysis according to the ASA classification[11] and the distribution of tumor stages showed no differences. Forty-one percent of the patients in the study had a complete resection of the tumor, while 59% had advanced tumors in which a complete resection seemed to be conditionally possible. If 42 patients who had preoperative radio-chemotherapy were included, only 39 of 137 patients (28.5%) with a carcinoma of the esophagus were diagnosed in a tumor stage that allowed a definite R_0-resection. This figure corresponds exactly to the rate of 28.2% (T1, T2) described by the Japanese Committee for Registration of Esophageal Cancer.[12]

The analysis of the operative and early postoperative data of our patients (Table II) shows that the overall time of anesthesia was longest for the esophagectomy and reconstruction with delayed urgency, as was expected. It is interesting that the average time of anesthesia of transmediastinal esophagectomy with direct reconstruction was not significantly less than the mean operation time of transthoracic esophagectomy with direct reconstruction. The average intraoperative transfusion was 2.75 units of packed red blood cells and was equal in all three groups. In accordance with our conviction that gastric tube construction is the best and most practical means of esophageal replacement,[4] this procedure was used in more than 80% of the patients. In patients with a prior gastric operation, a colon interposition was chosen. As expected, the time of postoperative respiration was longest in the patients with delayed reconstruction. This prolonged time of prophylactic postoperative respiration did not coincide with a higher complication rate. On the average, patients after esophagectomy remained in the surgical intensive care unit (ICU) or in the intermediate care unit for about 10 days.

Summary

This study demonstrates a further improvement of the results after esophagectomy, obviously as a result of a greater experience and standardization of the procedure. It has to be pointed out once again, however, that the patients in the study represent a selected group because they had no preoperative radio- and/or chemotherapy. The analysis of postoperative complications (Table III) shows that leakage of the cervical anastomosis, an incidence of 16.8%, still remains a significant problem. Usually these anastomotic leaks heal once sufficiently drained, without residual salivary fistula. However, three patients with a cervical leak (18.8%) became septic. This was due mostly to spread of the infection into the area of esophagectomy in the posterior mediastinum. To prevent these septic complications, it is important to recognize this leakage without delay and open the cervical wound to achieve optimal drainage. Two of these three patients died because of their septic complications.

The overall complication rate of 25.3% demonstrates that esophagectomy and reconstruction of the food passage still carry a high risk of complications, and supports our experience that patients after esophagectomy are primarily endangered by surgical complications. Thus, a thorough preoperative analysis of risk factors, and postoperative intensive therapy combined with prophylactic artificial respiration are appropriate to reduce mortality resulting from organ failure.[13]

The overall 30-day mortality rate of 2.1% is very low, and the surgical mortality without time limitation of 4.2% has to be considered favorable. These data are similar to the data published by other experienced centers,[2] and demonstrate that, with good preoperative selection, patients with completely resectable tumors can be operated on with a mortality rate of less than 5%. There were no differences among the study groups with transthoracic esophagectomy and the group of transmediastinal esophagectomy patients as to the rate of postoperative complications and postoperative mortality, and no one of these procedures can be considered superior. This study shows that transmediastinal esophagectomy does not entail a smaller risk and that postoperative complications and respiratory disorders appear at the same rate as after transthoracic esophagectomy. Therefore, the indication for transmediastinal esophagectomy is determined by the tumor location and in some cases also by the tumor type.

Reconstruction with delayed urgency did not produce advantages in comparison to direct reconstruction in our patients. On the other hand, it does not represent a disadvantage for the patient if the reconstruction is performed with a delay of 2 to 3 days. This procedure may be indicated in case of intraoperative complications during esophagectomy, in high-risk patients, in case of intraoperative radiation therapy, or because of organizational reasons. Therefore, delayed reconstruction of the esophagus following transthoracic en bloc esophagectomy should be part of the entire treatment spectrum of esophageal surgery.

References

1. Adolf J, Bartels H, Siewert JR: Transthoracic esophagectomy combined with regional lymphadenectomy and reconstruction with delayed urgency versus transmediastinal esophagectomy and immediate reconstruction: Effect on cardiopulmonary function. In: Diseases of the Esophagus, Siewert JR, Hölscher AH (eds), Berlin, Springer-Verlag, 1988, p 232.
2. Siewert JR, Hölscher AH, Roder J, Bartels H: En-bloc Resektion der Speise-rohre beim Oesophaguscarcinom. Langenbecks Arch Chir 373:367, 1988.
3. Siewert JR: Die Chirurgie des Oesophaguscarcinoms. Z Herz- Thorax- Gefässchir 2:123–130, 1988.
4. Hölscher AH, Voit H, Buttermann G, Siewert JR: Function of the intrathoracic stomach as esophageal replacement. World J Surg 12:835, 1988.
5. Liebermann-Meffert D, Siewert JR: Vascularisation of the gastric tube used for esophageal replacement. Presented at the Fourth World Congress of the International Society for Diseases of the Esophagus, Chicago, Sept. 6, 1989.
6. Siewert JR, Hölscher AH, Horvath OP: Transmediastinale Oesophagektomie. Langenbecks Arch Chir 367:203, 1986.
7. Bartels H, Siewert JR: Postoperative Intensivuberwachung nach Oesophagektomie. Z Herz- Thorax- Gefässchir 2:131, 1988.
8. Sganga G, Siegel JH, Colemann B, et al: The physiologic meaning of the respiratory index in various types of critical illness. Circ Shock 17:179, 1985.
9. Siewert JR, Adolf J, Hölscher AH, Hölscher M, Weiser HF: Ösophaguskarzi-nom: Transthorakale Ösophagektomie mit regionaler Lymphadenektomie und Re-konstruktion mit aufgeschobener Dringlichkeit. Dtsch Med Wochenschr 111:647, 1986.
10. Siewert JR, Hölscher AH: Treatment of dysphagia in esophageal carcinoma: Transthoracic en-bloc esophagectomy and reconstruction 48 hours later. Dysphagia 2:222, 1988.
11. American Society of Anesthesiologists (ASA): New classification of physical status. Anesthesiology 24:111, 1963.
12. Japanese Committee for Registration of Esophageal Carcinoma: A proposal for new TNM classification of esophageal carcinoma. Jpn J Clin Oncol 14:625, 1985.
13. Elman A, Giuli R, Sancho-Garnier H: Risk factors of pulmonary complications following oesophagectomy in carcinoma of the esophagus. In: Diseases of the Esophagus, JR Siewert, AH Hölscher (eds), Berlin, Springer-Verlag, 1988, p 224.

30

Postoperative Nutritional Status in Patients with Esophageal Carcinoma

Nobutoshi Ando, Yohtaroh Shinozawa,
Yukihiko Ikehata, Tai Ohmori, Osahiko Abe

Introduction

Esophageal reconstruction using colon interposition has been claimed to be superior to reconstruction using a gastric tube in terms of providing nutrition due to preservation of the stomach. However, colon interposition has the disadvantage of being more complicated technically. In order to objectively analyze which technique affords superior postoperative nutritional status, this prospective study was carried out and the first follow-up report,[1] including patients up to the 18th postoperative month, was presented in 1986. In this chapter, subsequent follow-up data and additional new data concerning motor function of the substitute organs are presented.

Materials and Methods

Beginning in July 1983, 33 patients with esophageal carcinoma who underwent curative resection by right thoracotomy and laparotomy were enrolled in this prospective controlled study. The eli-

Ferguson MK, Little AG, Skinner DB: Diseases of the Esophagus, Vol. I: Malignant Diseases. Futura Publishing Company, Inc., Mount Kisco, NY, © 1990.

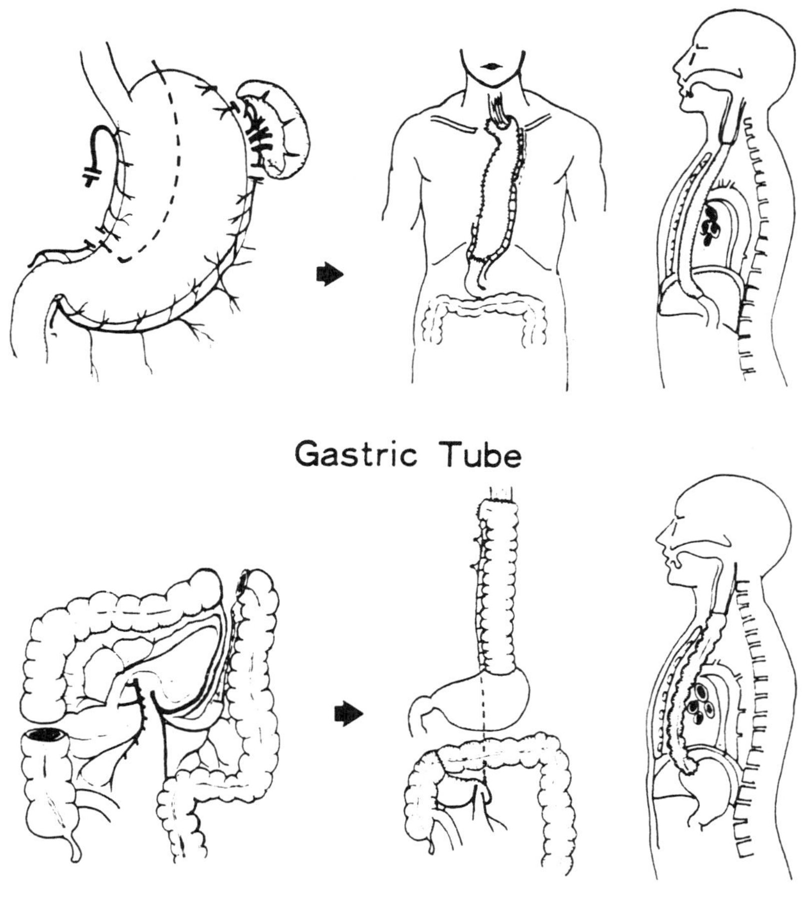

Figure 1: Retrosternal reconstruction using the gastric tube and colon interposition.

gibility criteria specified that the subjects were younger than 70 years old, and did not have concurrent severe metabolic disorders such as diabetes mellitus or liver cirrhosis. The subjects were divided to two groups based on the substitute used for reconstruction, one receiving a gastric tube and the other colon interposition. In both groups, retrosternal routes were used for reconstruction. In the cases undergo-

Table I
Patient Characteristics

		Stomach (18 cases)	*Colon (15 cases)*
Evaluable		16 cases	14 cases
Mean age (years)		61.2	59.3
Male:Female		15:1	13:1
Operating time (min)		435	598
Reconstruction time (min)		196	375
Bleeding (ml)		720	1440
Postoperative	Radiation	6 cases	6 cases
adjuvant	Chemotherapy	8	5
treatment	None	2	3

ing colon interposition, the right half of the colon with the left colic artery as the vascular pedicle was interposed between the cervical esophagus and the stomach (Fig. 1). Patients in whom severe postoperative complications occurred or recurred within 6 months after surgery were excluded from the evaluation.

Postoperative comparative studies between two groups were carried out at 3-month intervals for nutritional parameters, including body weight, total protein, serum albumin, rapid turnover proteins, lipids, calorie intake, and immunological parameters. Furthermore, motor function studies of the substitutes, such as radionuclide transit study[2] using pudding labeled by 5 mCi ^{99m}Tc or manometric study by the open-tip method were examined in five patients surviving more than 1 year postoperatively in each group.

Results

Eighteen patients in the group having a gastric tube and 15 patients in the group using colon interposition entered the study, and 16 cases and 14 cases were evaluable, respectively. Background factors such as mean age and male-female ratio were comparable in each group (Table I). Esophageal reconstruction using colon interposition requires much more time than that using a gastric tube. Therefore, operating time in the colon group was longer than that in the stomach group. Postoperative adjuvant radiotherapy or chemotherapy including cisplatin was performed in all but three patients in each group.

Preoperative mean body weight was 54.3 kg in the stomach group

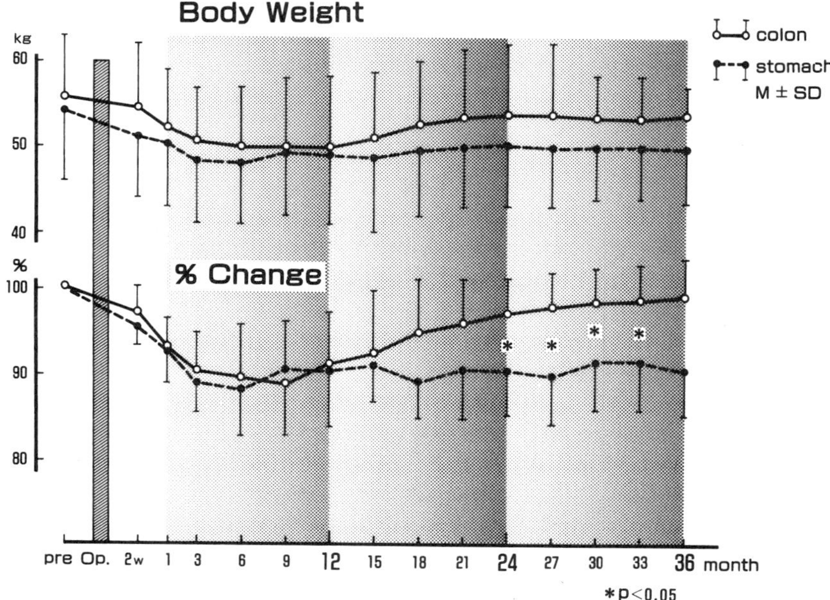

Figure 2: Changes in body weight.

and 56.0 kg in the colon group. Gradual loss of body weight was observed up to 6 months after surgery in both groups (Fig. 2). Thereafter body weight tended to gradually increase, but recovery to preoperative levels was not noted in either group.

Expressing the changes in body weight as a percentage of the preoperative value, body weight decreased to 89% of the preoperative value 6 months after surgery in both groups. Thereafter, in the colon group, gradual recovery was observed, returning to 99% of the preoperative value 30 months postoperatively. In the stomach group, slight recovery to over 90% was observed 9 months after surgery, but no changes in body weight were observed thereafter. Significant differences between the groups were observed from 24 to 33 months after surgery.

Total protein (TP) decreased to 6.8 g/dl in the stomach group and to 6. 6 g/dl, in the colon group 2 weeks after surgery (Fig. 3). Thereafter, TP increased to more than 7.0 g/dl in each group and significant differences between the groups were not observed. Serum albumin

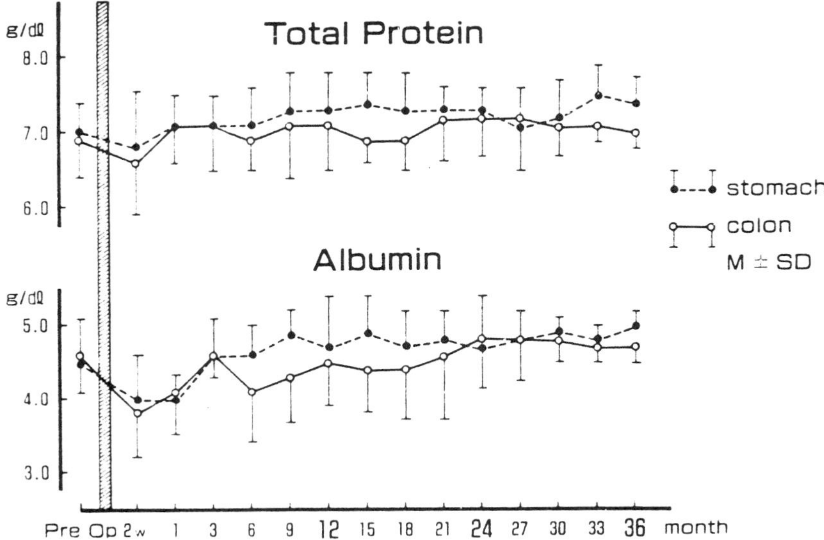

Figure 3: Changes in total protein and serum albumin.

decreased to 4.0 g/dl in the stomach group and to 3.8 g/dl in the colon group 2 weeks after surgery. Thereafter, albumin increased to more than 4.5 g/dl in each group and significant differences between the groups were not noted.

Among rapid turnover proteins, pre-albumin and retinol-binding protein did not recover to preoperative values (Fig. 4). The postoperative decrease in pre-albumin in the colon group was more marked than that in the stomach group. Significant intergroup differences in rapid turnover proteins were not observed. Marked intergroup differences in lipids such as total cholesterol, triglycerides, and free fatty acids were not noted (Fig. 5). Marked intergroup differences in PPD skin test reactivity were not noted. Lymphocytes (%) decreased 2 weeks after surgery in each group. Thereafter, marked differences between each the groups were not seen.

Mean value of transit time was 478 seconds in the stomach group and 108 seconds in the colon group (Fig. 6). Segmental contraction-like movements of the substitute following dry swallowing, not peristalsis, were observed in four of six patients who were studied in the colon group but were not observed in the stomach group.

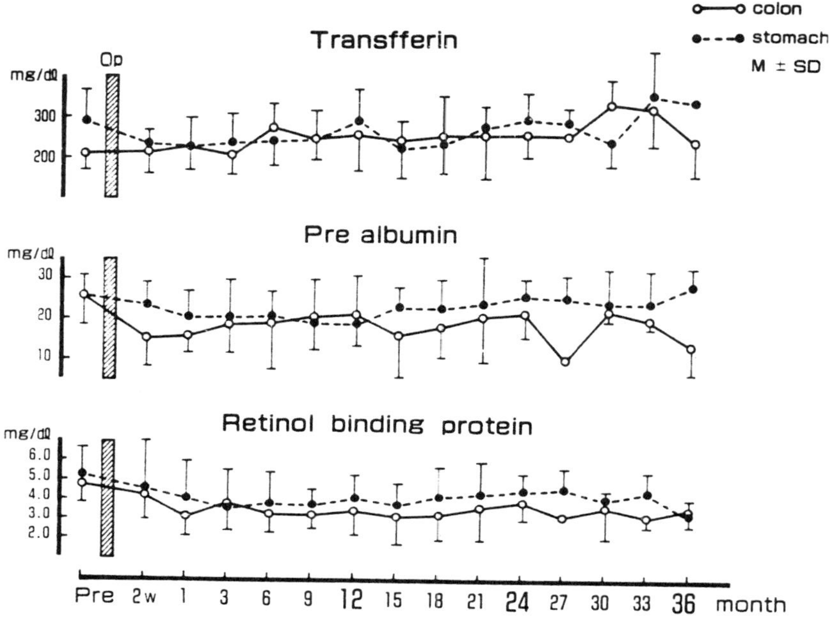

Figure 4: Changes in rapid turnover proteins.

Percent change in body weight in patients surviving longer than 3 years after surgery was calculated (Fig. 7). The nadir was 94% of the preoperative value and recovery to more than 98% was noted 24 months after surgery in the colon group. In the stomach group, the nadir was 89% and thereafter no changes in body weight were observed.

Discussion

In the first report, in which 25 evaluable cases were followed-up for up to 18 months postoperatively, postoperative recovery of body weight was found to be poorer in the colon group than in the stomach group. In this report, in which 30 evaluable cases were followed-up for up to 36 months after surgery, postoperative recovery of body weight was more marked after 18 months postoperatively in the colon

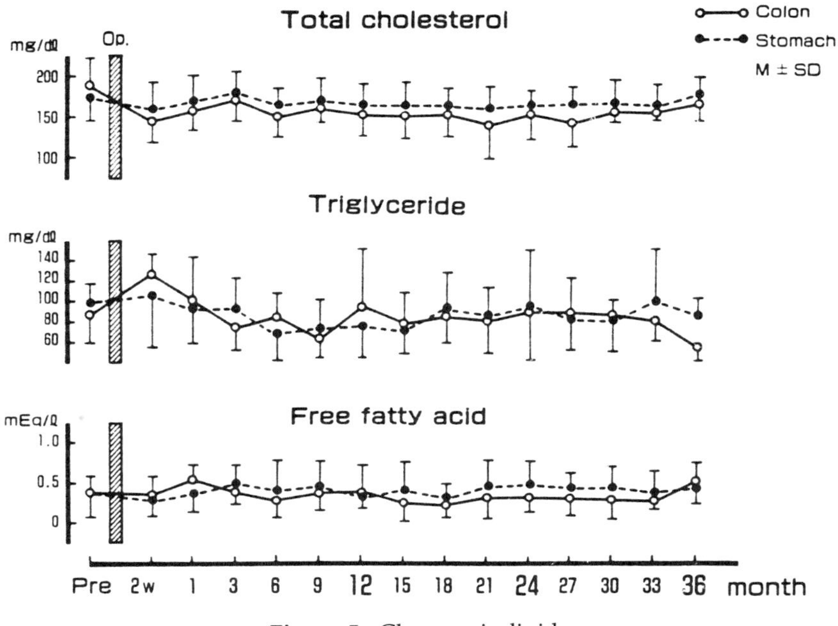

Figure 5: Changes in lipids.

group than in the stomach group. However, significant intergroup differences were not observed in nutritional parameters such as total protein, serum albumin, lipids, and rapid turnover protein except pre-albumin. Radionuclide transit studies of the substitutes more than 1 year after surgery revealed that the transit time through the interposed colon was shorter than that through the gastric tube. Therefore, satisfactory recovery of body weight in the colon group is most likely due to satisfactory transit of food through the substitutes.

For percent change in body weight in survivors beyond 3 years after surgery, recovery was more satisfactory in the colon group than in the stomach group, and the patients in the colon group were comparatively young, which may explain this difference. Based on the result of this study, colon interposition for esophageal reconstruction is indicated for the patients expected to be cured who are younger than 55 years old. Following this controlled study, colon interpositions were recently carried out in four patients who were eligible for this operation; body weight in these patients recovered to the preoperative value within 6 months after surgery.

	Transit Time
Gastric tube	478 sec
Colon interposition	108 sec

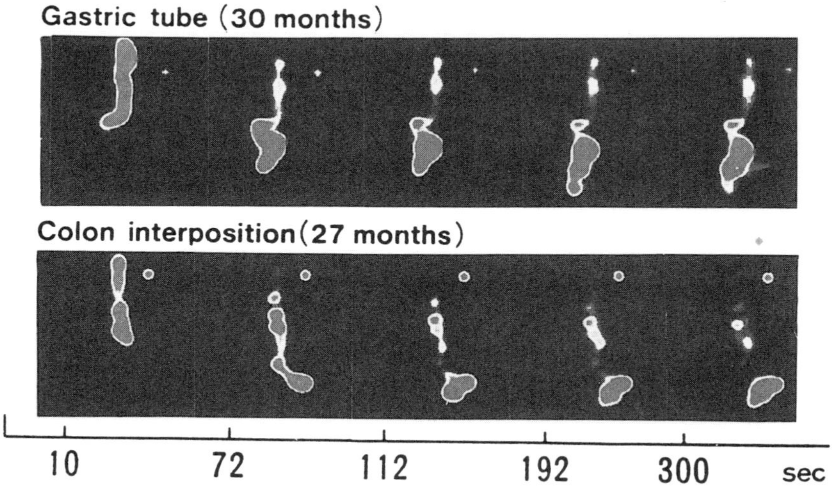

Gastric tube (30 months)

Colon interposition (27 months)

10 72 112 192 300 sec

Figure 6: Radionuclide transit study through the substitute.

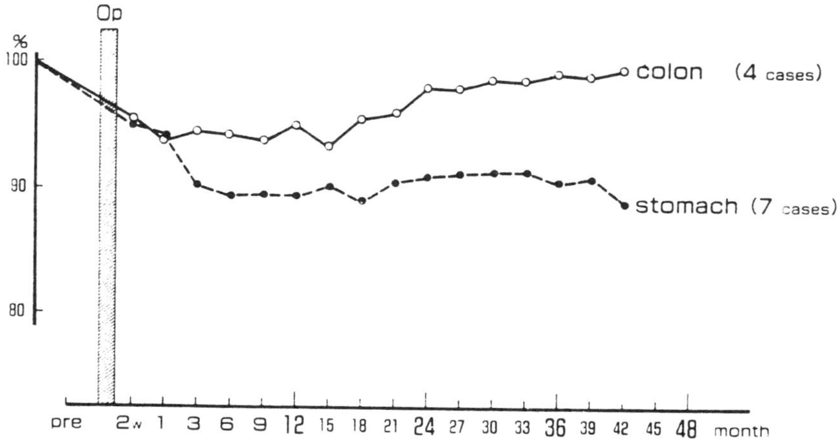

Figure 7: Percent changes in body weight in long-term survivors.

References

1. Ando N, Ikehata Y, Abe O, et al: Prospective studies on postoperative nutritional status in patients with esophageal carcinoma as evaluated from various substitutes for reconstruction. In: Diseases of the Esophagus, Siewert JR, Hölscher AH (eds), Berlin, Springr-Verlag, 1988, p 674.
2. Llamas-Elvira JM, Martinez-Parades M, Sopena-Monforte R, et al: Value of radionuclide esophageal transit in studies of functional dysphagia. Br J Radiol 59:1073, 1986.

IV.

Multimodality Therapy: Editors' Overview

Resection has been the mainstay of therapy for cancer of the esophagus for the past 50 years. Despite recent improvements in surgical techniques and patient care, poor overall long-term results following resection mandate the use of additional forms of therapy in most patients. Such modalities include radiation therapy, chemotherapy, immunotherapy, and other less common treatments. Radiation therapy alone has been used for many years for management of esophageal cancer. Most tumors are initially responsive, but the recurrence rate is high, there is a significant incidence of benign complications, and this modality by itself has no effect on distant disease. Single-agent chemotherapy has been used sporadically without significant success since the 1960's. The chapters in this section outline new techniques for utilizing these and other modalities, and the results reported suggest that further investigation of these techniques may prove fruitful in the near future.

In Chapter 31, Huang and his coauthors address the controversial issue of whether preoperative irradiation improves surgical results in carcinoma of the esophagus. They report results of an impressive prospective study of 360 patients with squamous cell carcinoma of the mid-esophagus, randomly assigned to irradiation of 40 Gy over 4 weeks followed by resection or resection alone. The results demonstrate a moderate benefit in patients irradiated preoperatively, who had a higher rate of resectability and a lower incidence of nodal metastasis, although these differences were not statistically significant. However, no improvement in long-term survival was provided by preoperative irradiation. Whether the irradiation treatment planning in this study was optimal remains to be seen, and it appears that the controversy regarding the utility of preoperative irradiation will continue.

The use of multiple-drug chemotherapy preoperatively or as a palliative measure has gained popularity in recent years. One difficulty that has become evident is assessment of response to chemotherapy. In Chapter 32, Walker et al. present data which show that current methods of assessing tumor response are inadequate. Computed tomography on occasion will demonstrate a complete response in patients in whom a tumor can be demonstrated pathologically, and, on the contrary, often underestimates the frequency of partial responses. A similar situation holds for barium contrast studies in evaluating response of esophageal cancer to chemotherapy. Considerable improvements in our ability to clinically assess esophageal cancer will be necessary before we can perform accurate posttreatment staging.

Selection of appropriate drug therapy for esophageal cancer patients is approached in a novel fashion by Ishigami and associates in Chapter 33. Using in vitro techniques, drug levels are measured in various tissues following intravenous, intra-arterial, and intramural injections. The sensitivities of esophageal cancer to various anticancer drugs are also measured in vitro. They report that tissue drug levels vary considerably, while there is equal or greater variation in the individual sensitivity of esophageal cancers to chemotherapeutic agents.

In Chapter 34, Peracchia and his co-workers report results of neoadjuvant chemotherapy for locally advanced esophageal squamous cell cancer using cisplatin and fluorouracil. The overall response rate was 50% (10% complete, 40% partial). Despite the fact that the patients were demonstrated to have tumor invasion into surrounding structures prior to chemotherapy, 42% underwent resection, of whom 80% had a complete resection. These data suggest that neoadjuvant chemotherapy may be able to substantially modify the natural outcome in a significant percentage of patients. In Chapter 35, Hirayama et al. describe their experience with adjuvant postoperative chemotherapy for patients with nodal metastases. Their results, using historical controls for comparison, suggest an improvement in 5-year survival in patients with extensive nodal involvement is offered by aggressive chemotherapy. These studies support further investigation into the role of neoadjuvant and adjuvant chemotherapy in the management of esophageal cancer.

In Chapters 36 and 37, the use of a new device for achieving local esophageal hyperthermia in the management of esophageal cancer is described. Matsuda et al. report results of a combination of hyperthermia, chemotherapy, and irradiation for preoperative treatment, while in a second group of patients with unresectable disease, this was used with palliative intent. The results suggest that hyperthermia, when combined with irradiation and chemotherapy, yields a higher response rate and improves survival when compared to the use of chemotherapy and irradiation alone. Fujimaki and co-workers describe the use of hyperthermia combined with irradiation and chemotherapy for nonresectable esophageal cancers. Their results echo those of Matsuda et al., demonstrating an overall response rate of more than 80%, with considerable palliative benefit. These findings indicate that further investigation of hyperthermia as adjuvant therapy for esophageal carcinoma is certainly warranted.

31

Combined Preoperative Irradiation and Surgery Versus Surgery Alone for Squamous Cell Carcinoma of the Midthoracic Esophagus:
A Prospective Randomized Study in 360 Patients

Guo Jun Huang, Xian Zhi Gu, Liang Jun Wang, Mei Wang, Da Wei Zhang, Wei Bo Yin, Ru Gang Zhang, Fu Sheng Liu, Zhen Yan Wang

Introduction

Reports on the value of combination therapy including preoperative irradiation and surgery for carcinoma of the esophagus have been controversial during the past three decades. In 1960, Clifton and associates[1] and Nakayama[2] reported independently the experiences with this combined treatment modality in 20 and 114 cases, respectively, coming to the same conclusion that preoperative irradiation inhibited tumor growth and raised the resectability rate. Huang and associates in 1962[3] and in 1981[4] reported respectively 113 and 408 selected cases of esophageal carcinoma treated by this combined ther-

Ferguson MK, Little AG, Skinner DB: Diseases of the Esophagus, Vol. I: Malignant Diseases. Futura Publishing Company, Inc., Mount Kisco, NY, © 1990.

apy with higher resectability rates than those of the cases treated contemporarily by surgery alone. Subsequent reports by Akakura and associates in 1963,[5] Nakayama and associates in 1974,[6] Marks and associates in 1976,[7] Parker and associates in 1982,[8] and Huang and associates in 1986[9] all indicated favorable results of this combined therapy in terms of resectability, long-term survivals, and other factors over those of either radiotherapy or surgery alone. More recent reports by Launois and associates in a prospective randomized study[10] and by Sasaki and associates in a retrospective analysis,[11] however, concluded that the survivals and other results obtained by combined preoperative irradiation and surgery were not superior to those from surgery alone.

This chapter is a further analysis of a prospective randomized study of combined preoperative irradiation and surgery for carcinoma of the esophagus preliminarily reported in 1986.[9]

Material and Methods

The present study was started in 1977 and included 360 patients eligible for analysis up to the end of 1987. Patients under 65 years of age with midthoracic (from the upper border of the aortic arch above to the inferior border of the inferior pulmonary vein below) esophageal squamous cell carcinoma not exceeding 7 cm in length (since 1984, this criterion was changed to a length of from 5 to 8 cm) by x-ray and with no contraindications to either surgery or radiation were randomized by envelope method into group A, to be treated by combined preoperative irradiation and subsequent surgery, or group B, treatment by surgery alone.

For group A patients, a linear accelerator was used almost exclusively with a total dose of 40 Gy divided into 20 fractions over 4 weeks. Irradiation was given through an anterior and a posterior portal, each 6 cm in width and about 22 to 25 cm in length from the upper margin of the manubrium sterni above to the tip of the xyphoid process below, covering the whole mediastinum and the celiac region. In group A, surgery was undertaken 2 to 4 weeks (average 18 days) after completion of irradiation. In both groups, a left posterolateral thoracotomy through the sixth rib bed or interspace was used exclusively. When the tumor was resectable, the stomach was used for esophageal replacement and in most cases, an intrapleural supra-aortic end-to-side manual esophagogastrostomy was done. Cervical

Table I
Clinicopathological Types of Tumors

Types	Group A		Group B	
	No. of Cases	%	No. of Cases	%
Medullary	129	76.8	131	68.2
Fungating	35	20.8	55	28.6
Intraluminal	3	1.8	4	2.1
Undetermined	1	0.8	2	1.0
Total	168		192	

Group A: Combined preoperative irradiation and surgery
Group B: Surgery alone

anastomosis was done in a small number of cases. In this study, it was mandatory to eradicate as completely as feasible all of the connective tissues and tumor-bearing tissues around the esophagus, and the draining lymph nodes of the perigastric group, the paracardiac, and the paraesophageal and mediastinal groups including the hilar, paratracheal, and subcarinal groups, along with the dissection and mobilization of the stomach and the esophagus. No special attempt was made, however, to routinely perform overextensive lymph node dissection or total esophagectomy.

Group A (combination therapy) consisted of 168 patients, 122 males and 46 females (2.7:1), with ages ranging from 28 to 65 years (average 52.3 years). In group B (surgery alone) there were 192 patients, 143 males and 49 females (2.9:1), with ages ranging from 30 to 65 years (average 53.7 years). The average lengths of the tumor were the same, or 6.1 cm, in both groups.

The clinicopathological typing of tumors of both groups is shown in Table I, from which it can be seen that medullary tumors were the most common in both groups, and that fungating tumors and intraluminal tumors, both known to be much more radiosensitive than medullary tumors, were more common in group B than in group A.

The postsurgical pathological staging of the two groups is shown in Table II, from which it can be seen that over 90% of cases in both groups had advanced disease (stages III and IV) with either extraesophageal invasion of tumor and/or regional or distant lymph node or organ metastases. Stage I disease was not seen in either group, and stage II disease was found in 7.7% of cases in group A and in 4.7% of cases in group B.

Table II
Postsurgical Pathological Staging of Diseases

	Group A		Group B	
Stages	*No. of Cases*	*%*	*No. of Cases*	*%*
I	0	0	0	0
II	13	7.7	9	4.7
III	121	72.0	150	78.1
IV	34	20.0	33	17.2
Total	168		192	

Group A: Combined preoperative irradiation and surgery
Group B: Surgery alone

Results

Of the 168 patients in group A, the tumor was resectable in 151, a resectability rate of 89.9%. The resection was classified as curative in 80.8% (122/151) and palliative in 19.2% (29/151) of the cases. In group B, the resectability rate was 83.3% (160/192) and the resection was curative in 77.5% (124/160) and palliative in 22.5% (36/160).

In group A, at operation the lungs and pleura were found to be little affected by the preoperative irradiation. In some instances only mild congestion and edema were seen over the irradiated mediastinal pleura. Usually there was some retraction and slight loss of luster of the mediastinal pleura overlying the tumor. Shrinkage of the tumor mass was noted in most cases. This was especially marked in cases where the postradiation esophagogram showed good radiation effects. Usually the tumor was much smaller in size and was softer in consistency with ill-defined boundaries. In some cases the tumor had regressed so much that it was indeed difficult for the exploring finger to exactly locate the lesion.[9]

The 30-day operative mortality rates for all operated cases were 3.0% (5/168) in group A and 3.6% (7/192) in group B, and for the resection cases the rates were 3.3% (5/151) in group A and 4.4% (7/160) in group B.

The incidence of intrathoracic anastomotic leakage was 0% (0/128) in group A and 2.3% (3/130) in group B, and that of cervical anastomotic leakage was 8.7% (2/23) in group A and 13.3% (4/30) in group B. It should be noted that practically all the intrathoracic anastomoses in group A were within the field of preoperative irradiation.

The incidence of residual tumor at cut edges of the esophagus was 0% (0/151) in group A and 1.9% (3/160) in group B. The incidence of lymph node metastasis was 25.8% (39/151) in group A and 38.8% (62/160) in group B, a difference of statistical significance ($P < 0.05$). In group A, degenerated tumor cells were seen sometimes in the lymph nodes, indicating the effect of radiation on metastatic lymph nodes.

The absolute 5-year survival rate calculated with all patients entered into each group (including unresectable cases and operative deaths) as denominator and number of known survivors as numerator was 35.4% (29/82) in group A and 34.2% (26/76) in group B. The 5-year survival rate of the resected cases excluding operative deaths was 38.7% (29/75) in group A and 39.4% (26/66) in group B. The median survival rate of all patients entered into each group was 17.3 months in group A and 13.6 months in group B, and that of the resected cases excluding operative deaths was 20.3 months in group A and 16.9 months in group B.

In group A, the 5-year survival rate was 50% (12/24) in patients with marked postradiation reaction of the resected primary tumor (i.e., tumor mass showing complete or nearly complete regression with microscopic findings consisting of either total disappearance of tumor cells or only remnants of degenerated tumor tissue), and was 31.8% (14/44) in those with mild or moderate reaction. It can be seen that the survival rates in both groups were encouraging but their differences were of no statistical significance.

Discussion

The present study was based on the rationale that preoperative irradiation reduces the viability of cancer cells inevitably disseminated during operative manipulation and hence the potential of cancer metastasis and implantation. It was also theorized that irradiation devitalizes or sterilizes microscopic tumor foci not accessible to surgical resection as well as tumor infiltration into adjacent vital organs, thus facilitating surgical resection and enhancing surgical results. In this study, strict randomization was used and the two groups were comparable with sufficiently large numbers of eligible cases for final analysis. It can be seen that the end-points in this study in terms of resectability, operative mortality, incidence of anastomotic leakage, incidence of residual tumor at cut edges, and incidence of lymph node metastasis are all superior in patients treated with combined therapy to those in the group treated by surgery alone, although many of the differences are not statistically significant. On the whole, these results indicate that preoperative irradiation causes definite regression of the tumor process, thus helping surgery in increasing the rate of resectability and the completeness of tumor extirpation. The degree of regression, however, for reasons not yet fully understood, differs from patient to patient, as does radiosensitivity from one tumor to another. The present study shows that, with the dose and rest intervals used in this trial, preoperative irradiation has no untoward effects on the healing power of the irradiated esophagus, and poses no difficulty to surgical manipulation or added risk to the patient. Whether or not a higher dose of preoperative irradiation, for example, 60 Gy, can bring about a more marked and uniform tumor regression without causing additional risk to the patient needs to be further investigated.

It is disappointing that preoperative irradiation in this study did not increase the 5-year survival rate over that by surgery alone. This is most probably due to the fact that radiotherapy is a local-regional treatment totally ineffective against any cancer outside the field of irradiation, which is a common situation in relatively advanced cases such as the majority of cases in the present series, and also a common cause of failure after either surgical or radiation therapy. Whether or not a larger field of irradiation than that used in this study, such as to further cover the cervical esophagus and the supraclavicular areas, in addition to a higher dose as suggested above, can be feasible and more beneficial remains to be answered.

It should also be pointed out that since the use of preoperative radiotherapy with its known cancericidal effect and its large field of irradiation covering the entire mediastinum and the celiac region as used in the present study did not increase the long-term survival over that by surgery alone, it follows that further enlarging the extent of surgical excision beyond that practiced in this study in an attempt to achieve this goal may not be rewarding.

Conclusion

Based on the present prospective randomized study on combined preoperative irradiation and surgery (group A) versus surgery alone (group B) for squamous cell carcinoma of the midthoracic esophagus in 360 patients, it is concluded that the early results in terms of resectability, operative mortality, incidence of anastomotic leaks, and incidence of residual tumor at esophageal cut edges are in favor of group A rather than group B, although the differences are not statistically significant. The incidence of lymph node metastasis is lower in group A than in group B ($P < 0.05$). These results serve to indicate that preoperative irradiation, with the dose and rest intervals used in this study, causes definite cancer regression within the field of irradiation with no untoward effects on the healing power of the irradiated esophagus or additional difficulty on surgical manipulation or added risk to the patients. The present study, however, failed to show any significant increase in long-term survival rates with the use of preoperative irradiation.

References

1. Clifton EE, Goodner JT, Bronstein E: Properative irradiation for cancer of the esophagus. Cancer 13:37, 1960.
2. Nakayama K: Combined surgical radiative treatment for cancerous lesions with particular interest in prevention of recurrence. Proceedings of the Japanese Cancer Association 19th General Meeting, 1960, p 214.
3. Huang GJ, Wang JZ, Liu YQ, et al: Preoperative irradiation for carcinoma of the esophagus: A report on the experiences in 113 cases. Shanghai Sci Tech Publ, Shanghai, 1962, p 1.
4. Huang GJ, Gu XZ, Zhang RG, et al: Combined preoperative irradiation and surgery in esophageal carcinoma: Report of 408 cases. Chin Med J 94:73, 1981.
5. Akakura K, Nakamura Y, Kakegawa T: The combined treatment for carcinoma of the esophagus with the radical resection and the preoperative irradiation. Keio J Med 14:145, 1963.
6. Nakayama K, Kinoshita Y: Surgical treatment combined with preoperative concentrated irradiation. J Am Med Assoc 227:178, 1974.
7. Marks RD Jr, Scruggs HJ, Wallace KM: Preoperative radiation therapy for carcinoma of the esophagus. Cancer 38:84, 1976.
8. Parker EF, Gregorie HB, Prioleau WH Jr, et al: Carcinoma of the esophagus: Observation of 40 years. Ann Surg 195:618, 1982.
9. Huang GJ, Gu XZ, Wang LJ, et al: Experience with combined preoperative irradiation and surgery for carcinoma of the esophagus. Gann Monograph on Cancer Res 31:159, 1986.
10. Launois B, Ben-Hassel M, Delarue D, et al: Perioperative treatment of esophageal cancer. In: Siewert JR, Hölscher AH (ed), Diseases of the Esophagus, Berlin, Springer-Verlag, 1988, p 308.
11. Sasaki T, Makuuchi H, Sugihara T, et al: Evaluation of preoperative irradiation therapy for carcinoma of the esophagus. In: Siewert JR, Hölscher AH (ed), Diseases of the Esophagus. Berlin, Springer-Verlag, 1988, p 313.

32

Assessment of the Response to Chemotherapy in Esophageal Cancer

Steven J. Walker, A. Steel, C. Edwards, M.H. Cullen, Hugoe R. Matthews

Introduction

The evaluation of chemotherapy in the management of any tumor is dependent on the methods available to identify a reduction in the bulk of the primary or secondary lesions. In the case of the esophagus, this is particularly difficult and the optimal method of measuring response has not been determined. Most reported studies have relied on computer-aided tomography (CT scanning), but two-dimensional measurements of tumor size on barium swallow have recently been recommended.[1] So far there have been no studies comparing one method with another.

Initial Observations

In 1986 at the Regional Department of Thoracic Surgery, East Birmingham Hospital, we embarked on a program of chemotherapy for esophageal carcinoma. The first trial involved a phase II study of preoperative chemotherapy using a single agent (Carboplatin) in pa-

Ferguson MK, Little AG, Skinner DB: Diseases of the Esophagus, Vol. I: Malignant Diseases. Futura Publishing Company, Inc., Mount Kisco, NY, © 1990.

tients with esophageal adenocarcinoma,[2] with CT scanning as the main indicator of response at the primary site. Fifteen patients entered this study and none showed any response to chemotherapy on CT scanning using the criteria of Miller et a1.[3] Eight of 15 patients underwent esophageal resection, and in four the gross specimen showed changes that were suggestive of at least a partial response of the tumor to chemotherapy, even though this had not been apparent on preoperative investigation.

The most obvious macroscopic changes that we noticed were: (1) partial destruction of the malignant edge of the tumor and a reduction in tumor bulk, and (2) appearance of a clean, healthy granulating floor to the ulcer instead of the usual slough and necrosis. Subsequent microscopic examination in seven of eight showed patients evidence of: (1) partial re-epithelialization of the mucosal surface, and (2) increased fibrous tissue formation. These features were appreciably different from those seen in many resected specimens from patients who had not undergone chemotherapy. We were forced to conclude that there had been some local response to chemotherapy although this had not been apparent on CT scanning.

In subsequent studies, we therefore decided to assess the response to chemotherapy by barium swallow as well as CT scanning, both before and after chemotherapy, and to document the appearance of the primary tumor by pinning out and photographing the freshly resected specimens, with detailed microscopic examination.

Patients

To date, a total of 20 patients with a localized esophageal carcinoma have undergone two courses of preoperative chemotherapy over a 6- to 8-week period with pre- and posttreatment assessment followed by subtotal esophagectomy[4] with detailed examination of the specimen. There were 18 male patients and two female patients; ages ranged from 49 to 74 years (mean 63 years). The histology and site of each tumor, the chemotherapy regimen used, and the number of patients in each group are shown in Table I.

For purposes of this study, a response was defined by any convincing reduction in the size of the primary tumor after chemotherapy. Shrinkage was referred to as a partial response, and gross disappearance of the tumor as a complete response.

Table I
Tumor Histology, Site, and Chemotherapy Regimen

Tumor	*Site*	*Chemotherapy Regimen*	*Patients*
Adenocarcinoma	Lower	Carboplatin	8
		FAM	7
Squamous carcinoma	Mid/lower	MIC	2
Small cell carcinoma	Mid/lower	Capomet	3
			20

FAM = 5-Fluorouracil, doxorubicin (Adriamycin), mitomycin-C.
MIC = Mitomycin-C, ifosfamide, cisplatin.
Capomet = Cyclophosphamide, doxorubicin, vincristine, methotrexate, etoposide.

Results

CT scans before and after chemotherapy were obtained in all 20 patients. Barium swallows after treatment were introduced later in the study and were obtained in eight patients. Pathological examination was performed in 19 cases (the remaining patient was operated on by another surgeon). The response rates as evaluated by the three principal methods of investigation are shown in Table II. The most notable finding was that a complete or partial response was found in only 50% of cases using CT scanning, compared to 75% using barium swallow, and 89% on pathological assessment.

Discussion

The results presented here represent simply an observation that there appears to be a discrepancy between the pathological appear-

Table II
Tumor Response to Chemotherapy

Evaluation	*No. of Patients*	*Complete*	*Partial*	*No Response*
CT scan	20	1 (5%)	9 (45%)	10 (50%)
Barium swallow	8	1 (12%)	5 (63%)	2 (25%)
Pathological	19	0	17 (89%)	2 (11%)

ance of the esophageal carcinoma and the response rates determined by CT scanning and barium swallow after chemotherapy. The specific pathological changes that result from chemotherapy have not yet been defined either in this or in any other studies. Nevertheless, we have observed marked changes in gross appearance of the tumors treated by chemotherapy, compared with the several hundred untreated specimens that we have examined in the past.

When a response was observed on CT scanning, it was always matched by a similar response on barium swallow and pathological examination of the resected specimen, but the converse did not apply. Responses were seen on barium swallow when they were absent on CT scanning, and some responses were also seen on pathological examination that were not present either on CT scanning or barium swallow.

On the basis of these observations, it would seem that neither CT scanning nor barium swallow is wholly adequate in assessing the response to chemotherapy in esophageal tumors, but we would agree with Agha et al.[1] that a barium swallow is a useful investigation in this context and may be superior to CT scanning. Whether the changes that we have noticed on pathological examination have any therapeutic significance is not clear, but they call into question existing methods of evaluating response if they do not truly reflect what is occurring at a cellular level in the primary lesion.

Miller et al.[4] have defined the response of tumors to nonsurgical treatment as:

Complete response – the disappearance of all known disease, determined by two observations not less than 4 weeks apart.

Partial response – a 50% or more decrease in tumor load of the lesions that have been measured to determine the effect of therapy by two observations not less than 4 weeks apart. In addition, there can be no appearance of new lesions or progression of any lesion.

No change – a 50% decrease in tumor size cannot be established nor can a 25% increase in the size of one or more measurable lesions be demonstrated.

Progressive disease – a 25% or more increase in the size of one or more measurable lesions or the appearance of new lesions.

Such criteria can only be applied, however, if the methods of measuring response in the tumor are sufficiently sensitive. Our observations suggest that with esophageal carcinoma, this may not be the case. We suggest that strict and specific criteria for a therapeutic response in esophageal carcinoma will have to be established before the results of chemotherapy in this disease can be reliably and accurately evaluated.

References

1. Agha FP, Gennis MA, Orringer MB, et al: Evaluation of response to preoperative chemotherapy in esophageal and gastric cardia cancer using biphasic esophagrams and surgical- pathological correlation. Am J Clin Oncol 9:227, 1986.
2. Steel A, Cullen MH, Robertson PW, et al: A phase II study of carboplatin in adenocarcinoma of the oesophagus. Br J Cancer 58:500, 1988.
3. Miller AB, Hoogstraten B, Staquet M, et al: Reporting results of cancer treatment. Cancer 47:207, 1981.
4. Matthews HR, Steel A: Left-sided subtotal oesophagectomy for carcinoma. Br J Surg 74:1115, 1987.

33

Adjuvant Chemotherapy for Esophageal Cancer in Consideration of the Sensitivities to Anticancer Drugs

Koichi Ishigami, Takuo Murakami, Masaaki Oka, Yasushi Masaki, Norio Matsumoto, Kiichi Honma, Hiroto Hayashi

Introduction

The results of surgical treatment of esophageal cancer have been unsatisfactory and discouraging in spite of recent surgical progress. For the purpose of improving these results, adjuvant chemotherapy was investigated.

Distribution of Anticancer Drugs in Body Fluids and Tissues[1,2]

The concentrations of anticancer drugs in various body fluids and tissues were determined by the "band culture method" invented by Okubo,[3] which employs a bioassay, a technique employing bacteria

Ferguson MK, Little AG, Skinner DB: Diseases of the Esophagus, Vol. I: Malignant Diseases. Futura Publishing Company, Inc., Mount Kisco, NY, © 1990.

Table I
Measurement of Anticancer Drug Concentrations Using the Band Culture Method

Anticancer Drug	*Strain of Test Organism*	*Medium*	*Incubation Time at 37°C (hrs)*	*Minimum Inhibition Concentration μg/ml*
BLM PEP	*B. subtilis* PCI 219 2.1×10^7/ml	Müller-Hinton medium	5 to 7	0.25 0.13
5-FU	*S. aureus* 209-P 6.5×10^7/ml	Müller-Hinton medium	7 to 9	0.025
MMC	*E. coli* B 1.0×10^7/ml	Nutrient agar	5 to 7	0.0025

BLM = Bleomycin, PEP = Peplomycin, 5-FU = 5-Fluorouracil, MMC = Mitomycin

as a test organism. This test is based on the antibacterial activity of anticancer drugs. Various conditions of measurement were determined by the preliminary investigations shown in Table I. The excised tissues were minced with scissors and homogenized in a Waring blender with two to four times the volume of physiological saline or pH 7.2 phosphate buffer solution. These homogenates were kept in a refrigerator at 4°C for 48 hours. The resultant supernatant fluids were used for the measurement of anticancer drug concentrations in various tissues.

Bleomycin (BLM) levels in the esophagus and regional lymph nodes in dogs increased 30 minutes following 0.5 mg/kg of intramural, intravenous, and selective intra-arterial injections, in decreasing order. BLM levels in the lung were uniformly lower than in the esophagus following intravenous, selective intra-arterial and intramural injections, in decreasing order (Fig. 1). Relatively high levels of BLM were detected in the esophagus, especially in the mucosal layer, in cancer patients 30 minutes following intravenous injection of 0.5 mg/kg of BLM. BLM levels in esophageal cancer were higher than those in the adjacent normal esophagus. A considerable amount of BLM remained in the esophagus in dogs even 25 hours after intravenous injection of 0.5 mg/kg of BLM (Fig. 2). This result is noteworthy because BLM is one of the concentration- and time-dependent anticancer drugs. BLM levels in esophageal cancers and regional lymph node

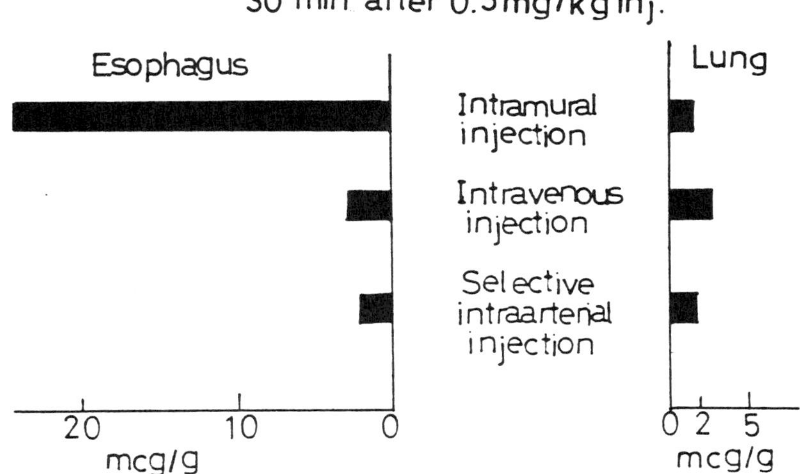

Figure 1: Bleomycin levels in the esophagus and lung in dogs following various routes of administration.

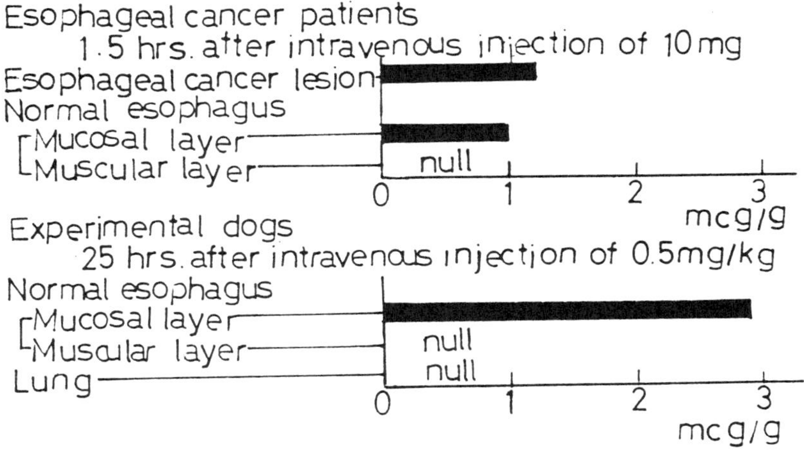

Figure 2: Bleomycin levels in each part of the esophagus.

Table II
Bleomycin (BLM) Levels in Esophageal Cancers and Regional Lymph Node Metastases in Cancer Patients 1.5 Hours After Intravenous Injection

Injection Dose (mg)	BLM Level (μg/g)	
	Main Lesions	Lymph Node Metastases
7.5	1.92–2.16	3.18
10	1.72–3.0	3.0
15	0.84–2.01	0.96–1.78

metastases about 1.5 hours after intravenous injection at a dose of 7.5, 10, and 15 mg were 0.84 to 3.0 and 0.96 to 3.18 μg/kg and were not in proportion to the administered doses (Table II). Blood levels of BLM in dogs that had undergone a single intramuscular injection at a dose of 1.0 mg/kg were higher than those in dogs that had undergone three intramuscular injections every 6 hours, each at a concentration of 0.33 mg/kg. On the other hand, BLM levels in the esophagus showed almost the same value in both groups, but those in the lung showed a lower value in the multiple injections of small doses than the single injection of a large dose (Fig. 3). To prevent pulmonary complications caused by BLM administration, multiple injections of small doses may be better than a single injection of a large dose.

The Sensitivities of Esophageal Cancer to Various Anticancer Drugs[1,4,5]

The sensitivities of esophageal cancer to various anticancer drugs were measured by the Inhibition of Nucleic Acid Synthesis (INAS) method invented by Higashi et al.,[6] using ^{3}H-thymidine for BLM, peplomysin (PEP), and cisplatin (CDDP) or ^{14}C-formate for 5-fluorouracil (5-FU) as a labeled precursor. Relatively uniform viable tumor tissues were obtained from fresh surgical specimens and sliced to about 500 μm in thickness. Tissue slices weighing 200 mg were preincubated with 0.5 ml anticancer drug solution and 1.8 ml TC 199-containing 20% calf serum for 4 hours, and followed by another 1-hour incubation with ^{3}H-thymidine or ^{14}C-formate at 6 μCi/ml as a labeled precursor. BLM solutions were added into the test mixtures

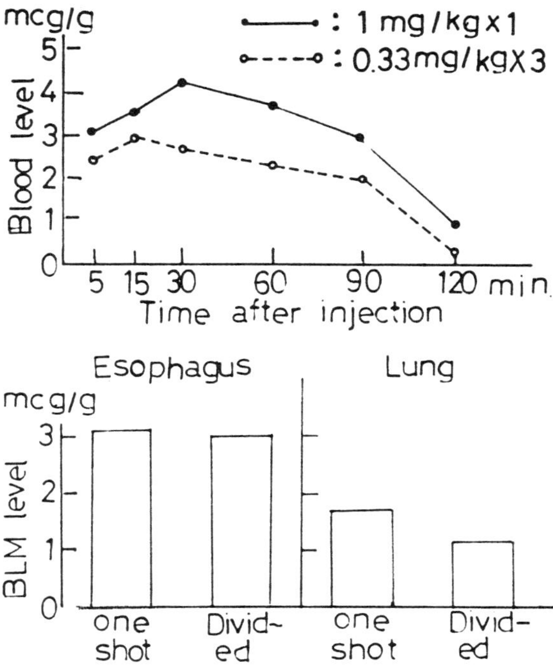

Figure 3: Comparison between single and multiple injections of bleomycin.

at a rate of 25, 5, 1, and 0.2 μg/ml, respectively, which corresponded to the peak blood levels following intravenous injection of normal doses. 5-FU solutions were added at a rate of 100, 10, and 1 mg/ml. The test mixtures were agitated and incubated at 37.5°C. After incubation for 5 hours, tumor tissues were removed. DNA was extracted from these tissues by the modified Schmidt-Thannhauser's method and its specific radioactivity was determined with a liquid scintillation spectrometer (Packard 3385). The quantity of DNA was determined by the diphenylamine method. Thereafter, the percent radioactivity (the ability of DNA synthesis) was determined by the following expression:

$$\begin{array}{c}\text{Percent radioactivity} \\ (\text{cpm}/\mu\text{g DNA})\end{array} = \frac{\text{Radioactivity of DNA (cpm/ml)}}{\text{Quantity of DNA } (\mu\text{g/ml})}$$

All of the test mixtures had duplicate controls. According to Higashi, the test was considered positive in the cases where DNA synthesis

Table III
Sensitivities of Esophageal Cancer to Various Anticancer Drugs

Anticancer Drug	No. of Patients	Sensitivity (+)	Sensitivity (−)	Positive Rate
BLM	77	43	34	56%
PEP	18	11	7	61%
CDDP	26	9	17	35%
5-FU	17	9	8	53%

Anticancer Drug	MultiSensitive Cases
BLM,CDDP,5-FU	3/25
BLM,CDDP	1/25
BLM,5-FU	1/25
CDDP,5-FU	4/25
Total	9/25

BLM = Bleomycin, PEP = Peplomycin, CDDP = Cisplatin, 5-FU = 5-Fluorouracil

of the tumor was inhibited below 70% of control; this standard value agreed with the results from clinical practice. The necessary concentrations of BLM for the main lesions in the sensitive cases were about 0.6 to 4 μg/ml, and those for the lymph node metastases were about 0.3 to 3 μg/ml.

Forty-three cases out of 77 (56%) were sensitive to BLM, 11 cases out of 18 (61%) to PEP, 9 cases out of 26 (35%) to CDDP, and 9 cases out of 17 (53%) to 5-FU. Sixteen cases out of 25 were sensitive to any of these drugs, and 9 cases out of 25 were sensitive to more than two drugs (Table III). This suggests that combination chemotherapy is effective in esophageal cancer patients. The well-differentiated squamous cell carcinomas showed a higher sensitivity rate than the moderately and poorly differentiated carcinomas and adenocarcinomas (Table IV). The sensitivities were higher in lymph node metastases than in main lesions, while cancer cells in the peripheral portions of the tumors showed higher sensitivities than those in the central portions.

Superficial and protruded types showed a higher sensitivity rate than the ulcerated type. Roentgenologically, the superficial and tumorous types showed a higher sensitivity rate than the serrated, fun-

Table IV
Results of Sensitivity Tests According to the Types of Histologic Findings

Histologic Findings	Sensitivity to BLM (+)		Sensitivity to BLM (−)		Total	
Well-differentiated squamous cell carcinoma	21		6		27	
Moderately differentiated squamous cell carcinoma	5	10	6	11	11	21
Poorly differentiated squamous cell carcinoma	4		2		6	
Adenocarcinoma	1		3		4	
Total	31		17		48	

BLM = Bleomycin, (p = 0.01)

neled, and spiral types. Patients who had not undergone preoperative treatment by radiotherapy or chemotherapy by means of BLM showed high sensitivity rates compared to patients who had undergone preoperative treatment with irradiation above 3,000 rads or administration of BLM above 60 mg.

The Results of Clinical Application of the Sensitivity Test[4,7]

The cumulative 4-year-survival rates in patients with esophageal cancer who had undergone curative resection and adjuvant chemoradiotherapy postoperatively, including 120 mg of intravenous BLM administration and 6,000 rads of T-shaped irradiation, were 50% in BLM-sensitive group and 28% in BLM-nonsensitive group (Fig. 4). No other differences were observed between these two groups as to the age and sex of patients or location and stage of lesions.

Conclusion

The sensitivities of esophageal cancer to various anticancer drugs showed considerable clinical variability and should be assessed prior to beginning adjuvant chemotherapy. Considering the sensitivity of

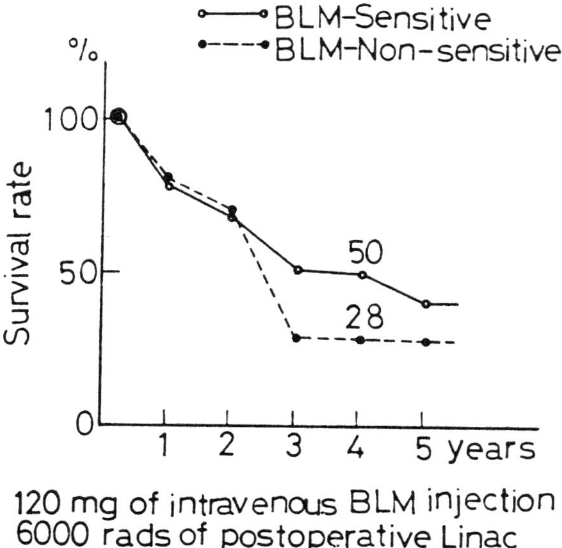

Figure 4: Cumulative survival rates in patients with esophageal cancers who had undergone curative resection and adjuvant chemoradiotherapy postoperatively.

esophageal cancer to BLM, the administration of BLM was thought to be almost adequate at the smallest among the doses of 5 to 15 mg. Adjuvant chemotherapy may contribute to improvement in the long-term results of radical operation for esophageal cancer.

References

1. Masaki Y: Studies on the sensitivities of esophageal cancer to anticancer agents and the supplementary chemotherapy combined with surgical treatment. Arch Jpn Chir 50:769, 1981.
2. Shibata G: Studies on supplementary chemotherapy combined with surgical treatment of carcinoma of the esophagus. Arch Jpn Chir 44:169, 1975.
3. Okubo H, Okamoto Y: Microassay of antibiotic levels in body fluids and tissues. Clin J Jpn 31:205, 1973.
4. Masaki Y, Ishigami K, Oka M, et al: Sensitivity of esophageal cancer to anticancer agents and supplementary chemotherapy combined with surgical treatment. Jpn J Cancer Chemother 13(Part II):1165, 1986.
5. Matsumoto N: A study of sensitivity of esophageal cancer to anticancer agents. Arch Jpn Chir 55:58, 1986.

6. Higashi H, Mori T, Takai S, et al: Selection of anticancer agents based upon inhibitory action on nucleic acid synthesis. Gekka Chiryo 33:253, 1975.
7. Hayashi H: Clinico-pathological studies and result of surgical treatment of esophageal cancer. Arch Jpn Chir 55:334, 1986.

34

Results of Surgery After Cisplatin and 5-FU Combination Chemotherapy for Locally Advanced Esophageal Squamous Cell Carcinoma

Alberto Peracchia, Pietro DeBesi, Carlo Castoro, Romeo Bardini, Antonella Ruffatto, Stefano Lazzaro, Silvia Toso

Introduction

The general prognosis of esophageal squamous cell carcinoma remains dismal. Neither new surgical procedures nor supervoltage radiotherapy have significantly improved long-term results for these patients, and 5-year overall survival rates do not exceed 10%.[1] Radical surgery remains a milestone among the therapeutic options against this tumor and must be performed when possible.[2] When surrounding organs are grossly involved by the primary tumor, palliation of dysphagia very often represents the only goal of treatment.[3]

In the recent past, our interest has been particularly devoted to this latter type of patient. This situation represents nearly 50% of our

Ferguson MK, Little AG, Skinner DB: Diseases of the Esophagus, Vol. I: Malignant Diseases. Futura Publishing Company, Inc., Mount Kisco, NY, © 1990.

experience, as nearly half of the almost 200 squamous cell esophageal cancer patients referred to our institution each year are not amenable to radical surgery. In this situation, alternative modalities such as radiotherapy and/or chemotherapy become essential weapons in our tactics. To this end, our group has adopted programs in which chemotherapy could play a major role in reducing the tumor mass with the aim of increasing its resectability. Prior to 1983, our antineoplastic treatment in advanced esophageal cancers consisted of a combination of cisplatin, bleomycin, and methotrexate, administered on an outpatient basis.[4] That combination was proved effective in one half of treated patients, but only 26% of them have really obtained an objective tumor regression. In early February 1983, we abandoned this chemotherapeutic approach for a new one consisting of cisplatin and fluorouracil, which had previously been shown to have a high response rate in epidermoid cancers of the head and neck, and was also tested in a small series of esophageal cancers.[5,6]

Materials and Methods

Between February 1983 and October 1988, 105 patients with esophageal cancer entered the study. All patients had histologically proven squamous cell carcinoma. Staging studies included barium swallow, upper aerodigestive tract endoscopy, CT scan, and esophageal ultrasonography demonstrating these to be locally advanced cancers (T4, any N, M0) following the TNM classification. Complete physical examination, ENT visit, and pulmonary function tests were obtained. Patients with severe cardiac, renal, or hepatic failure were excluded from the study.

The extreme ages at the time of study entry were 36 and 72 (mean, 56 years). The male:female ratio was 3:1. Karnofsky performance scores ranged from 60 to 90 (average, 80). No previous treatment had been performed in any patient. The patients were also instructed about the objective of the study in accordance with our institution policy and gave informed consent.

The treatment schedule consisted of 100 mg/m^2 of cisplatin in a 2-hour infusion on day 1, and of 1000 mg/m^2 of fluorouracil as a continuous 5-day infusion, along with allopurinol in a daily oral dosage of 600 mg.[7] Cisplatin was delivered along with adequate prehydration and posthydration; this regimen was repeated 3 or 4 weeks later if hematologic surveillance and renal function allowed it.[8] Antiemetics were administered with the above regimen consisting of metoclopramide given 30 minutes prior to the cisplatin infusion and repeated at 2-hour intervals as required.[9] The treatment was discontinued in case of progressive disease or major toxicity after the first course.

The response to chemotherapy was assessed after a minimum of two courses, repeating the initial staging procedures to evaluate possible surgery. Response was defined as clinically "complete" when total disappearance of sizable lesions occurred. "Partial" remission was defined as 50% volume reduction, whereas patients showing disease regression less than 50% were considered "nonresponders." The time to progression and overall survival were measured from the first day of treatment.

Results

The clinical objective response rate among all the patients was equal to 50% (10% complete and 40% partial). The side effects of chemotherapy for the entire patient population were primarily gastrointestinal and hematologic ranging from grade 1 to grade 3 of the World Health Organization scale. Moderate to severe nausea and vomiting were present in more than one half of patients after cisplatin infusion despite antiemetic medication. All patients experienced alopecia of varied degrees. Increase in the serum creatinine to >50% above baseline occurred in a few patients. Chemical phlebitis due to continuous fluorouracil infusion and mild stomatitis were frequently observed but were never dose-limiting. All but two treatment-related complications were considered reversible: one patient died because of persistent renal damage, probably related to cisplatin infusion and a second patient died of septicemia due to gram-negative organisms. Forty-four (42%) patients out of 105 underwent surgery after chemotherapy. The site of primary tumor in this group was as follows: cervical esophagus – 28%, upper thoracic – 36%, middle thoracic – 32%, and lower thoracic – 4%, respectively. Fifty-five percent of these patients had gross tracheobronchial invasion, 15% had laryngeal nerve palsy, and the remaining had mediastinal tumor spread. After surgery, 35 patients (80%) were classified as radically resected, whereas 9 (20%) had palliative resections. Pathological examination demonstrated a complete response in three cases (6.8%), while lymph node metastases were proved in 48% of cases.

Hospital mortality occurred in five patients (11.4%) and anastomotic leaks in 4 (9.1%). This incidence of death and leaks is not different from that seen in patients who underwent esophageal resection through a thoracotomy and reconstruction with a cervical anastomosis. The actuarial survival among operated patients was 76.8% at the first year and of 51.2% at the second; this latter figure was maintained during the third year. Two patients are alive and free of disease more than 4 years after operation.

Discussion

Patients with locally advanced esophageal cancers (T4) are usually considered poor candidates for radical surgery. These patients are usually eligible for palliation only, such as palliative resection, bypass, intubation, and laser therapy or radiotherapy.[10,11] In our experience, these palliative procedures lead to a median survival of only 7.8, 6.2, 4, and 4.1 months, respectively.[12] Radiotherapy has not shown any improvement in overall survival.[13] Chemotherapy, even when effective, did not improve survival in our previous experience, but only showed reduction of tumor mass.

Since 1983, we used cisplatin and fluorouracil as initial treatment for T4 esophageal cancers with the aim of reducing the tumor mass and followed by resection with radical intent.[14] Out of 105 patients, 35 (33%) underwent radical resection. The conversion to potentially radical surgery from palliative surgery has largely increased survival: one half of our resected patients are alive after 3 years. However, these data concern only the 44 resected cases, and long-term follow-up is not yet available to assess the full effects this program might have on survival.

The treatment-related morbidity and mortality rates were not negligible, but compare favorably to those observed in similar cases palliatively treated with intubation, laser, or surgical bypass.[12]

Our results cannot be compared with those of other authors[16,17] who report the use of chemotherapy in a neoadjuvant fashion. Our patients have been staged as having T4 primary tumor, while most cases in the literature appear to be operable at presentation.

In conclusion, we think that in locally advanced esophageal cancers for which conventional methods can only give transient relief of symptoms, combination chemotherapy is able to substantially modify the natural outcome. Such protocols should remain investigational until the hypotheses above are confirmed in a larger series.[18]

References

1. Kelsen DP, Ahuja R, Hopfan S, et al: Combined modality therapy of esophageal carcinoma. Cancer 48:31, 1981.
2. Skinner DB, Dowlatshahi KD, De Meester TR: Potentially curable cancer of the esophagus. Cancer 50:2571–2575, 1982.
3. Boyce HW Jr: Palliation of advanced esophageal cancer. Semin Oncol 11:186–195, 1984.
4. De Besi P, Salvagno L, Endrizzi L, et al: Cisplatin, bleomycin and methotrexate in the treatment of advanced oesophageal cancer. Eur J Cancer Clin Oncol 20:743–747, 1984.
5. Kish J, Drelichman A, Jacobs J, et al: Clinical trial of cisplatin and 5-FU infusion as initial treatment for advanced squamous cell carcinoma of the head and neck. Cancer Treat Rep 66:471–474, 1982.
6. Hellerstein S, Rosen S, Kies M, et al: Cis-Diaminedichloroplatinum (II) and 5-fluorouracil combined chemotherapy of epideroid esophageal cancer. Proc ASCO C-497, 1983.
7. De Besi P, Chiarion Sileni V, Salvagno L, et al: Phase II study of cisplatin, 5-FU, and allopurinol in advanced esophageal cancer. Cancer Treat Rep 70:909–910, 1986.
8. Vogl SE, Zaravinos T, Kaplan BH: Toxicity of cis-diaminedichloroplatinum (II) given in a two-hour out-patient regimen of diuresis and hydration. Cancer 45:11–15, 1980.
9. Gralla RJ, Itri LM, Pisko SE, et al: Antiemetic efficacy of high dose metoclopramide: Randomized trials with placebo and prochlorperazine in patients with chemotherapy-induced nausea and vomiting. N Engl J Med 305:905–909, 1981.
10. Orringer MB: Pallitive procedures for esophageal cancer. Surg Clin North Am 63:941–950, 1983.
11. Buset M, des Mares B, Baize M, et al: Palliative endoscopic management of obstructive esophagogastric cancer: Laser or prosthesis. Gastrointest Endosc 33:357–361, 1987.
12. Segalin A, Little AG, Ferguson MK, et al: Surgical and endoscopic palliation of esophageal carcinoma. Ann Thorac Surg 48:267, 1989.
13. Earlam R, Cunha-Melo JR: Oesophageal squamous cell carcinoma: II. A critical review of radiotherapy Br J Surg 67:457–461, 1980.
14. De Besi P, Chiarion-Sileni V, Salvagno L, et al: Systemic chemotherapy with cisplatin, 5-fluorouracil and allopurinol in the management of advanced epidermoid esophageal cancer. Recent Results Cancer Res 110:196–197, 1988.
15. Peracchia A, Bardini R, Toso S, De Besi P: Chimiotherapie preoperatoire et progres en chirurgie. Pathol Biol 37:142–143, 1989.
16. Bains M, Kelsen D, Beattie E, et al: Treatment of esophageal carcinoma by combined preoperative chemotherapy. Ann Thorac Surg 34:521–528, 1982.
17. Schlag P, Herrman R, Raeth V, et al: Neoadjuvant chemotherapy in esophageal cancer results of a phase II-trial (Abs) ECCO-4, 117, 1987.
18. Kelsen D: Multimodality therapy of esophageal carcinoma: Still an experimental approach. J Clin Oncol 5:530–531, 1987.

35

Postoperative Aggressive Chemotherapy for Thoracic Esophageal Carcinoma with Lymph Node Metastasis

Katsu Hirayama, Tetsuro Nishihira,
Michihiko Kitamura, Takashi Akaishi,
Ryuzaburo Shineha, Yasuaki Watanabe,
Akihiko Okayama, Yuji Goukon, Shozo Mori

Introduction

With the remarkable improvement of operative procedures and postoperative care, radical surgery for carcinoma of the thoracic esophagus can now be performed with safety.[1] However, long-term survival is still poor even in patients with curative resection of the primary lesion.[2] The prognosis of thoracic esophageal cancer patients without node metastasis has improved markedly with the administration of postoperative radio-chemoimmunotherapy, indicating that such therapy prevents the recurrence of micrometastasis after curative surgery.[1,2] However, the prognosis of thoracic esophageal cancer patients with node metastases is poor regardless of radical surgery including lymphadenectomy and the use of postoperative combined therapy. Therefore, for the purpose of obtaining better survival, a

Ferguson MK, Little AG, Skinner DB: Diseases of the Esophagus, Vol. I: Malignant Diseases. Futura Publishing Company, Inc., Mount Kisco, NY, © 1990.

new therapeutic regimen employing aggressive chemotherapy has been attempted since 1980,[3,4] using a dose twice that of the conventional regimen. In this chapter, we describe the long-term evaluation of such treatment and discuss its effectiveness in comparison with that of other therapies.

Materials and Methods

Patients with thoracic esophageal cancer presenting from 1975 to 1987 underwent routine postoperative adjuvant therapies. During this period, resection was performed in 375 (77.2%) of 486 patients with carcinoma of the thoracic esophagus; curative resection was done in 310 patients. Death within 30 days after operation occurred in 10 patients. All patients underwent radical surgery for cancer of the thoracic esophagus which was completely macroscopically resected. The same procedure was also employed for lymph node dissection with right thoracotomy. Reconstruction of the esophagus was performed mainly with gastric tube or, in some cases, with pedicled jejunum through the retrosternal route or the retromediastinal route.

Selection of postoperative combined therapy was done in accordance with the degree of lymph node metastasis confirmed with microscopic examination of surgical specimens. Postoperative radiochemoimmunotherapy was performed in combination with prophylactic T-shaped irradiation to the neck and mediastinum to a total dose of 4,000 rads (200 rads each, five times a week) and chemoimmunotherapy (FT-207, pepleomycin, OK-432 and/or PSK).

Patients with positive node metastases underwent one of two protocols. PAM therapy consisted of 5 mg/day of pepleomycin as synchronizer continuously infused for 4 days, and 2 mg/kg of adriamycin given on the fifth day. Three to 4 weeks later, pepleomycin and mitomycin C (0.5 mg/kg) were given. This regimen was repeated once, the doses being twice as high as the conventional doses for Japanese patients. PAM therapy was attempted in 24 patients. F-CAV therapy was composed of 5-FU, cisplatin, adriamycin, and vindesine. The total dose and schedule for administration are shown in Figure 1. It was attempted in 17 patients.

Evaluation was based on a historical control study, and 5-year survival rates were calculated using the Kaplan-Meier method,[5] and included deaths due to unrelated diseases. The terms regarding lymph node metastasis used in this text are in accordance with the guidelines specified by the Japanese Society for Esophageal Diseases.[6]

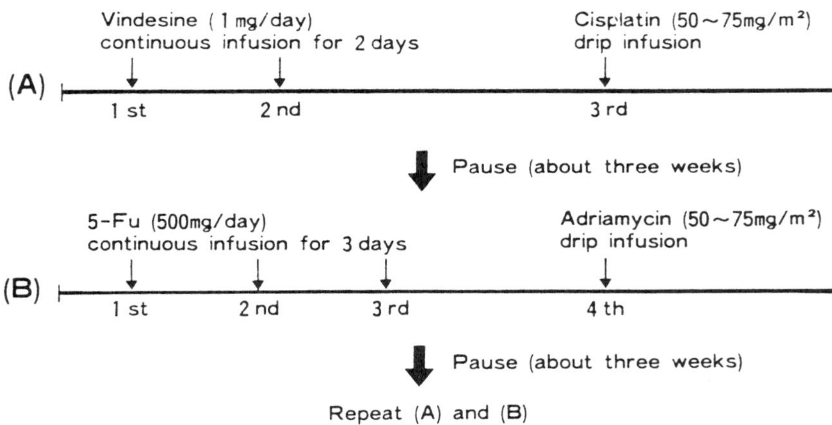

Figure 1: Schedule of postoperative aggressive chemotherapy for thoracic esophageal cancer patients with lymph node metastases.

Results

The prognosis of thoracic esophageal cancer patients with curative resection correlated with the degree of lymph node metastases. Patients with negative lymph nodes had a 45.1% 5-year survival rate, even when they had no postoperative combined therapies. This was elevated to 50.3% with postoperative radiotherapy, and to 73.5% with postoperative radio-chemoimmunotherapy. Patients with regional lymph node metastasis [n1(+), n2(+)] showed a 24.0% 5-year survival rate without postoperative combined therapy. Survival was lowered with postoperative radiotherapy, but was elevated to 34.2% with radio-chemoimmunotherapy. Patients with distant lymph node metastasis [n3(+), n4(+)] had a very poor prognosis without postoperative combined therapy. They showed no improvement in long-term prognosis even with postoperative prophylactic irradiation or radio-chemoimmunotherapy. Only two patients with postoperative radiotherapy survived for more than 2 years (Fig. 2).

The 5-year survival rate of patients with n1(+), n2(+) treated with aggressive chemotherapy was 35.0%, which was almost similar to the corresponding rate (34.2%) for patients treated with radio-chemoimmunotherapy. The outcome of the patients with n3(+), n4(+) who underwent aggressive chemotherapy is shown in Figure 2. The 1-, 2-, 3- and 5-year survival rates were 55.9%, 40.6%, 30.5%, and

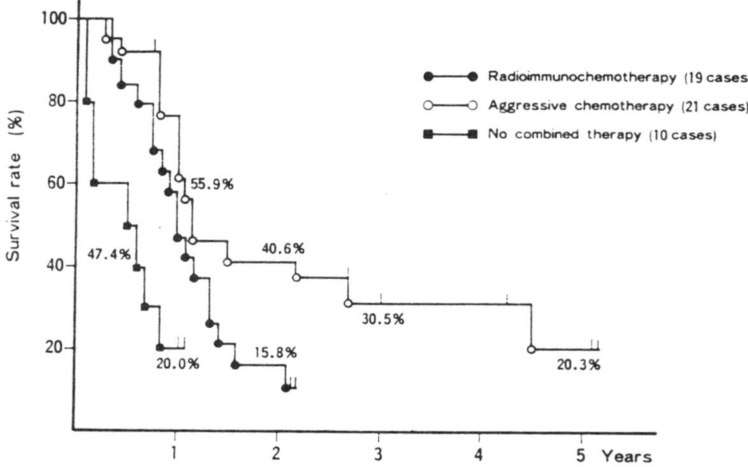

Figure 2: Survival rate of thoracic esophageal cancer patients with distant lymph node metastases after curative surgery.

20.3%, respectively. The 2-year survival rate of the 19 patients who received radio-chemoimmunotherapy was 15.8%, and there were significant differences in survival rates between aggressive chemotherapy and radio-chemoimmunotherapy ($p = 0.002$). As shown in Figure 3, there was no significant difference in prognosis between PAM and F-CAV treatment.

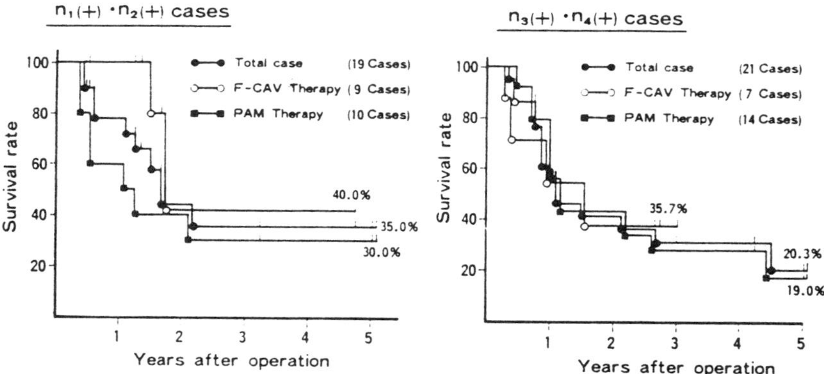

Figure 3: Survival of thoracic esophageal cancer patients undergoing post-operative aggressive chemotherapy.

Side effects such as nausea, anorexia, alopecia, and severe bone marrow suppression were commonly observed during chemotherapy. However, the intensity of such symptoms was milder with F-CAV than with PAM treatment. The frequency of organ dysfunction with each treatment was nearly the same. Active enteral and parenteral nutritional support of 40 to 45 kcal/kg daily was absolutely necessary to complete the regimens. The rate of completion of PAM and F-CAV was 71% and 74%, respectively.

There was a higher rate of recurrence in the neck and/or mediastinum in patients who received aggressive chemotherapy than in those who underwent postoperative prophylactic radiotherapy.

Discussion

The primary aim of the present study was to clarify whether or not appropriate adjuvant chemotherapy can improve the prognosis of patients with positive lymph node metastases. Postoperative radio-chemoimmunotherapy improved the 5-year survival rate of patients without lymph node metastases to 73.5% compared with 45.1% of patients not receiving any postoperative combined therapy. In cases of n1(+) and n2(+), the 5-year survival rate of patients treated with aggressive chemotherapy (35.0%) was similar to the corresonding rate (34.2%) for patients treated with radio-chemoimmunotherapy. In cases of n3(+) and n4(+), remarkable improvement of the prognosis of patients who received aggressive chemotherapy was noted compared with the prognosis of patients who received radio-chemoimmunotherapy.

Thus far there has been scant evidence in the literature that adjuvant chemotherapy is effective in prolonging the survival of esophageal cancer patients with lymph node metastasis. The present study strongly suggests that the prognosis of patients with node metastasis can be improved to some extent if aggressive chemotherapy is applied. It has also been shown that active nutritional support is necessary to overcome the inevitable severe side effects.

References

1. Nishihira T, Watanabe T, Kasai M, et al. Long-term evaluation of patients treated by radical operation for carcinoma of the thoracic esophagus. World J Surg 8:778–785, 1984.

2. Kasai M, Mori S, Watanabe T: Follow-up results after resection of thoracic esophageal carcinoma. World J Surg 2:543–551, 1978.
3. Nishihira T, Hirayama K, Kasai M, et al. Postoperative aggressive chemotherapy with nutritional support in cases of thoracic esophageal cancer with distant lymph node metastasis. In: Cancer Chemotherapy: Challenges for the Future, Kimura K (ed), Tokyo, Excerpta Medica, 1985, pp 165–173.
4. Nishihira T, Hirayama K, Mori S, et al. Aggressive adjuvant therapy prolongs survival of patients with metastatic carcinoma of the thoracic esophagus. Dis Esoph 1989 (in press).
5. Kaplan EL, Meier P: Nonparametric estimation for incomplete observation. J Am Stat Assoc 53:457–460, 1958.
6. Japanese Society for Esophageal Diseases: Guidelines for the clinical and pathologic studies on carcinoma of the esophagus. Jpn J Surg 6:69–86, 1976.

36

Histopathologic and Long-Term Effects of Hyperthermia Combined with Chemotherapy and Irradiation for Esophageal Carcinoma

Hiroyuki Matsuda, Shin-ichi Tsutsui, Masaaki Nagamatsu, Shinji Ohno, Masaki Mori, Hiroyuki Kuwano, Keizo Sugimachi

Introduction

It has been shown that hyperthermia is particularly effective for the treatment of carcinoma, when applied concomitantly with irradiation and chemotherapy[1,2] However, the clinical application of hyperthermia in cases of esophageal carcinoma presents problems because an appropriate apparatus for selective application of heat to the esophageal lesion has not been available. We designed an endotract electrode for radiofrequency delivery,[3] and clinically applied hyperthermia combined with chemotherapy and irradiation, so called hyperthermo-chemo-radiotherapy (HCR therapy) to patients with both resectable and nonresectable carcinoma of the esophagus. We report herein the histopathological effectiveness of hyperthermia in resected

Ferguson MK, Little AG, Skinner DB: Diseases of the Esophagus, Vol. I: Malignant Diseases. Futura Publishing Company, Inc., Mount Kisco, NY, © 1990.

specimens and the long-term results on survival in cases of both resectable and nonresectable carcinoma of the esophagus.

Methods and Patients

Hyperthermia for esophageal carcinoma was clinically applied using a radiofrequency system with an endotract electrode. A thin, long electrode placed in the esophagus and a broad, wide counter electrode placed on the body surface make localization of the electromagnetic field at the esophagus feasible and properly heats the lesion. The temperature of the endotract electrode is controlled by a water cooling system within a balloon.[3]

Eighty-eight patients were given preoperative hyperthermia combined with chemotherapy and irradiation (HCR therapy) and another 122 were treated with irradiation and chemotherapy preoperatively (CR therapy). In the majority of patients, the operation was carried out in one stage. Subtotal esophagectomy and lymph node dissection were performed through a right thoracotomy, and esophageal reconstruction was done with a gastric tube through the antesternal route. The regimen of preoperative HCR therapy in patients with resectable carcinoma was as follows: irradiation (1.5–2.0 Gy daily) with Co-60 or x-ray given 5 days a week. Two fractions a week were combined with chemotherapy and hyperthermia (42.5–45°C for 30 minutes) plus 5 mg of bleomycin, given intravenously within 1 hour after the irradiation.

The histopathological effectiveness of the preoperative therapy was evaluated according to guidelines for clinical and pathological studies on carcinoma of the esophagus.[4] Lesions in which viable neoplastic cells were destroyed were defined as Ef_3, and lesions in which most of cancer cells were extensively damaged, despite a few viable cells, were defined as Ef_2. All others were categorized as Ef_1. Treatment for the lesions showing Ef_2 or Ef_3 was considered effective.

There were another 124 patients, none of whom underwent resection for esophageal carcinoma. These patients were divided into two groups according to treatment status: 36 received HCR therapy, and the other 88 were treated with CR therapy but not with hyperthermia. Far advanced tumorous processes and associated severe diseases were the main reasons why resection could not be done. There were no significant differences between the groups with regard to prognostic factors such as age, sex, site of carcinoma, and TNM stage.

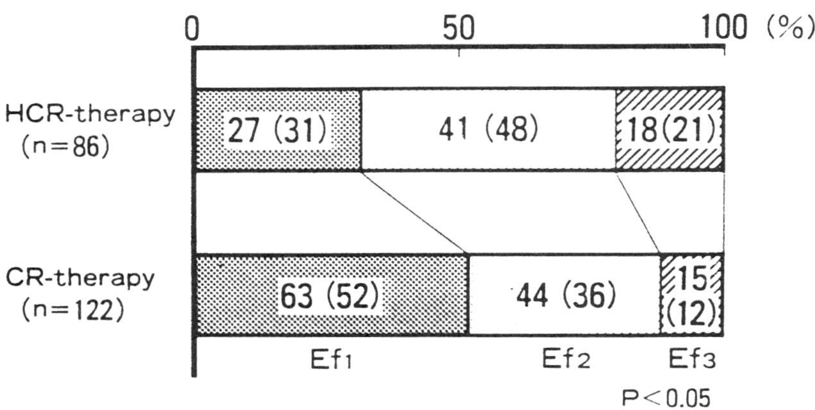

Figure 1: Histopathological effectiveness in the resected cases. In the resected specimens, preoperative HCR resulted in a significantly higher histopathological effectiveness rate (69%, n=86) compared with that in cases treated by CR (48%, n=122) ($p<0.05$). Lesions in which viable neoplastic cells were destroyed were defined as Ef_3, and lesions in which most of the cancer cells were extensively damaged, despite of a few viable cells, were defined as Ef_2.

For patients with nonresectable carcinoma of the esophagus, the same regimen of HCR therapy was prescribed and was continued as many times as possible. There was no statistical difference among the groups with regard to doses of irradiation and chemotherapy.

Results

In the resected cases, preoperative HCR resulted in a significantly higher histopathological effectiveness rate (69%, n=86) compared with that in cases treated by CR (48%, n=122) ($p<0.05$) (Fig. 1).

Survival rates of patients given preoperative HCR therapy, and the control group (preoperative CR therapy) are shown in Table I. Three-year survival rates in the HCR group and the control group were 31.3% and 19.4%, respectively. Survival rates of patients given HCR therapy were significantly better than those of patients given CR therapy preoperatively ($p<0.05$, generalized Wilcoxon test). In particular, for the patients classified as TNM stages III and IV, a significantly longer survival was obtained with preoperative HCR.

Table II shows survival rates of patients with nonresectable carcinoma of the esophagus. Survival rates at 12 months in patients given

Table I
Survival Rates of Surgically Treated Patients

Groups*	No. of Patients	Survival Rate (%) 1 Year	2 Years	3 Years
HCR	88	71.3	47.0	31.3
CR	122	47.6	25.9	19.4
(TNM stages III, IV)				
HCR	37	68.1	35.0	30.0
CR	69	31.6	17.3	8.6
			(Kaplan-Meier procedure)	

* HCR: patients given preoperative hyperthermia combined with chemotherapy and irradiation.
CR: patients treated with irradiation and chemotherapy preoperatively, but not hyperthermia.

HCR and CR were 35.1% and 10.2%, respectively, and rates at 24 months were 9.6% and 1.1%, respectively. There is a statistical difference favoring HCR therapy, as compared with CR therapy ($p<0.05$). In particular, for the patients classified as TNM stages I and II, a significantly longer survival was obtained with HCR in these nonresectable cases.

Table II
Survival Rates of Patients with Unresectable Carcinoma

Groups*	No. of Patients	Survival Rate (%) 0.5 Years	1 Year	1.5 Years	2 Years
HCR	36	62.9	35.1	24.6	9.6
CR	88	52.3	10.2	1.1	1.1
(TNM stages I, II)					
HCR	14	85.7	63.5	47.6	35.7
CR	29	70.0	20.7	3.5	3.5
				(Kaplan-Meier procedure)	

* HCR: patients given preoperative hyperthermia combined with chemotherapy and irradiation.
CR: patients treated with irradiation and chemotherapy preoperatively, but not hyperthermia.

Discussion

As we have already reported,[5] when cancer cells of the esophagus are extensively damaged preoperatively, the 5-year survival rate of patients treated with surgery was 45.1%. Therefore, it is very important to enhance the direct effect of irradiation to cancer cells before the surgery. Our data on histopathological and long-term effects of hyperthermia combined with chemotherapy and irradiation suggest that proper hyperthermia combined with radiation and chemotherapy shows great promise for treating patients with esophageal carcinoma. As local hyperthermia has no severe side effects, this treatment is thought to be an interesting modality to be considered in patients with a malignant lesion such as carcinoma of the esophagus.

References

1. Dewey WC: Interaction of heat with radiation and chemotherapy. Cancer Res 44:4714, 1984.
2. Manning MR, Cetas TC, Miller RC, et al: Clinical hyperthermia: Results of a phase 1 trial employing hyperthermia alone or in combination with external beam or interstitial radiotherapy. Cancer 49:205, 1982.
3. Sugimachi K, Inokuchi K, Kai H, et al: Endotract antenna for application of hyperthermia to malignant lesions. Gann 74:622, 1983.
4. Japanese Society of Esophageal Disease: Guidelines for clinical and pathological studies on carcinoma of the esophagus. Jpn J Surg 6:69, 1976.
5. Sugimachi K, Matsufuji H, Kai H, et al: Preoperative irradiation for carcinoma of the esophagus. Surg Gynecol Obstet 162:174, 1986.

37

Adjuvant Hyperthermia in Nonresectable Esophageal Carcinoma

Masao Fujimaki, Hiroshi Katoh, Kenji Tazawa, Iwao Yamashita, Takashi Sakamoto, Akira Yamada

Introduction

The multidisciplinary treatment approach is extremely important in advanced nonresectable cases of esophageal carcinoma. The effectiveness of hyperthermia was demonstrated in a basic study carried out on three cell lines established from human esophageal carcinoma in the authors' department. With the development by Sugimachi of a hyperthermia applicator for use in the esophageal lumen in 1983,[1] it became possible to perform hyperthermia at selected sites. Since 1985 hyperthermia has been applied in combination with radiotherapy and chemotherapy in cases requiring preoperative treatment and in nonresectable cases.[2] This chapter describes the effectiveness of hyperthermia in multidisciplinary treatment.

Materials and Methods

Hyperthermia was performed in 12 cases of advanced esophageal carcinoma (Table I). Ages ranged from 55 to 81, the average age being

Ferguson MK, Little AG, Skinner DB: Diseases of the Esophagus, Vol. I: Malignant Diseases. Futura Publishing Company, Inc., Mount Kisco, NY, © 1990.

Table I

Case No.	Sex	Age	Location	Tumor Length	Radiologic Findings	Endoscopic Findings	Stage
1	M	81	Imlu	10 cm	spiral	elevated	IV A_3
2	M	65	ImEilu	17 cm	funneled	depressed	IV A_3
3	M	59	Eilm	9.5 cm	funneled	elevated	IV $N_4(+)$
4	M	61	ImEi	11 cm	serrated	depressed	IV $N_4(+)$
5	M	71	Iulm	7.5 cm	spiral	depressed	IV A_3
6	M	72	ImEi	12.2 cm	spiral	depressed	IV A_3
7	M	67	Im	4.0 cm	tumorous	elevated	IV $N_4(+)$
8	M	77	Imlu	10.0 cm	spiral	depressed	IV A_3
9	M	60	Ph			depressed	IV $N_4(+)$
10	M	55	Imlu	14.0 cm	serrated	depressed	IV $N_4(+)$
11	M	75	ImEilu	7.0 cm	spiral	depressed	IV A_3
12	F	55	Ce	5.0 cm	spiral	depressed	IV A_3

Ph = pharyngeal, Ce = cervical, Iu = upper thoracic, Im = middle thoracic, Ei = lower thoracic.

66.5, and the male:female ratio was 11:1. The tumor was in the hypopharyngeal region in one case, cervical esophagus in one, and the remaining 10 were in the thoracic esophagus. The length of the tumors varied from 4.0 cm to 17.0 cm, with an average of 9.7 cm. Apart from the single hypopharyngeal case, the roentgenological findings showed tumorous type in one case, serrated type in two cases, spiral type in six, and funnel type in two cases. The endoscopic findings showed protruding type tumors in three cases, and depressed type in nine cases. Biopsy or resected specimens revealed three cases to be well-differentiated, six moderately, and two poorly differentiated squamous cell carcinomas. There was one case of small cell carcinoma. All 12 cases were advanced, and prior to treatment the esophageal submucosal esophagography, CT, and fiberoptic bronchoscopy showed seven cases to be A_3 and five to be $N_{4(+)}$. Cases 7 and 11 complained of hoarseness which was attributed to swelling of the upper mediastinal lymph nodes. Hypercalcemia was recognized in case 1 before treatment.

As is shown in Figure 1, the therapeutic strategy consisted of twin portal irradiation of 2 Gy per day, 5 days per week for a total of 15 sessions (30 Gy), combined with a total of 75 mg bleomycin (10 doses of 7.5 mg delivered in continuous 24-hour subcutaneous infusions) and twice-weekly hyperthermia for a total of six sessions.

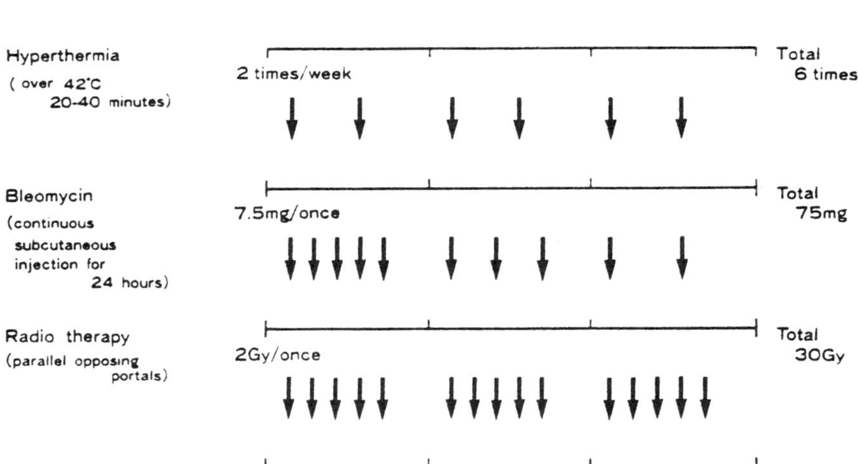

Figure 1: Protocol for combined chemotherapy.

For hyperthermia, two extracorporeal applicators (IH-500T model RF, 13.56 MHz, Japan Crescent Inc., Tokyo, Japan) were placed on the anterior and posterior chest wall and an intraesophageal applicator (Second Department of Surgery Toyama Medical and Pharmaceutical University Model) was inserted into the esophagus for internal hyperthermia. In the case of the hypopharyngeal tumor, the applicator could not be inserted and hyperthermia was carried out with a Thermotron RF8. A temperature sensor was placed on the surface of the tumor and a temperature of more than 42°C maintained for 20–40 minutes was considered sufficient for effective hyperthermia.

Evaluation of effectiveness was performed by endoscopic and roentgenologic examination 1 month after the completion or cessation of treatment.

Results

The results are shown in Table II. Hyperthermia was performed between two and nine times, 4.9 times on average. The temperature and RF wave output changes during the treatment of case 11 are shown in Figure 2. The hypercalcemia that had been recognized prior

Table II

Case No.	No. of Hyperthermia	Combined Therapy	Local Response	Operation	Prognosis (cause of death)
1	5	R: 30 Gy	NC	by-pass	6M dead (cancer)
2	9	R: 80 Gy, BLM: 140 mg, CDDP: 500 mg FT-207: 263 25 g	CR	(−)	3Y 4M alive
3	3	R: 30 Gy, BLM: 75 mg, CDDP: 100 mg	PR	blunt dissection	4M dead (intra-abdominal bleeding)
4	4	R: 30 Gy, BLM: 75 mg	CR	esophagectomy	1Y 1M dead (bone and skin metastasis)
5	5	R: 30 Gy, BLM; 75 mg	PR	esophagectomy	6M dead (pneumonia)
6	2	R: 60 Gy, O-BLM: 300 mg	PR	(−)	1Y dead (cancer)
7	2	R: 60 Gy, BLM: 90 mg, CDDP: 200 mg	CR	(−)	1Y 4M dead (cancer)
8	8	R: 45 Gy, BLM: 75 mg, CDDP: 100 mg	PR	(−)	10M dead (cancer)
9	6	R: 36 Gy, BLM: 90 mg, CDDP: 100 mg	PR	cervical esophagectomy	10M dead (cancer)
10	5	R: 64 Gy, BLM: 75 mg, CDDP: 24 mg	NC	(−)	3M dead (cancer)
11	9	R: 45 Gy, BLM: 65 mg, CDDP: 150 mg	CR	(−)	9M dead (liver metastasis)
12	5	R: 30 Gy, BLM: 75 mg	CR	cervical esophagectomy	1Y 2M alive

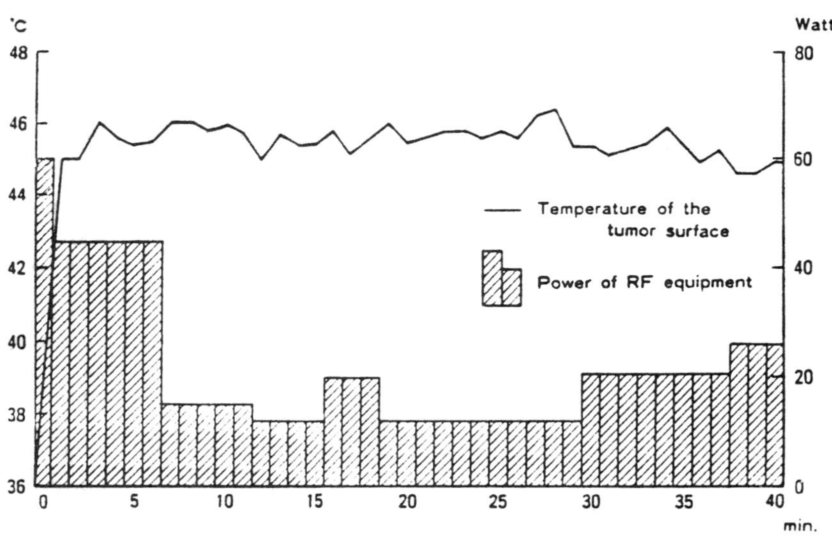

Figure 2: Esophageal temperature changes during hyperthermia.

to commencement of treatment in case 1 was seen to improve and the hoarseness in cases 7 and 11 caused by the mediastinal lymphadenopathy disappeared after treatment. The dysphagia that had been present prior to treatment in all cases disappeared in all but one case. According to the results of evaluation of local effects, there were five complete responses (CR), five partial responses (PR), and no change (NC) in two cases. If effectiveness is considered to be the total of CR and PR cases, then the overall effectiveness was 83.3%. After treatment, surgical resection was performed in six cases, including bypass in one, thoracic esophagectomy in three (one case of blunt dissection), and cervical esophagopharyngolaryngectomy in two cases. The postsurgical evaluation of effectiveness using the resected specimens was Ef_3 in two cases, Ef_2 in two cases, and Ef_1 in one case.

Concerning posttherapeutic courses, the two NC cases succumbed 3 and 6 months later. The six PR cases succumbed at 4, 6, 10 (two cases), 12, and 13 months. Case 4 showed CR and underwent thoracic esophagectomy. The resected specimen revealed Ef_3, but viable cells were recognized in one portion of the dissected cervical lymph nodes and widespread bone and skin metastases were present 13 months later when he died. Case 11 was a case of small cell carcinoma and showed CR. At 9 months, the general condition was good when multiple liver metastasis suddenly appeared and he succumbed within a short time. The other two CR cases are still alive, apparently disease-free, and the longest survivor has had a posttreatment course of 3 years and 4 months.

During hyperthermia itself, no change in general condition was noted, but during the period of treatment leukocytopenia due to bone marrow suppression was recognized as a complication in three cases and transient renal dysfunction was recognized in one case in which CDDP was also administered. There was one case of radiation gastritis and another case with bilateral blindness caused by fungal uveitis.

Discussion

Although the results of treatment of esophageal carcinoma have improved in association with developments in surgical technique, the results in advanced cases are not yet satisfactory. The 12 cases described in the present paper were all stage IV cases treated by a combination of radiotherapy, chemotherapy, and hyperthermia. A CR was obtained in five cases and a PR in five cases, yielding an overall effective rate of 83.3%. Improvements in the hyperthermia applicator made it safe and simple to maintain the tumor surface temperature between 42°C and 45°C and hyperthermia in the future is planned with temperatures around 45°C (Fig. 2).

Complications included leukocytopenia as a result of bone marrow suppression in three cases (25%), but all cases recovered after being placed in a clean room for 10–14 days. However, there were other serious complications, consisting of one case of bilateral blindness due to fungal uveitis and one case of impaired passage of food as a result of radiation gastritis. These aspects will require careful consideration in the future.

Cases 4 and 11 showed CR but these succumbed due to hematogenic metastasis at 11 and 9 months, respectively. This emphasizes the importance of treatment of widespread hematogenic and lymphatic metastasis in advanced esophageal carcinoma. Case 2 showed local recurrence at 1 year after treatment, but further combined treatment, including hyperthermia, once more obtained CR. These results indicate the effectiveness of hyperthermia in long-term multidisciplinary treatment of advanced esophageal carcinoma.

References

1. Sugimachi K, Inokuchi K, Kai H, Sogawa A, Kawai Y: A newly devised endotract antenna for hyperthermotherapy for cancer patients. Gann 74:622–624, 1983.
2. Fujimaki M, Soga J, Kawaguchi M, Maeda M, Sasaki K, Tanaka O, Muto T: Role of preoperative administration of bleomycin and radiation in the treatment of esophageal cancer. Jpn J Surg 5:48–55, 1975.
3. Japanese Society for Esophageal Disease: Guidelines for the Clinical and Pathologic Studies on Carcinoma of the Esophagus, 7th ed, Kanehara, Tokyo, 1989.

V.

Palliative Therapy:
Editors' Overview

The previous two sections dealt, rather optimistically, with methods for achieving a potential cure in patients with esophageal cancer. Unfortunately, the vast majority of patients will present with disease at such an advanced state that no thought of cure is possible, or they will experience progressive disease despite all efforts to forestall it. Providing palliative therapy for these patients remains an important function of surgical and medical oncologists. Historical techniques for palliating malignant obstruction consisted primarily of a feeding gastrostomy with or without a diverting cervical esophagostomy. These methods resulted in little improvement in either quality of life or duration of survival. True palliation of malignant obstruction was first achieved with regularity through the use of intubation techniques. This section outlines improvements in both equipment for and methods of intubation, and illustrates newer laser modalities that provide complementary benefits in these patients.

The first three chapters compare intraluminal palliative methods for obstructing esophageal cancer. In Chapter 38, Fuchs and co-workers present a randomized comparison of endoscopic laser therapy versus endoscopic intubation for obstructing esophageal carcinoma. Laser therapy employed the Nd-YAG laser in a retrograde fashion without the use of contact fibers, while intubation was performed using the Celestine-Medoc tubes. The data demonstrate no significant advantage of one technique over the other, and show that the typical degree of palliation is not very substantial. Similar findings are reported in Chapter 39 by Juettner et al. who compare sequential therapy of dilation, Nd-YAG laser therapy, and prothesis insertion with intraluminal irradiation using high-dose rate ^{192}Ir. Their data demonstrate that no single palliative technique is optimal for every patient, and that complication rates are substantial even for the least aggressive techniques. Finally, Moraldi and his co-workers present results of a prospective randomized study comparing Nd-YAG laser therapy to intubation for management of nonresectable obstructing cancers. In contrast to the previous reports, they find that the incidence of morbidity and mortality is greater in patients undergoing intubation than those having laser therapy. Although neither treatment appears to provide a survival advantage, they recommend that Nd-YAG laser be the first choice of palliative therapy in patients with obstructive symptoms due to nonresectable esophageal cancer. With the wide variety of palliative techniques currently available, it is clear that further prospective randomized studies will be necessary before an algorithm for optimal patient care can be constructed.

In the mid-1980's, exciting new therapeutic possibilities became available with the introduction of commercial high-powered medical Nd-YAG lasers. Substantial experience is now extant, demonstrating important clinical benefits with this technique. In Chapter 41, Norberto and his colleagues present results of one of the largest series ever published of patients with inoperable esophageal cancer treated with Nd-YAG laser therapy. Their findings, which should serve as a standard for palliative laser therapy, demonstrate substantial benefit in most patients accompanied by an acceptable degree of morbidity and mortality. They caution, however, that laser therapy should be used in concert with other therapeutic modalities for optimal management of obstructing cancers.

In addition to the exciting introduction of YAG laser therapy in the mid-1980's, a second laser modality was pioneered which is still in a decidedly investigative form. Using low-power laser light, photoactive compounds are stimulated to release toxic oxygen metabolites into cancerous tissues causing selective death of neoplastic cells. This process is termed "photodynamic therapy," or PDT. In Chapter 42, Monnier and his colleagues report results of PDT in 25 patients with early stage pharyngo-esophageal carcinomas. Their findings support the potential clinical benefit of photodynamic therapy in treating superficial squamous cell cancers. Unfortunately, technical problems in the therapy remain to be solved, including establishing accurate laser light dosimetry and improving selective retention of the photosensitive compound by neoplastic cells. As there are a large number of photoactive compounds available, the prospect of being able to selectively kill tumor cells while leaving the normal tissues undamaged through this method remains quite real, and exciting improvements are on the horizon.

In Chapter 43, Peracchia et al. describe recommendations for management of one of the most vexing problems associated with esophageal cancer, malignant respiratory tract fistula. A number of palliative techniques for these patients are available, but the most effective ones in their hands appear to be gastric bypass and intubation, selected according to the general condition of the patient. With continued improvements in intubation techniques, this method of management will likely become the first choice of therapy in the future for patients with malignant esophageal-respiratory fistula.

38

Randomized Comparison of Endoscopic Palliation of a Malignant Esophageal Stenosis

K.-H. Fuchs, S. Freys, H. Schaube, A.-K. Eckstein

Introduction

Unfortunately, in most patients with cancer of the esophagus and cardia curative resection is not possible because of advanced disease. Even palliative resection is limited to the few patients with fairly restricted tumor invasion and acceptable general condition. The majority of patients with cancer of the esophagus in an unselected clinic population will depend on palliation via "minimal invasive surgery," endoscopic procedures, and/or radiotherapy. The advantage of palliative irradiation is the low incidence of early complication in contrast to most endoscopic techniques. Nevertheless, a variety of endoscopy-related palliative procedures with or without combination of minimal surgery have been developed and introduced in the past decade. The two major competing procedures are endoscopic tube implantation (ETI) and endoscopic laser therapy (ELT). Both techniques have been shown to be successful in treating malignant stenosis.[1–4]

It has been reported that the combination of ELT and afterloading irradiation appears to be advantageous in comparison to ELT alone.[5] Bader states that endocavitary afterloading irradiation prolongs the effect of laser therapy. The purpose of this study is to compare ETI

Ferguson MK, Little AG, Skinner DB: Diseases of the Esophagus, Vol. I: Malignant Diseases. Futura Publishing Company, Inc., Mount Kisco, NY, © 1990.

and ELT, the latter in combination with afterloading irradiation, as to their applicability, their early and late complication rate, their effect on the patients' quality of life, and their cost-benefit ratio.

Material and Methods

All patients referred to the Endoscopic Unit of the Department of General Surgery at the University Hospital Kiel from January 1, 1987, to December 31, 1988, for palliative treatment with inoperable cancer of the esophagus or cardia were evaluated. The data obtained from 82 patients (51 male, 31 female) were prospectively registered and documented. The spectrum of palliative treatment of cancer of the esophagus and cardia in our unit includes: endoscopic tube implantation (ETI), endoscopic laser therapy (ELT), percutaneous endoscopic gastrostomy (PEG), transnasal feeding tube (TFT), radiotherapy (RT), and endoscopic bougienage (EB). Since it was the aim of this study to compare laser therapy versus tube implantation, those patients who met the following criteria were randomized to an ELT or to an ETI group: (1) dysphagia allowing intake of semi-solid food at best, (2) tumor anatomy allowing either procedure, and (3) absence of fistulae. All other patients were comprised in an escape group, presenting with either tumor invasion in the upper esophagus from pharyngeal, laryngeal, bronchial or mediastinal tumors, esophagotracheal fistula formation, esophageal squamous cell carcinoma with dysphagia limited to solid food only with good prospects for successful radiotherapy, or an extremely poor general condition only allowing minimal manipulation. The patient characteristics of the ELT, ETI, and the escape group are listed in Table I.

Only 23 patients met the criteria to be randomized. After their randomization, three patients initially started on ETI had to be withdrawn from this therapy because of a high risk of tube dislocation. Therefore, we finally treated 14 patients with ELT and nine patients with ETI.

ELT was performed using the neodymium YAG laser (MBB Medizin-technik GmbH München); depending on the grade of stenosis, the laser probe was passed through an Olympus GIF-Q 10 or GIF-1T 10 fiberoptic endoscope. Endoscopic tumor resection with the laser was performed at a distance of approximately 0.5 to 1 cm from the tumor tissue, with a pulse duration of 0.5 to 5 seconds using energies between 60 and 100 watts. The tumor was vaporized from its distal

Table I
Patient Characteristics

Groups		Randomized Group	Escape Group
Total Number		23	59
Age		72 (44–89)	68 (42–90)
Sex		♂:14/♀:9	♂:37/♀:22
Previous treatment	irradiation	3	14
	surgery	6	18
Type of Malignant Stenosis	pharyngeal/laryngeal cancer	—	8
	esophageal squamous cell carcinoma	8	33
	lung cancer/mediastinal metastases	—	9
	cancer of the cardia	9	5
	gastric cancer	6	4

to its proximal edge in order to minimize the risk of perforation. The aim is a lumen width of approximately 15 mm. In unusual cases of short and tight stenoses or polypoid tumor growth, we started the laser resection at the proximal end. All laser sessions were performed under general anesthesia. After completion of the laser therapy requiring courses of one or more laser sessions depending on the extent of the stenosing tumor masses, a combined afterloading irradiation therapy was performed by the Department of Radiology at the University of Kiel. The regular course is a percutaneous irradiation of 30 Gy in 3 weeks, followed by 3 days of two afterloading irradiation sessions 9 weeks apart. If the patient's condition allowed it, another percutaneous treatment of 20 Gy was added. Depending on the patient's general condition and distance from home, a hospital admission was sometimes necessary.

ETI was performed using Celestine-Medoc tubes in three different lengths (12, 15, and 21 cm). After initial endoscopic measurement of the tumor and simultaneous determination of the extent of malignant stenosis, the chosen tube was mounted together with a Bristol applicator on an Olympus GIF-XQ 10 endoscope with the tube being attached to the applicator by the help of an inflatable cuff.

In both randomized groups and the escape group, the following parameters were registered for each patient before and after treat-

Table II
Therapeutic Management of Escape Group

Total Number	*ELT* *6*	*ETI* *8*	*PEG* *8*	*TFT* *7*	*RT* *19*	*EB* *11*	*Total No.* *59*
Pharyngeal/laryngeal cancer	1		4	2		1	8
Esophageal squamous cell carcinoma	3	3	1	4	19	3	33
Lung cancer/mediastinal metastases		2	3	1		3	9
Cancer of the cardia	1	1				3	5
Gastric cancer	1	2				1	4
Food passage: much improved	1	4			3	2	10
Food passage:	4	1			7	8	20
improved	1	2	7	6	3		19
same		1		1	3	1	6
worse							
Change in food passage not known			1		3		4

ment: history and physical examination, nutritional status, symptoms, degree of dysphagia, type and extent of malignant stenosis, and quality of life according to the Visick classification. Follow-up examinations were performed at 2-month intervals so far as the general condition of the patient allowed transportation to our unit. If a trip to the hospital was impossible for the patient, information about the clinical situation was gathered from the patient, the patient's family, or the family doctor by telephone interview.

Patients who could not be randomized, thus entering the escape group, were treated by either ELT, ETI, PEG, TFT, RT, or EB (see Table II for management and results).

Results

In the two randomized groups (ELT and ETI), we found no significant difference in the age distribution. The ELT group consisted of 11 male and 3 female patients while the ETI group consisted of 3 male and 6 female patients. There was an almost equal distribution with regard to the histologic type of neoplasms treated: 5 patients

Table III
Results of Palliative Treatment

Groups	Therapy	Total No.	Complications: Early	Complications: Late	Hospitalization in days: Median (Range)	Survival Time in Weeks: Median (Range)
RANDOMIZED	ELT	14	—	2 re-stenosis	14 (3–77)	17 (0–45)
	ETI	9		2 tube dislocation 1 tumor overgrowth 2 bolus obstruction	7 (2–80)	12 (0–52)
ESCAPE	ELT	6	1 perforation	2 re-stenosis	21 (14–49)	10 (4–28)
	ETI	8	3 perforation	1 tube dislocation	14 (0–77)	8 (1½–28)
	PEG	8	—	—	14 (0–112)	16 (1–52)
	TFT	7	—	1 aspiration pneumonia	28 (3–56)	8 (1–24)
	RT	19	—	5 esophageal-tracheal fistula	0 (0–98)	28 (1–36)
	EB	11	2 perforation	—	10 (0–42)	32 (16–120)

with squamous cell carcinoma and 9 patients with adenocarcinoma were treated by ELT, while 3 patients with squamous cell carcinoma and 6 patients with adenocarcinoma were palliated by ETI. Tumor consistency in both groups was classified to be either polypoid and firm or exophytic and soft at a ratio of 10:4 in the ELT group and 7:2 in the ETI group. There was no significant difference in the size of tumors treated. The median length of tumors in the ELT group was 7.5 cm with a range from 2 to 13 cm, while neoplasms in the ETI group had a median size of 4 cm with a maximal range from 2 to 7 cm. The median duration of the history of the disease was found to be 3 months (range: 1–24 months) in the ELT group and 5 months (range: 3–14 months) in the ETI group with a median weight loss of 10 kg (range: 1–40 kg) before treatment in the ELT group and 8 kg (range: 2–18 kg) in the ETI group, respectively.

Looking at the different parameters that were determined by the two types of therapy (Table III), the length of initial hospitalization was 14 days (range: 3–7 days) in the ELT group compared to 7 days (range: 2–80 days) in the ETI group. In addition, 10 ELT patients required an additional hospitalization or frequent hospital visits to the Department of Radiology for their course of combined afterloading irradiation. In six ELT patients and in two ETI patients, a second and third hospitalization in the Surgical Department were necessary in order to treat complications. Complications and other results are listed in Table III.

The results in improvement of food passage by the two treatments were almost equal. While 2 of 14 patients in the ELT group and 1 of 9 patients in the ETI group did not show any change in their ability to swallow food, 12 of 14 ELT patients and 8 of 9 ETI patients noted an improvement. Five of the ELT patients were even able to switch from a liquid diet to solid food, and three ETI patients could be started on a semi-solid diet even though there was no passage of food possible before therapy.

The median survival time in both therapeutic groups did not show a significant difference with 17 weeks (range: 0–45 weeks) in the ELT group and 12 weeks (range: 0–52 weeks) in the ETI group. There was an equal distribution with regard to the number of weeks during which the patient's quality of life was improved by the chosen therapeutic scheme, with 8 weeks (range: 0–40 weeks) in the ELT group and 4 weeks (range: 0–46 weeks) in the ETI group. The highest quality of life reached after treatment according to the Visick classification amounted to four cases with Visick III, seven cases with Visick IV, and three cases with Visick V in the ELT patients, while in the ETI group two patients reached Visick III, three patients obtained Visick IV, and four patients were left with Visick V. Results of therapeutic management in the escape group are shown in Table III.

Discussion

Modern operative endoscopy has enlarged the spectrum of palliative therapy for advanced carcinoma of the esophagus and cardia. Although the most successful means of palliating an esophageal carcinoma is resection, in most patients, tumor spread and poor general condition limit the extent of procedure that the patient is able to tolerate.[6] The major problem of patients with malignant stenosis of the esophagus and cardia is dysphagia associated with weight loss, malnutrition, and decreased quality of life, the latter also caused by social isolation. Since we cannot expect endoscopic techniques to prolong life, the aim of palliation is the normalization of the patient's daily life as much as possible.

The major competing palliative techniques are ETI and ELT. Very few comparative studies have been finished.[7,8] One prospective trial showed superior palliation of dysphagia and even longer survival provided by laser compared to ETI.[7] When planning this randomized trial on ETI versus ELT combined with afterloading irradiation, the selection of patients for randomization created serious problems because of the heterogeneity of the population. Individual problems such as the patient's family living a long distance from the hospital, and associated factors such as previous irradiation and concomitant diseases are difficult to press into a rigid randomization plan. With only 19 out of 82 patients being candidates for irradiation alone as optimal palliation, a total of 63 patients needed endoscopic palliative therapy. Still, it was surprising to us that only 23 patients met the criteria for being accepted into the randomization group within 2 years. The fact that three patients from the ETI group were withdrawn because of high risk of dislocation indicates that even this extensive selection was not sufficient enough to generate a completely homogeneous patient group.

The comparison of ETI and ELT did not show a significant difference in survival time. Survival depends primarily on the patient's general condition and cannot be significantly influenced by different palliative procedures. In our experience, the early as well as the late complication rate was similar in both groups, if re-stenosis in the ELT group was judged as a late problem. The latter should be counted as such, since a re-stenosis after ELT has a similar impact on the patient's quality of life as a dislocation after ELT. It is interesting that most of the complications and late problems after ELT, i.e., three re-stenoses and one fistula, had to be treated by tube implantation. The food passage improvement did not differ significantly between the two trial groups (Table III). The ability to pass food by natural means into the stomach is the important aim of the therapy and this was achieved in most patients. Nevertheless, when we evaluated the ability of food passage again after 2 months, very few patients were able to eat regular solid meals.

The authors are aware that the Visick classification was initially not designed for evaluation of the patients that were studied in this trial. Nevertheless, Visick criteria were used because they are easy to evaluate and many readers are familiar with them. There were no differences between the two groups regarding the highest grade of Visick classification reached in the posttherapeutic period. But if we look at the duration of hospitalization and the time during which the patient's quality of life was improved by the palliation, we notice differences between the two groups of treatment. There is a substantial difference in hospitalization between ELT and ETI patients in our department, i.e., 14 versus 7 days (median values). The difference reaches statistical significance if the additional hospitalization of approximately 4–6 weeks or the frequent daily hospital visits at the Department of Radiology for the afterloading therapy are taken into account. This aspect gains even more importance if the patient's home is several travelling hours away from the hospital. Therefore, from these data we conclude that no single palliation procedure has a superior effect on survival, food passage, or quality of life compared to other techniques. Depending on the situation of an individual patient, one or another endoscopic palliation procedure must be chosen to help the patient in the best way and to improve the patient's life in the shortest possible time, taking into account the patient's possible survival time. Thus patients in poor condition should have a tube implantation, since this procedure has the lowest duration of hospitalization and gives the patient as much time as possible at home. Patients in good condition, preferably with a short stenosis, are good cases for laser therapy.

References

1. Manegold BC: Palliative tumor therapie in der endoskopie. In: Operative Endoskopie, Stuttgart, F.K. Schattauer, 1979.
2. Tytgat GNJ, den Hartog Jaeger FCA, Bartelsman JFWM: Endoscopic prosthesis for advanced esophageal cancer. Endoscopy 18:32–39 (Supplement 3), 1986.
3. Sandler R, Poesel H, Spuhler A: Therapie gastrointestinaler tumoren mit laser. Internist 26:22–28, 1985.
4. Fleischer D, Sivak MV Jr: Endoscopic Nd:YAG laser therapy as palliation for esophagogastric cancer. Gastroenterology 89:827–831, 1985.
5. Bader M, Dittler HJ, Ultsch B, Ries G, Siewert JR: Palliative treatment of malignant stenoses of the upper gastrointestinal tract using a comination of laser and afterloading therapy. Endoscopy 18:27–31, 1986.
6. DeMeester TR, Barlow AP: Surgery and current management for cancer of the esophagus and cardia. Curr Prob Surg 25:580, 1988.
7. Carter R, Smith J: Esophageal carcinoma: A comparative study of laser recanalization versus intubation in the palliation of gastroesophageal carcinoma. Lasers Med Sci 1:245–251, 1986.
8. Lux GG, Ell C: Tumor stenoses of the upper gastrointestinal tract: Therapeutic alternatives to laser therapy. Endoscopy 18:37–43 (Supplement 1), 1986.

39

Comparison of Intraluminal Palliation Methods for Cancer of the Esophagus and the Esophagogastric Junction

F. M. Juettner, B. Pakisch, P. H. Kohek,
G. Stuecklschweiger, E. Poier, G. B. Friehs, A. Hackl

Introduction

Palliative treatment for cancer of the esophagus or of the esophagogastric junction should be rapidly effective in restoring the ability to swallow without the need for long hospitalization or multiple repetitive treatment sessions, and should have a low rate of complications. We compared various intraluminal palliation methods of esophageal cancer regarding their efficacy in palliation, the duration, the palliative effect, their rate of complications, and their practicability.

Patients and Methods

We reviewed 193 patients with cancer of the esophagus and/or the esophagogastric junction, who, due to generalized spread of their disease, local extent, or general condition, were not candidates for a

Ferguson MK, Little AG, Skinner DB: Diseases of the Esophagus, Vol. I: Malignant Diseases. Futura Publishing Company, Inc., Mount Kisco, NY, © 1990.

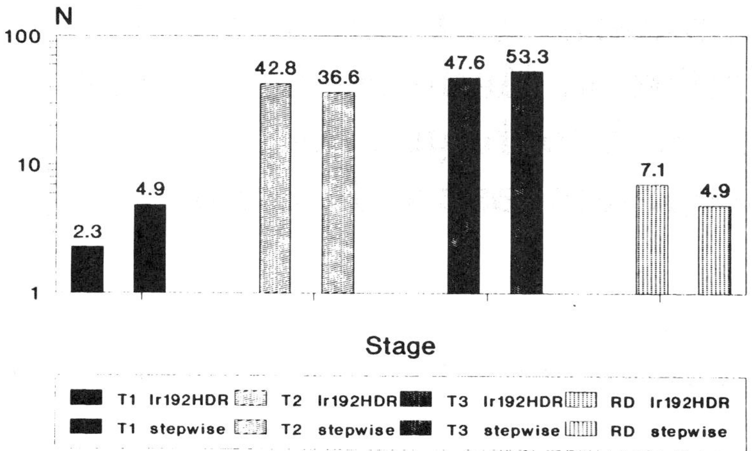

Figure 1: Treatment distribution by stage.

combined modality treatment with curative intention. We compared two treatment series that had been applied at different times in our department, depending on the technical facilities available. The distribution of age, performance status, tumor stage (see Fig. 1) and tumor localization did not differ significantly in two series. In both groups, treatment was not begun until dysphagia for semi-solid food was experienced. All intraluminal interventions were done under short-term intravenous anesthesia combined with topical anesthesia.

In the first series of 142 patients, we applied a stepwise schedule including dilation (Gilliard's device), combined bougienage, and retrograde or primary antegrade Nd-YAG noncontact laser obliteration (CBL), and endoprosthesis insertion (Wilson-Cook's device) by the push method. The succeeding palliative step was only taken if no satisfactory result had been achieved by the preceding one, or if the time interval between necessary interventions became shorter than 14 days.

In a second series, Ir-192 high dose rate intraluminal afterloading (Ir-192 HDR) was administered in a total of 51 patients. Initial dilation or CBL were done only if the degree of stenosis did not allow the insertion of the outer afterloading catheter (diameter: 8 or 6 mm, Selectron and Microselectron device, respectively, Nucletron Inc.; source activity: 2–10 Ci). We administered 3–5 Gy per session calculated at a 1-cm distance from the surface of the source. Two sessions were done during the first week. If necessary, further afterloading treatments were applied after 3 weeks.

In patients with a severely compromised general condition, only dilation and/or CBL were done if additional treatment was needed. In patients with a fair general condition, Ir-192 HDR was combined with external irradiation using the multiple field technique to administer a total dose of 60 Gy. Dilation and/or CBL were also optional in this group.

Results

Dilation as the initial treatment modality was done in 136 patients, and in 54 of them it was found to be a sufficient therapy until death. The average number of treatment sessions per patient was 8.7 at a frequency of 2.3 sessions per month. Total occlusion of the esophageal lumen necessitated primarily antegrade CBL in six cases. As the second step, retrograde CBL was applied in 73 patients. In 43 of the 79 CBL cases, no change to another treatment modality became necessary. The average treatment number per patient after the initial CBL series was 5.9 at a frequency of 1.6 sessions per month. However, in lesions with a long craniocaudal extent, three or four CBL sessions were necessary to achieve initial patency of the lumen. In nine patients, endoprosthesis followed the dilation procedures, since angulation (N = 7) or fistulization (N = 2) did not allow the use of CBL. The implantation of an endoprosthesis as the last and final modality was done in 36 cases. Obstruction or dislocation of the tubes necessitated additional interventions in 12 patients. The average treatment number per patient after the implantation of the tube was 1.3 at a frequency of one treatment session every 3 months. For the whole series of sequential palliation, the average number of interventions per patient was 6.4 at a frequency of 2.1 intraluminal treatments per month.

In the Ir-192 HDR group, pre-irradiation dilation or CBL were necessary in 22 patients (average: 1.1 intervention/patient). A total of 114 afterloading sessions were done (average: 2.24 interventions/pa-

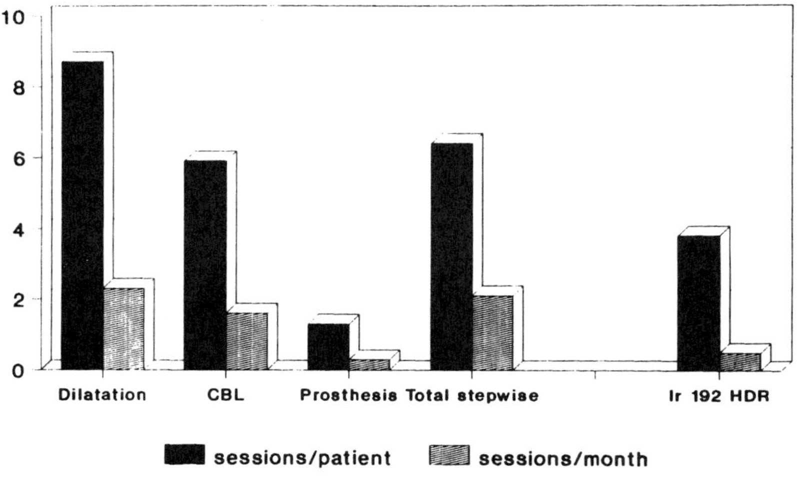

Figure 2: Frequency of therapeutic interventions.

tient; range: 1–4). Cumulative Ir-192 doses, calculated at a 1-cm distance from the surface of the source, ranged from 3 to 21 Gy (average: 12 Gy/patient). Dilation or CBL during or following the afterloading treatment series was necessary in 38 patients (1.4 interventions/patient). The total number of intraluminal interventions per patient averaged 3.8, corresponding to one intraluminal treatment session every 2 months. In 27 patients, additional external beam irradiation was delivered (18–60 Gy). The number of necessary intraluminal interventions was not significantly influenced by additional external irradiation (Fig. 2).

In the first group, a satisfactory ability to swallow all types of properly chewed food was obtained in 123/136 patients following dilation, in 69/73 patients following retrograde CBL, and in 4/6 patients following antegrade CBL. Placement of an endoprosthesis resulted in satisfactory palliation in 41/45 cases. In the Ir-192 HDR group, satisfactory palliation was achieved in 28 cases after one and in 16 cases after two afterloading sessions. The remaining seven patients needed three afterloading sessions to experience a relief from dysphagia.

The mean duration of satisfactory palliation before another treatment session or before a switch to the next option was required ranged from 1 to 3 weeks following dilation, 1 to 5 weeks following CBL, and 20 to 25 weeks after the implantation of an endoprosthesis. With the help of intraluminal afterloading therapy alone, treatment-free intervals lasted from 12 to 24 weeks, and increased up to 10 to 72 weeks if combined with external irradiation.

In the presence of endophytic tumors that caused a "ball-valve like" stenosis, in case of an additional extraluminal obstruction, or in tumors with excessive length, dilation did not show any benefit. In the presence of an esophageal fistula, both CBL and dilation were used only to open a passage for the endoprosthesis. The practicability and efficacy of both CBL and endoprosthesis were limited by anatomical features such as excessive length of the lesion, tumors beginning at the cricoid, and angulation of the esophagus, respectively. Ir-192 HDR afterloading, with and without external irradiation, was effective and practicable in all sites and in the presence of both intra- and extraluminal obstruction. In case of even the slightest evidence of invasion of the tumor into neighboring organs, however, fistulization inevitably occurred.

The rate of complications following dilation was 3.7%, 13.9% after CBL, 39% after endoprosthesis, and 19.6% after Ir-192 HDR (see Fig. 3). For the types of complications found, see Table I. In the first 4 to 8 hours following dilation or CBL, pain was experienced in 73% of the patients. Most of them were also alarmed about the short intervals between the necessary repetitive treatments, which tended to become shorter from one session to the next. Patients with endoprostheses complained about regurgitation if the prosthesis had to be placed in the distal third of the esophagus through lesions that involved the cardia. Most of them also objected to the absolute need to ingest only purèed food. A sensation of a retrosternal lump was experienced in most patients after tube implantation in the middle third, but it usually subsided after 2 to 7 days.

The least degree of discomfort and the best quality of life were evident following Ir-192 HDR alone, whereas additional external irradiation caused temporary radiation sickness and mild esophagitis in 63.3%. Benign stenoses that often necessitated dilation occurred in all patients following afterloading treatment. Another cause for intraluminal re-intervention was intraluminal tumor regrowth, which up to this time has been observed in eight patients.

The mean survival after stepwise dilation, laser obliteration, and endoprosthesis insertion was 6 months, compared with 8.6 months

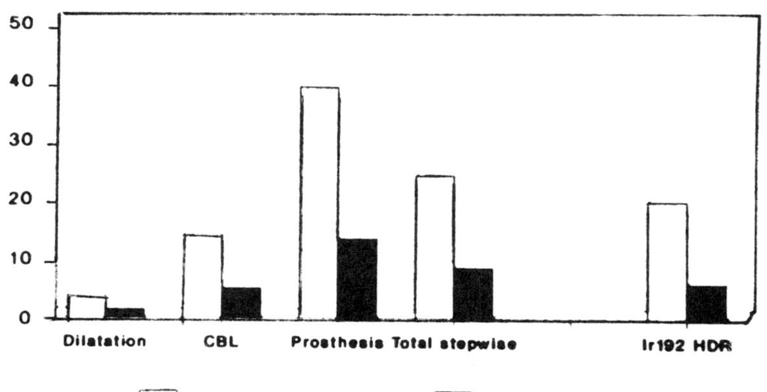

Figure 3: Incidence of complications following palliative therapy.

Table I
Complications After Intraluminal Palliation of Esophageal Cancer

Type of Therapy	*Type of Complication*	*Number of Cases*
Dilation	perforation	4
	bleeding	1
CBL	perforation	5
	stricture	2
	penetration/mediastinitis	2
	fistula	2
Endoprosthesis	perforation	4
	dislocation	8
	obstruction	6
Ir-192 HDR	fistula	1
	bleeding	3
	stricture/ulcer	6

No patient had more than one complication.

for all Ir-192 HDR cases ($p < 0.05$). All patients died from local or distant spread of esophageal cancer.

Discussion

The average overall 5-year survival rate of patients with esophageal cancer has been reported as 5%.[1] It is commonly agreed that only an aggressive, combined-modality treatment can improve these poor results. Not all patients, however, are possible candidates for such an approach. Palliation still plays a major role in the treatment of esophageal cancer.[2] The "ideal" palliative treatment must provide rapid relief from symptoms while the rate of complications and the degree of discomfort for the patient should be as low as possible. A short time of hospitalization without the need for repetitive treatments is also desirable, both from the patient's point of view and from a cost-effectiveness viewpoint.

None of the modalities used in our patients has been found to meet all these requirements, though each of them has specific value of its own. Dilation or CBL alone cause few complications[3] but carry the problem of a high frequency of necessary interventions. In contrast, the comparably lower rate of interventions in endoprosthesis therapy goes along with a high rate of complications and mortality.[4] Dilation and CBL alone provided sustained palliation only in some cases, and thus further steps, such as endoprosthesis insertion, were necessary in most patients.[5,6] Though this sequential process showed satisfactory palliative effects, both the total number of necessary interventions for the individual patient and the rate of complications were high. The quality of life was reduced both by frequent interventions and by the pain caused by intraluminal manipulations. Moreover, many patients were not satisfied by the palliation provided by an endoprosthesis, as the need for puréed food interfered with their social life.

The dose distribution of intraluminal high dose rate irradiation shows a high dose close to the surface of the source with a rapid falloff in the periphery. This results in a palliative effect by destruction of tumor in a radius of about a 1-cm distance from the source. It has to be considered, however, that with a dose of 5 Gy calculated at 10 mm from the surface of the source, as in our patients, the dosage to tissue adjacent to the source is as high as 35–40 Gy. This may result in side effects such as ulcers or strictures, which were frequently found in our patients. Thus, additional treatment for stricture was necessary in many cases. Similar findings have been reported in the literature.[7–9] The use of external beam irradiation in combination with Ir-192 HDR may achieve a cure in small lesions of localized disease, but in general its effect must be considered to be palliative.[10] The mean survival in the Ir-192 HDR group was higher than in the sequential therapy group. We were not able, though, to determine the rate of tumor response in our patients because radiation-induced artifacts did not allow an exact evaluation by imaging methods, and biopsies were inconclusive. The rate of complications and mortality was lower than in the sequential therapy group, and this was also true for the number and frequency of necessary interventions. Subjectively, the intraluminal treatment caused little discomfort.[11]

Though Ir-192 HDR intraluminal irradiation is far from being an ideal palliation method, we now use it as the primary therapeutic option in incurable patients. We restrict the use of dilation and laser obliteration to the rare cases in which no guidewire can be passed over the stenosis, and to local recurrences after Ir-192 HDR in which no further radiation dosage is possible. Endoprostheses are used only in case of esophagotracheal fistulae and in stenoses after Ir-192 HDR which are not otherwise manageable.

References

1. National Cancer Institutes: 1986 Annual cancer statistics review. Division of Cancer Prevention and Control, NIH Publication No. 87-2889, Bethesda, MD, 1987.
2. Burdette WJ: Palliative operation for carcinoma of cervical and thoracic esophagus. Ann Surg 173:714, 1971.
3. Celestin LR, Campbell WB: A new and safe system for esophageal dilatation. Lancet 1:74, 1981.
4. Angorn IB: Intubation in the treatment of carcinoma of the esophagus. World J Surg 5:535, 1981.
5. Pietrafitta JJ, Dwyer RM: Endoscopic laser therapy of malignant esophageal obstruction. Arch Surg 121:395, 1986.
6. Ghazi, A, Nussbaum M: A new approach to the management of malignant esophageal obstruction and esophagorespiratory fistula. Ann Thorac Surg 40:337, 1985.
7. Hishikawa Y: Radiation treatment of esophageal carcinoma using a high dose rate remote afterloader. Radiat Med 1:237, 1983.
8. Hagenmueller F, Sander C, Sander R, et al. Laser and endoluminal 192-iridium radiation. Endoscopy 19:16, 1987.
9. Hishikawa Y, Kamikonya N, Tanaka S, et al. Radiotherapy of esophageal

carcinoma: Role of high dose rate intracavitary irradiation. Radiother Oncol 9:13, 1987.
10. Beatty JD, DeBoer G, Rider WD: Carcinoma of the esophagus: Pretreatment assessment, correlation of radiation treatment parameters with survival and identification and management of radiation treatment failure. Cancer 43:2254, 1979.
11. Rowland CG, Pagliero KM: Intracavitary irradiation in palliation of carcinoma of esophagus and cardia. Lancet I:981, 1985.

40

A Prospective Randomized Study of Nd:YAG Laser Therapy versus Intubation for Cancer of the Esophagus and Cardia

A. Moraldi, C. Iascone, M. Zerilli, P. Ginevri, R. Pasquali Lasagni, N. Campioni, C.U. Casciani, S. Stipa

Introduction

Most patients with cancer of the esophagus and gastric cardia cannot be radically treated and palliation is often the only therapeutic alternative. Dysphagia is by far the most common local symptom, and the goal of all current treatments is to palliate the obstruction which is the cause of severe nutritional depletion and recurrent aspiration with subsequent pneumonitis. Since palliative surgery has particularly high mortality and morbidity rates, other modalities such as surgical or endoscopic intubation must be considered.

Recently endoscopic laser therapy for treatment of malignant esophageal obstruction has been proposed as a valid alternative to relieve dysphagia because of its low morbidity and mortality rates. For these reasons we did a prospective randomized trial in patients

Ferguson MK, Little AG, Skinner DB: Diseases of the Esophagus, Vol. I: Malignant Diseases. Futura Publishing Company, Inc., Mount Kisco, NY, © 1990.

with inoperable cancer of the esophagus and gastric cardia comparing the results of surgical and endoscopic intubation with laser therapy in terms of mortality, morbidity, time of hospitalization, and the ability to restore esophageal patency with normal swallowing.

Materials and Methods

From November 1987 to May 1989, 51 patients with nonresectable cancer of the esophagus and gastric cardia were seen, of whom 28 were eligible for a prospective randomized study comparing endoscopic Nd:YAG laser therapy versus surgical or endoscopic intubation. This study included patients with advanced local or metastatic disease and high-risk patients (poor general condition, cardiorespiratory insufficiency, renal failure, liver cirrhosis, etc.). There were 23 male and 5 female patients with a mean age of 64 years (range 44–92). Mean length of tumors of the cardia was 4 cm and for esophageal cancers was 7 cm, with no difference between the groups of patients (intubated or laser treated). Surgical intubation by Haring tubes was performed in six patients with adenocarcinoma of the lower third of the esophagus or cardia, while endoscopic intubation using Wilson tubes was done in eight patients with squamous cell carcinoma of the thoracic esophagus. Laser therapy was performed in six patients with adenocarcinoma of the lower third of esophagus or cardia and in eight patients with squamous cell carcinoma of the thoracic esophagus. The laser source was both a contact neodymium:YAG laser (Surgical Laser Technology—maximal power output of 60 watts) and noncontact neodymium:YAG laser (Medilas 2—maximal power output of 100 watts). Eight out of 14 patients who underwent laser therapy were previously dilated by Celestin or Savary-Gilliard dilators to allow a safer treatment, eventually by a retrograde technique.

Patients submitted to endoscopic intubation and laser therapy were treated by local anesthesia (tetracaine tablets) and general sedation by diazepam. Laser therapy was usually performed without necessity of hospitalization. Laser sessions were done twice a week, with a 3-day interval between treatments.

Results

Successful surgical intubation was carried out in all six patients with cancer of the cardia, while recanalization after laser therapy was effective in five out of six patients. We had two complications in the surgical group (one wound infection and one subphrenic abscess) and none in the laser group; no mortality was observed. Late complications consisted of food impaction in one patient 2 months after intubation. All patients were able to tolerate a normal diet until their death. Median survival for the surgical group was 4.5 months and 1 month after laser therapy.

The eight patients with cancer of the thoracic esophagus were successfully intubated. Three major complications in patients treated by endoscopic intubation were observed: one perforation, one hemorrhage, and one respiratory distress syndrome. All of these patients died after 5, 12, and 2 days, respectively. Of eight patients undergoing laser therapy, one patient developed a tracheo-esophageal fistula 3 days after laser therapy and was treated by endoscopic intubation. Late complications in thoracic esophageal cancer patients consisted of occlusion of the prosthesis secondary to tumor growth in one patient. All patients were totally free of dysphagia except two cases treated by laser who required a semi-solid diet. One case was retreated by laser therapy 4 months after the first successful treatment. Median survival was 5.5 months in patients after endoscopic intubation and 6.5 months in patients after laser therapy.

Mean hospital stay for surgically intubated patients was 14 days whereas for those treated by endoscopic intubation it was 1 week. Two laser sessions were typically required for patients with cancer of the gastric cardia and three sessions were required for patients with cancer the of thoracic esophagus. The mean total energy necessary to complete the treatment was 7,200 joules (4,500 to 13,400) for cancer of cardia and 8,900 joules (4,400 to 25,000) for cancer of thoracic esophagus.

Discussion

Since most of the patients with esophageal carcinoma cannot undergo curative resection because of advanced disease, palliation is extremely important because it remains the only therapeutic alternative. Palliation should relieve dysphagia and restore esophageal patency, allowing the patient to eat and drink normally. The ideal palliative technique provides normal swallowing by a method that is quick, safe, with a short hospital stay, and has a low complication rate. There are three choices of palliation: surgery, intubation, and laser therapy. Surgery is an excellent method of palliation because it usually relieves dysphagia completely, but has particularly high mortality and morbidity rates. Complications in these patients with a low life expectancy will often prolong the hospital stay until death. Therefore, the risk-benefit ratio has to be considered and surgical treatment must be compared with the other modalities.

Surgical intubation in our total experience of more than 80 cases[1] has low morbidity and mortality rates as shown by this small series. But the international literature usually reports a high complication rate (hemorrhage, perforation, reflux esophagitis, aspiration pneumonitis) and postoperative mortality.[2] For these reasons surgical intubation has been generally abandoned for easier and more attractive endoscopic methods. This technique is usually performed without general anesthesia, requires a short hospital stay and provides an immediate improvement in swallowing. The early complication rate is lower than with the surgical method but a high mortality rate still persists (up to 27%)[3] as our experience has shown.

The relatively new laser therapy avoids some of the problems of intubation and offers good relief from dysphagia. An international inquiry from Ell and Demling[4] reported a successful rate of 83% in 1,184 patients with inoperable cancer of the esophagus and cardia, with a 4.1% complication rate (12.8% after radiotherapy); mortality rate was 1%. Very good results are reported by Norberto and others[5] in 111 cases of cancer of the esophagus and cardia with complete palliation in 90% of the patients treated, a 7.6% complication rate and only one death. In our total experience of almost 40 cases treated by laser, we have only one complication (perforation with tracheo-esophageal fistula), no mortality, and an overall success rate of 85%. In this series we report one failure, 11 patients out of 14 with complete palliation, and two patients with mild dysphagia requiring a semi-solid diet.

It is interesting to note that functional results may be impaired by associated motility disturbances, even if patency is fully restored. The possible explanations are: laser treatment after radiotherapy, very high lesions involving an apparently tumor-free esophagopharyngeal junction, and strictures involving the esophageal muscle for a long segment. Severe anorexia, pain, and a bad "performance status" may contribute to worse functional results.[6] According to our experience, laser therapy is the treatment of choice because of its high success rate, low morbidity, no mortality, and no hospitalization. Intubation may be a complementary technique in those stenotic tumors where the extrinsic component becomes prevalent, for rapidly growing tumors which would require very frequent laser sessions, and is the treatment of choice for esophagobronchial fistulae.

References

1. Campioni N, Filippetti M, Pasqualetti AM, et al: Complicanze del trattamento palliativo delle stenosi esofagee neoplastiche mediante endoprotesi. Nostra esperienza Il Gastroenterologo 3:81, 1984.
2. Watson A: Study of the quality and duration of survival following resection, endoscopic intubation and surgical intubation in oesophageal carcinoma. Br J Surg 69:585, 1983.
3. Diamantes T, Mannell A: Oesophageal intubation for advanced oesophageal cancer: The Baragwanath experience, 1977–1981. Br J Surg 70:555, 1983.
4. Ell C, Demling L: Laser therapy of tumor stenoses in the upper gastrointestinal tract: An international inquiry. Laser Surg Med 7:491, 1987.
5. Norberto L, Cusumano A, Segalin A, et al: La terapia del carcinoma inoperabile esofago-cardiale. VIII Congr Coll Int Chir Dig 3:541, 1987.
6. Mellow MH, Pinkas H: Endoscopic laser therapy for malignancies affecting the esophageal and gastroesophageal junction. Arch Intern Med 145:1443, 1985.

41

Short- and Long-Term Results After Nd:YAG Laser Therapy of Inoperable Esophageal and Cardia Cancer

Lorenzo Norberto, Alberto Ruol, Andrea Segalin, Marco Baessato, Antonino Cusumano, Romeo Bardini, Luigi Bonavina, Alberto Peracchia

Introduction

Endoscopic neodymium:yttrium aluminum garnet (Nd:YAG) laser therapy has been shown to be a technically feasible treatment for patients with nonresectable carcinoma of the esophagus and of the gastric cardia. Since the initial experience of Fleisher,[1,2] several series have suggested the effectiveness of this therapeutic option in relieving dysphagia and improving the quality of life for these patients.[3–5] Moreover, in patients with carcinoma of the cervical esophagus or with angulated and/or complete strictures, Nd:YAG laser therapy could represent the only therapeutic option other than a feeding gastrostomy or jejunostomy.[6]

The aim of this study was to evaluate the impact of Nd:YAG laser palliation on the quality of the remaining life of patients with esophageal and cardia carcinomas.

Ferguson MK, Little AG, Skinner DB: Diseases of the Esophagus, Vol. I: Malignant Diseases. Futura Publishing Company, Inc., Mount Kisco, NY, © 1990.

Materials and Methods

In the years between 1980 and 1988, 1,519 patients with primary squamous cell carcinoma of the esophagus and 339 patients with adenocarcinoma of the gastric cardia were admitted to the 1st Department of Surgery of the University of Padova.

In this study we analyzed 84 patients with inoperable esophageal and cardia cancers treated with Nd:YAG laser therapy. The patients were followed up monthly or every 2 months until death. The first Nd:YAG laser session was performed during a short period of hospitalization; after the recanalization, the treatment was continued on an outpatient basis. All of the patients were treated with local pharyngeal anesthesia and premedication with intravenous sedation. A Cooper Lasersonics Model 8000 laser, with power output set to deliver 50 to 100 watts at the fiber tip, was used. The tumor was dilated by means of the Savary or American Endoscopy dilators and the retrograde laser technique was employed in most cases.[7] Laser energy was applied using a quartz fiber passed through the operating channel of an Olympus GIF-XP10 endoscope, and it was delivered in 0.5-second pulses at a distance of 0.5 to 1.5 cm from the tumor.

A prospective computerized data collection, including data on age, sex, concomitant diseases, histology, site and stage of the tumor, and hospital morbidity and mortality was performed, and a complete follow-up to December 1988 was obtained. Information on diet, weight, general status, and Karnofsky Performance Index was specifically sought during each follow-up visit. The quality of the palliation was scored from 1 to 5 and evaluated according to the following functional parameters: ability to swallow before and after follow-up laser sessions (5 = normal diet, 4 = occasional dysphagia, 3 = semiliquid diet, 2 = liquid diet, 1 = total dysphagia), weight (5 = increase, 3 = stable, 1 = loss), general status (5 = excellent, 4 = good, 3 = fair, 2 = poor, 1 = terminal), Karnofsky Performance Index (5 = 100–90%, 4 = 80–70%, 3 = 60–50%, 2 = 40–30%, 1 = 20–10%).

The mean age was 64 years (range 40–88); 75 patients were males and nine females. The tumor involved the cervical, upper thoracic, middle thoracic, lower thoracic esophagus, and cardia in 11, 18, 23, 12, and 20 cases, respectively. The histologic type of the tumor was available in 79 cases; there were 57 squamous cell carcinomas, 20 adenocarcinomas, one anaplastic carcinoma, and one mixed adenosquamous carcinoma. The indications for palliative laser treatment were a locally advanced or metastatic tumor in 34 patients, and poor surgical risk in 50. The length of the tumor ranged between 1 and 18 cm, with an average of 6.4 cm and a median of 6 cm.

The mean and the median number of spots and joules per session was 177.8 and 149.0 (range 3–999), and 5,179 and 4,720 (range 231–17,230), respectively. Overall, two sessions (range 1–4) of laser therapy were necessary for recanalization. During the follow-up, the mean number of laser sessions per patient was 3.4 (range 1–17) at an average interval of 2 months.

Results

Hospital Morbidity and Mortality

Five early perforations (5.9%) occurred during the first recanalization laser session and were related to the technique. These patients were treated with palliative esophagectomy and gastric pull-up in one case, pulsion intubation in one, and conservative management (with one death) in three cases. Two bleeding episodes occurred; one patient was treated with endoscopic diathermy and the other with a Nd:YAG laser session, both followed by pulsion intubation. Overall, three hospital deaths occurred (3.5%); they were due to perforation, respiratory failure, and cachexia with pneumonia.

Late Complications

Four perforations (4.7%) occurred during the follow up and were probably related more to tumor progression than to the laser treatment or tumor dilation. These 4 patients were treated with pulsion intubation in 2 cases and conservative management in 2 cases. Furthermore, 6 patients developed an esophagotracheobronchial fistula which was probably related to tumor progression or post-radiation tumor necrosis. Five of these 6 patients underwent pulsion intubation.

Follow-up

During the follow up, a variety of therapeutic procedures was performed to improve the quality of palliation and possibly also the life expectation: endoscopic dilations in 25 patients, photodynamic

Table I
Average Scores of Functional Parameters Evaluated During the Follow-up of the Patients Treated with Nd:YAG Laser

Follow-up:	*1 mo.*	*3 mos.*	*6 mos.*	*9 mos.*	*12 mos.*	*18 mos.*	*24 mos.*
Swallowing	3.4–4.0	3.3–3.8	3.3–3.8	3.5–3.9	4.2–4.3	4.0–4.3	3.5–4.2
Weight	3.2	2.9	2.7	2.8	3.2	2.9	3.0
General status	4.1	3.9	4.0	4.0	4.3	4.0	4.3
Karnofsky PI*	3.7	3.5	3.8	4.0	4.1	4.1	4.2

* PI = Performance Index
See text for details on scoring.

therapy in five, pulsion intubation in seven, feeding gastrostomy in one, endoscopic diathermy in two, radiation therapy in 24, and chemotherapy in 20.

In 70 patients with an evaluable follow-up until death or of at least 1 year, the quality of the palliation was studied according to the ability to swallow, the patient's weight, general status, and the Karnofsky Performance Index. All of these functional parameters were evaluated monthly or bimonthly and scored 1 to 5; the average scores are reported in Table I. An analysis of the functional parameters was also performed according to the location of the tumor, i.e., cervical esophagus versus thoracic esophagus versus cardia, and according to the length of the tumor, i.e., <7 cm versus >7 cm. In the above categories, the quality of palliation was not significantly different, although it was slightly worse in tumors located in the cervical esophagus and in tumors longer than 7 cm. The mean survival of the 32 patients who died during follow-up was 8.6 months (range 1–38); 38 patients are alive between 1 and 22 months (mean 6.8).

Discussion

An aggressive surgical approach should still be considered the treatment of choice for esophageal and cardia carcinomas. Unfortunately, in the Western hemisphere tumors are typically advanced at the time of diagnosis. Therefore, treatment is frequently palliative and associated with one of the worst prognoses of all solid tumors. A variety of surgical and endoscopic procedures are used to palliate symptoms in patients whose stage of disease is too extensive for curative therapy or whose physiological condition is too poor to permit extensive surgery. The aim of palliative treatment should be to improve the major symptoms and to delay related complications due to disease progression. The treatment should be as simple as possible and with minimal morbidity and mortality, to allow patients to remain outside of the hospital and enjoy their short life span.

The selection of the method of palliation is difficult and, at the present, no technique is suitable for all patients. The choice between palliative resection, bypass operations, tumor intubation, endoscopic laser therapy, feeding gastrostomy or jejunostomy and chemotherapy or radiotherapy depends on the site and extent of the tumor, the general condition of the patient, and the experience and aggressiveness of the physician.

Endoscopic Nd:YAG laser therapy has been shown to be a useful therapeutic option in situations where choices are limited. Patients with inoperable carcinoma of the cervical esophagus or of the gastric cardia[6] or with inoperable but nonstenosing carcinoma of the intrathoracic esophagus[8] may be candidates for Nd:YAG laser therapy. We think that in the above patients, the other forms of surgical and endoscopic palliation are far from satisfactory. Palliative surgical resection and bypass operations have significantly greater hospital morbidity and mortality rates and require longer hospitalization periods. Tumor intubation is contraindicated in tumors of the cervical esophagus and in nonstenosing tumors of the intrathoracic esophagus, and is frequently unsatisfactory in angulated cardia tumors. Finally, feeding gastrostomy or jejunostomy should always be reserved as the last resort since it actually worsens the quality of life of the patient.

Several studies have reported a dramatic improvement of dysphagia after YAG laser therapy.[3,4,6] However, the real impact of Nd:YAG laser therapy on the quality of life of these patients is difficult to evaluate and was seldom analyzed in the previous literature. After initial palliation, the follow-up of the patient is of great importance because a good initial functional result does not predict an effective palliation lasting until death from generalized disease. In fact, early recurrence of symptoms requires repetition of the procedure or the selection of a different form of palliation, which means an important burden to the patient and an increased risk of complications. Rutgeerts et al.,[6] in a series of 34 patients, reported an initial technical success of 94%, but the dysphagia-free interval after the first laser session was only 4 weeks long. In the series of Ahlquist et al.[5] and Mathus-Vliegen et al.,[8] swallowing ability was improved in 80% of the patients; these authors reported that a single laser treatment provided adequate palliation in more than half of the patients until death. However, the number of patients was small, 25 and 15 respectively, and the criteria for the follow-up were not standardized.

In our experience, good initial functional results were obtained in 83% of the patients, but repeated laser sessions were needed in almost all of the long-term survivors at a median interval of 8 weeks. In agreement with Rutgeerts et al.,[6] we found an increased difficulty to perform repeated laser treatments because of the increased tumor load and an increasing debility of the patient. Moreover, in some patients, the functional results were jeopardized by extrinsic growth of the tumor, and by fistulization in the mediastinum or in the respiratory tract. All of these situations required other forms of palliation such as esophageal intubation. In disagreement with Lightdale et al.,[4] the level and the histologic type of the tumor did not significantly influence the quality of palliation.

Conclusion

Endoscopic Nd:YAG laser therapy is an effective and perhaps the only palliative modality in a number of patients with inoperable esophageal and cardia cancers. It entails acceptable morbidity and mortality rates, and produces satisfactory functional results. However, its exact place in the palliative treatment of inoperable esophageal and cardia carcinomas has yet to be defined. All potential therapeutic modalities should be considered in an integrated fashion.

References

1. Fleisher D, Kessler F: Endoscopic Nd:YAG laser therapy for carcinoma of the esophagus: A new form of palliative treatment. Gastroenterology 85:600, 1983.
2. Fleisher D, Sivak MV: Endoscopic Nd:YAG laser therapy as palliative treatment for advanced adenocarcinoma of the gastric cardia. Gastroenterology 15:353, 1984.
3. Fleisher D, Sivak MV: Endoscopic Nd:YAG laser therapy as palliation for esophagogastric cancer. Gastroenterology 89:827, 1985.
4. Lightdale CJ, Zimbalist E, Winawer SJ: Outpatient management of esophageal cancer with endoscopic Nd:YAG laser. Am J Gastroenterol 82:46, 1987.
5. Ahlquist DA, Gostout CJ, Viggiano TR, Blam RK, Pairolero PC, Hench

VS, Zinsmeister AR: Endoscopic laser palliation of malignant dysphagia: A prospective study. Mayo Clin Proc 62:867, 1987.
6. Rutgeerts P, Vantrappen G, Broeckaert L, Muls M, Geboes K, Coremans G, Janssens J: Palliative Nd:YAG laser therapy for cancer of the esophagus and gastroesophageal junction: Impact on the quality of remaining life. Gastrointest Endosc 34:87, 1988.
7. Pietrafitta JJ, Dwyer RM: New laser technique for the treatment of malignant esophageal obstruction. J Surg Oncol 35:157, 1987.
8. Mathus-Vliegen MH, Tytgat NJ: Laser photocoagulation in the palliative treatment of upper digestive tract tumors. Cancer 57:396, 1986.

42

Photodynamic Therapy (PDT) of 25 Early Pharyngo-Esophageal Carcinomas: Results and Complications

Philippe Monnier, Marcel Savary, Charlotte Fontolliet, Georges Wagnières, Hubert Van den Bergh, A. Chatelain

Introduction

Some porphyrins have a natural tendency to concentrate more in malignant tumors than in normal tissue.[1] Such porphyrins, which alone are quite harmless, can become very toxic when exposed to light. Thus a tumor which is enriched in porphyrin can be destroyed by applying light, whereas the surrounding normal tissue, which contains little porphyrin, survives. The possibilities of a new cancer therapy based on this selective tumor destruction, via the intravenous injection of a porphyrin mixture and exposure to red light,[1–11] are currently being developed.

Figge and co-workers[12] appear to be the first to have mentioned the potential of cancer therapy with porphyrins and metalloporphyrins. In 1960, Lipson[13–15] enhanced the localization properties of porphyrins in tumors by the synthesis of a hematoporphyrin derivative (HpD). The introduction of lasers to the market in the 1970s gave a new boost to photodynamic therapy, when Dougherty,[16] Dia-

Ferguson MK, Little AG, Skinner DB: Diseases of the Esophagus, Vol. I: Malignant Diseases. Futura Publishing Company, Inc., Mount Kisco, NY, © 1990.

mond,[17] and Kelly and Snell[18] reported on the use of a combination of HpD and light for selective tumor destruction.

Since the early 1980s, PDT has been used in clinical experiments as a new treatment modality against cancer. For ethical reasons, present clinical investigations deal only with severe obstructing tumors of the esophagus and bronchi. The main relevance for the use of PDT, however, is not as a palliative treatment in end-stage disease. Its final goal is aimed at the selective and curative endoscopic treatment of early carcinomas, particularly in the aerodigestive tract. ENT cancer patients, suffering from a symptomatic primary cancer, often present with synchronous second primaries in the pharynx, esophagus, or bronchi. These second primaries, detected during the systematic pretherapeutic endoscopy, are staged as early cancers (in situ, microinvasive, or submucosal carcinomas) in about 90% of the cases.[19] Conventional invasive treatments (surgery, chemotherapy, radiotherapy) applied simultaneously to the primary and second primary tumors often lead to high morbidity and mortality in these patients, due to a poor general condition. In this regard, ENT cancer patients are an ideal group to test the full potentiality of PDT in early cancers.

Materials and Methods

In this study, the main symptomatic ENT cancer governing the overall oncological prognosis was treated by conventional means. Early second primary cancers were treated by PDT only. All patients were volunteers, older than 40 years of age, and gave their written informed consent before receiving the HpD injection. We used a HpD, manufactured by Ciba-Geigy, Switzerland, chromatographically comparable to Photofrin I. It was administered intravenously slowly over 1 hour at a dose of 3 mg/kg body weight in a 500 cc saline solution. PDT was carried out 72 hours after the HpD injection. An argon pumped dye laser supplied the red light energy at 630 nm. The radiation dose (50 mW to 120 mW/cm^2 during 20 minutes) was between 60 and 150 joules/cm^2.

Homogenous light distribution at the tumor site was a main concern to us. The Swiss Institute of Physics in Lausanne manufactured red light diffusing cylinders allowing homogenous light distribution over the entire irradiation surface (Fig. 1a,b). At first, we used a 360° window for circular irradiation. However, the lack of selectivity of HpD induced circular necrosis and subsequent strictures. Following

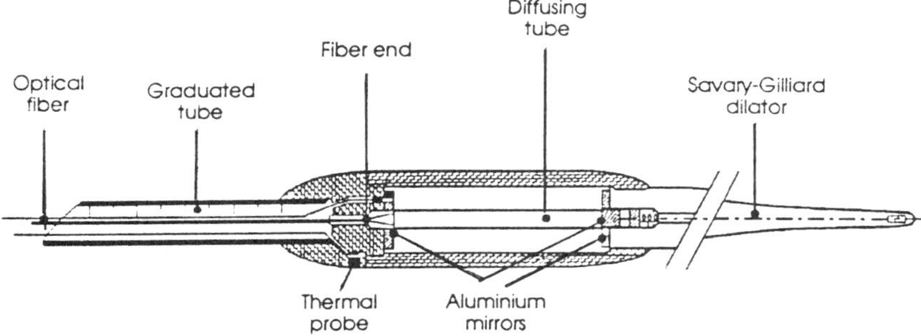

Figure 1a: Light-diffusing cylinder for pharyngeal and esophageal PDT. A diagram showing the cylinder fixed on a Savary-Gilliard dilation bougie, which facilitates its insertion into the esophagus. The light-scattering medium is made of a transparent elastomer loaded with varying concentrations of titanium oxide particles to obtain an homogenous light distribution over the whole length of the cylinder.

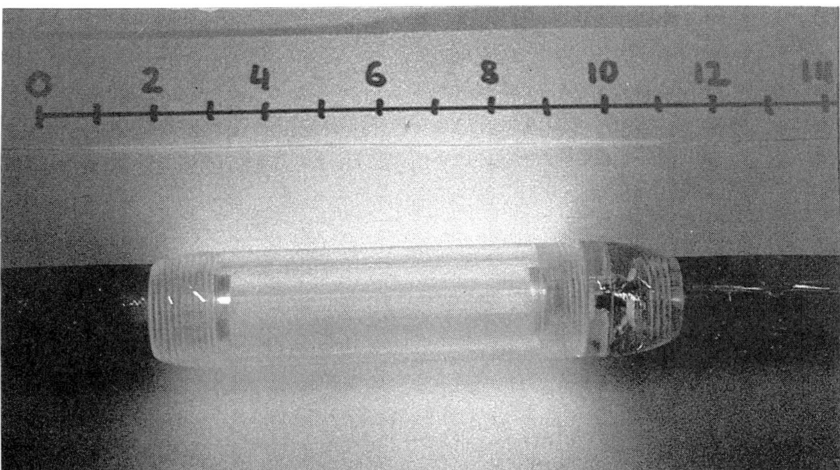

Figure 1b: Light-diffusing cylinder for pharyngeal and esophageal PDT. Detail of the red light distribution for a 3.5–cm-long cylinder. Several different cylinders have been manufactured, the outer diameter varying from 15 to 20 mm and the length from 3.5 to 7 cm.

Table I
Pretherapy Staging of Early Pharyngo-Esophageal Carcinomas: Prospective Study of 50 Cases

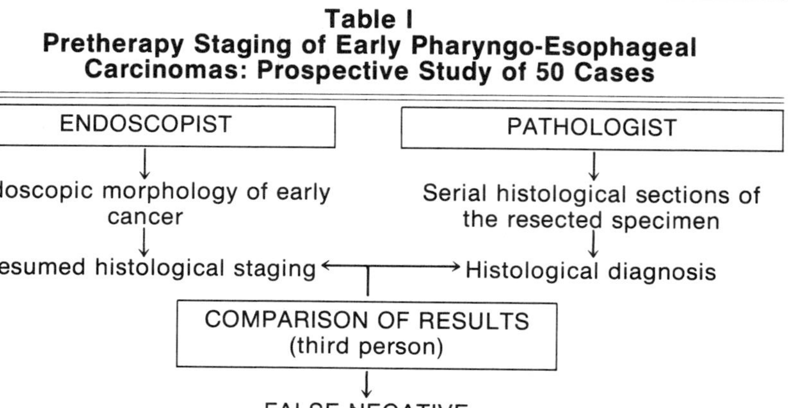

this observation, we used only semi-circular (180° window) cylinders of varying lengths, according to the extent of the early carcinoma to be treated.

The pretherapy staging of early carcinomas was based on biopsy, cytology, and endoscopic morphologic criteria for the extent of parietal carcinomatous invasion.[20,21] In a prospective study on 50 cases,[22] the author established a visual staging of early carcinomas. The lesions were resected in toto and submitted to serial histologic sections, the pathologist being unaware of the endoscopic staging. Endoscopic and histologic stagings were compared by a third person. Taking into account the false negative results (underestimation of an early carcinoma), the error by endoscopic visual staging was only 4% (Table I). According to this endoscopic staging, we have treated 25 "early" carcinomas: 10 in the pharynx and 15 in the esophagus (Table II).

Treatment evaluation was based on the following information: 6/10 early pharyngeal and 2/15 early esophageal carcinomas were resected 10 days (four pharyngeal lesions) and 3 months after PDT (two pharyngeal and two esophageal lesions). These specimens were submitted to serial histologic sections, and treatment was considered curative if no residual tumor could be found in the specimen. In the remaining 17 cases (4 pharyngeal, 13 esophageal carcinomas), no re-

Table II
PDT of 25 Early Pharyngo-Esophageal Carcinomas

Endoscopic Staging	
Carcinoma in situ	5
Microinvasive carcinoma	14
Submucosal carcinoma	6
Total	25

section was carried out. Follow-up endoscopies were routinely done at 10 days, 3 months, and subsequently every 6 months with systematic biopsies and brushings for cytology taken. Patients were considered disease-cured if endoscopy, biopsies, and brushings for cytology were all negative.

To assess the selectivity of tumor necrosis by PDT, a control zone of 1 cm^2 normal buccal mucosa was irradiated at the same light dose as the early pharyngeal or esophageal cancer. We used either a cylinder with a 1 cm^2 square-window or a frontal irradiator (spot size 1 cm^2). The radiation dose varied from 50 mW/cm^2 to 200 mW/cm^2 for 20 minutes (60 to 240 $joules/cm^2$). Our hope was to establish a therapeutic ratio showing necrosis at the tumor site and none on the normal buccal mucosa. A control group of 10 patients who did not receive HpD were also irradiated at a light dose of 240 $joules/cm^2$ to ensure that necrosis was not caused by a thermal effect (Table III).

Results

Following PDT, all tumors showed necrosis, the selectivity of which was far from being optimal (Fig. 2a–c). This clinical impression was confirmed by the results obtained from normal buccal mucosa irradiation. Four days after PDT, all 25 patients showed necrosis at the irradiation site, even with light doses as low as 60 $joules/cm^2$ (Fig. 3a,b). In contrast, no lesion was found in the control group without HpD at a light dose of 240 $joules/cm^2$. This is clear evidence that thermal effects did not play a role in the induction of necrosis in patients receiving HpD.

The overall results are displayed in Table IV. When analyzing

Table III
Red Light (630 nm) Irradiation of Normal Buccal Mucosa (spot size 1 cm²)

No. of Patients	*Experimental Conditions*	*Light Dose*	*Results (4 days post-PDT)*
25	72 hours post-HpD injection	60 J–240 J/cm²	25 necrosis
10	without HpD	240 J/cm²	0 necrosis

these data, one has to remember that a long follow-up is necessary to assess whether an in situ carcinoma is cured. The results may be considered satisfactory for in situ and microinvasive carcinomas. Further studies need to be carried out to evaluate PDT for submucosal carcinomas. In the pharynx, three out of four nonresected early cancers did not recur after 58, 26, and 26 months, respectively. One recurrence (positive biopsy) was detected 6 months following PDT. Among the six resected specimens, two showed residual tumor at the borders or at the base of the necrosis, 10 days post-PDT. It was not possible, however, to assess histologically whether these residual cancerous cells were viable or not. In the esophagus, 3/15 early carcinomas recurred, two of which had been staged submucosal at endoscopy. Considering the short time elapsed between PDT and recurrence, these two cases were probably underestimated as far as their parietal invasion was concerned. Ten patients are disease-free 6 to 58 months following PDT (mean, 19.9 months).

We encountered three severe complications: one esophageal stricture and two esophageal fistulae. The esophageal stricture was induced by a circular necrosis when still using 360° irradiation cylinders at the beginning of our study. It was successfully treated by dilation. Esophageal fistulae were due to overtreatment with light doses exceeding 200 joules/cm². One of these two patients died. The death rate was 1/25 (4%).

Discussion

According to our experience, the tumor selectivity of HpD (Photofrin II as well as Photofrin I) is very poor in the digestive tract lined with squamous cell epithelium. Light dosimetry is often inaccurate

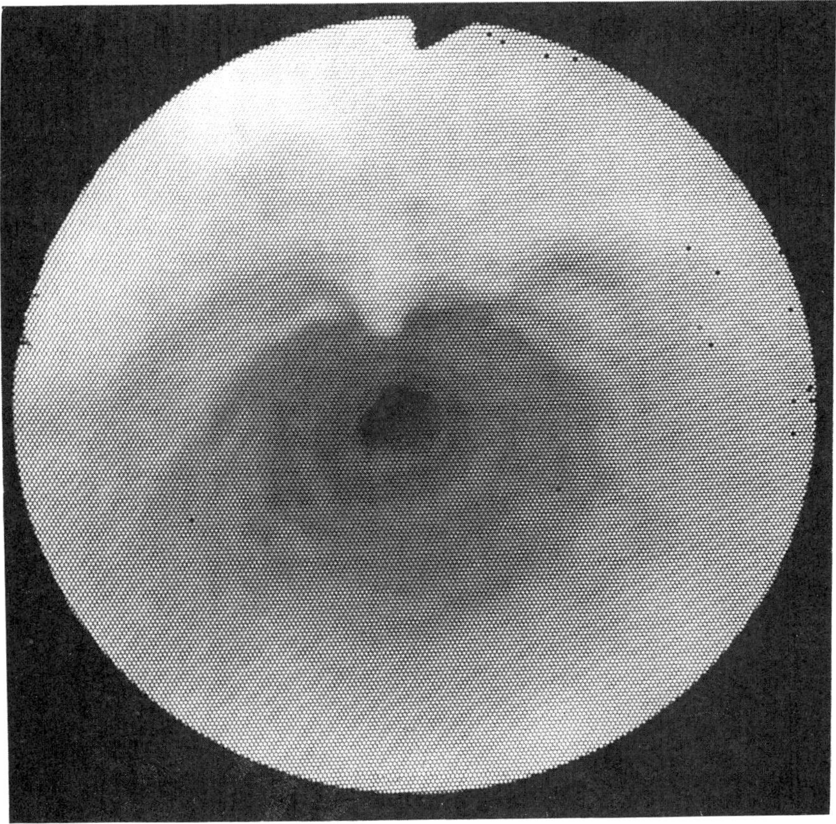

Figure 2a: Submucosal squamous cell carcinoma of the esophagus in an ENT cancer patient presenting with four other synchronous cancers. Pretherapy endoscopic view. The slightly exophytic and infiltrating lesion is located on the anterior wall of the cervical esophagus. It was staged submucosal at endoscopy.

when the tumor is irradiated with a fiber passed through the biopsy channel of an endoscope.[23–25] Considering that light intensity varies as the square of the distance, one clearly understands that without a light-diffusing cylinder closely applied to the esophageal mucosa, light dosimetry is merely speculative. Furthermore, directing the red light towards the tumor only induces pseudoselectivity, since normal surrounding tissues only are less irradiated. At follow-up endoscopy, one may have a false impression of a selective necrosis.

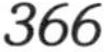

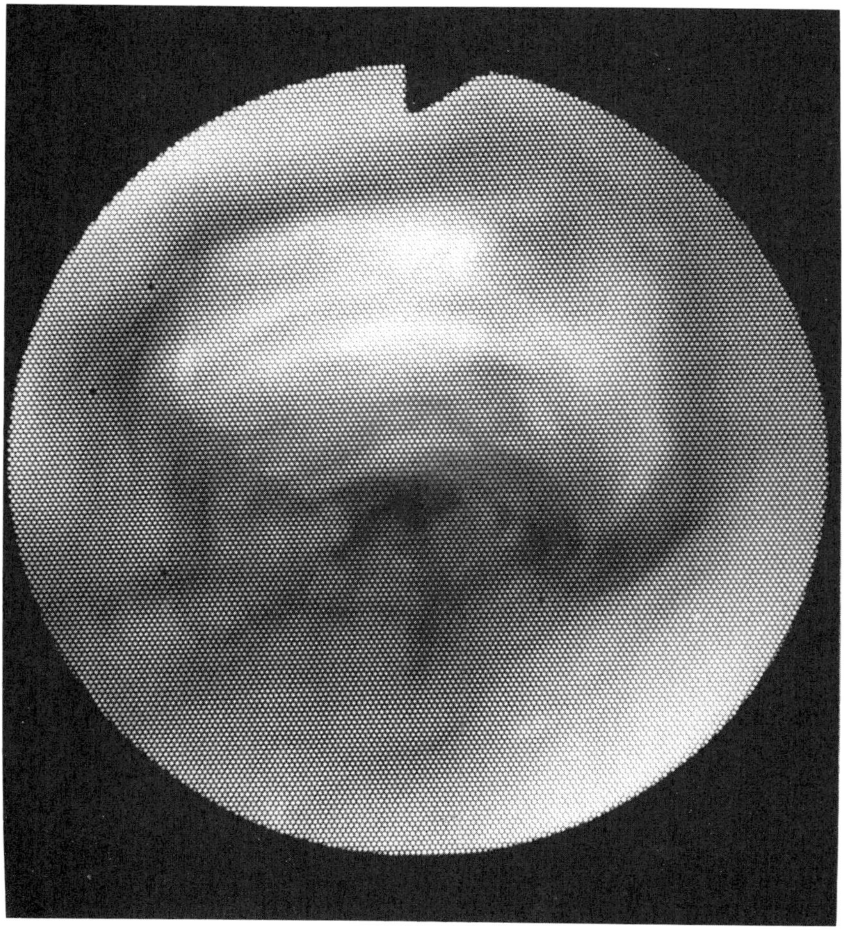

Figure 2b: Same patient as in Figure 2a. Endoscopy 10 days post-PDT (120 joules/cm^2). The necrosis is not limited to the tumor but shows the exact rectangular shape of the irradiation window of the cylinder.

Two major problems remain: the capability of precisely measuring the in-depth parietal extent of early cancers, and the lack of selectivity of the photosensitizing agent (HpD). At the present time, neither computed tomography nor endoscopic ultrasonography are able to differentiate an intramucosal from a submucosal carcinoma. In the near future, this problem will certainly be solved.

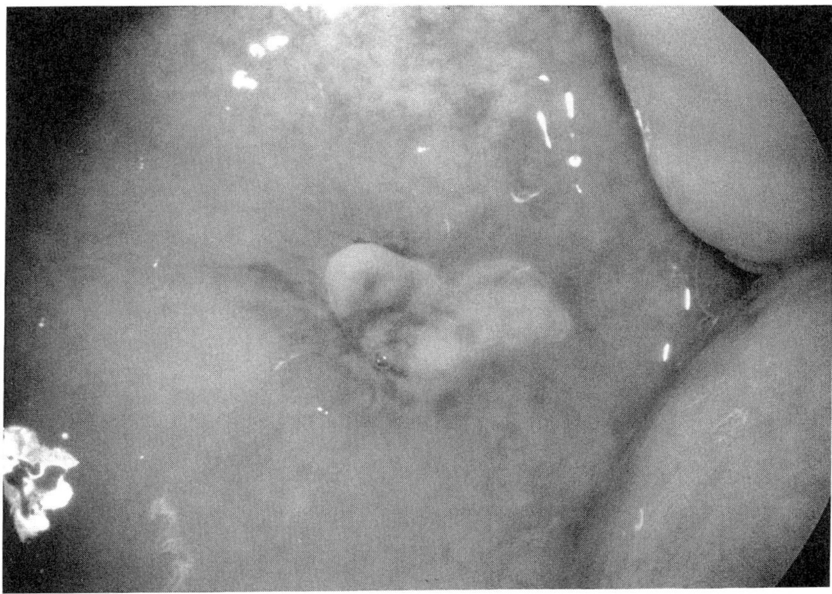

Figure 2c: Same patient as in Figures 2a and b. Resected specimen 3 months post-PDT. No residual tumor could be found on serial histologic sections. The muscularis mucosa and submucosa have been replaced by dense scar tissue, while the muscularis propria is preserved.

For the past 10 years, a tremendous amount of information has been accumulated on porphyrins, but little progress has been achieved in tumor selectivity. Dihematoporphyrin ether or ester (DHE) is probably the substance mainly responsible for the photosensitizing activity of the HpD mixture. However, in our clinical experiments, DHE also induced necrosis of normal buccal mucosa at a light dose of only 60 joules/cm^2. Further reducing the light dose would lead to insufficient irradiation to induce complete tumor necrosis. Two of our early carcinomas, showing residual tumor at the base of the necrosis on the resected specimen, had received a light dose of 100 joules/cm^2.

Conclusions

PDT is efficient at destroying in situ and microinvasive carcinomas of the pharynx and esophagus, but the selectivity of HpD is

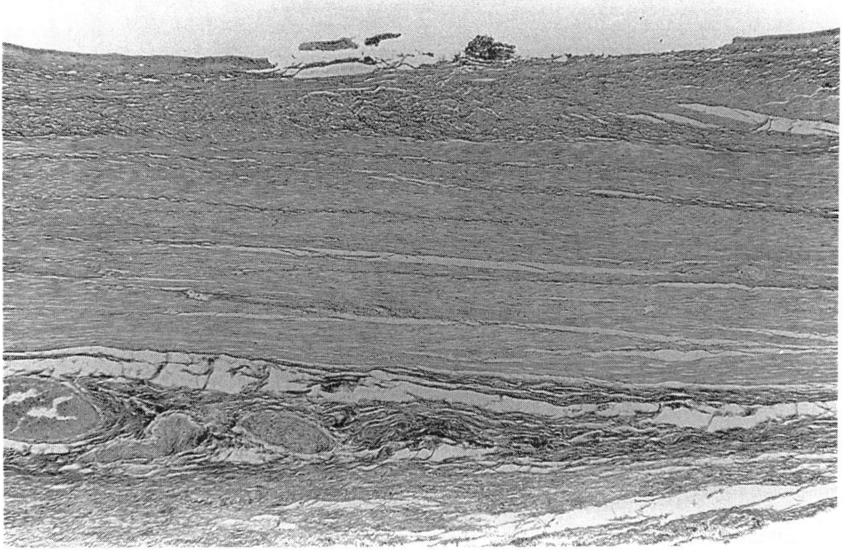

Figure 3a: Irradiation zone of a normal buccal mucosa 72 hours after HpD injection. Experimental conditions. The spot size (1 cm^2) and distance from the tip of the fiber to the mucosal surface are precisely measured with a caliper rule. In this case, the light dose was 80 mW/cm^2 for 20 minutes = 100 joules/ cm^2.

not sufficient. With light-diffusing cylinders, the problem of a homogenous light distribution in the esophagus is solved. At the present time, early cancers can only be treated using a fenestrated irradiating cylinder to avoid circular necrosis and subsequent stenosis in the esophagus or the pharynx. The lack of selectivity of HpD is also responsible for the high rate (12%) of complications encountered in our series. The only hope for the future lies in the synthesis of a more selective and more stable photosensitizer than HpD. Otherwise, this elegant and promising technique will never be applicable in everyday clinical endoscopy.

AKNOWLEDGMENTS: The authors are grateful to E. Profio, G. Jori, T. Dougherty, W. Potter, A. Oseroff, B. Henderson, J.E. Van Lier, and R. Tyrell for many helpful discussions. We are also grateful to the Swiss Fonds National (PN 18), CIBA-GEIGY, the Swiss Cancer League, the Vaudoise, Valaisanne, and Genevoise Cancer Leagues, the Fondation Dreyfuss (Lausanne), the Fondation E. Muschamp, the Ecole Polytechnique Federale of Lausanne, the University of Lausanne, and the CHUV Hospital for financial support.

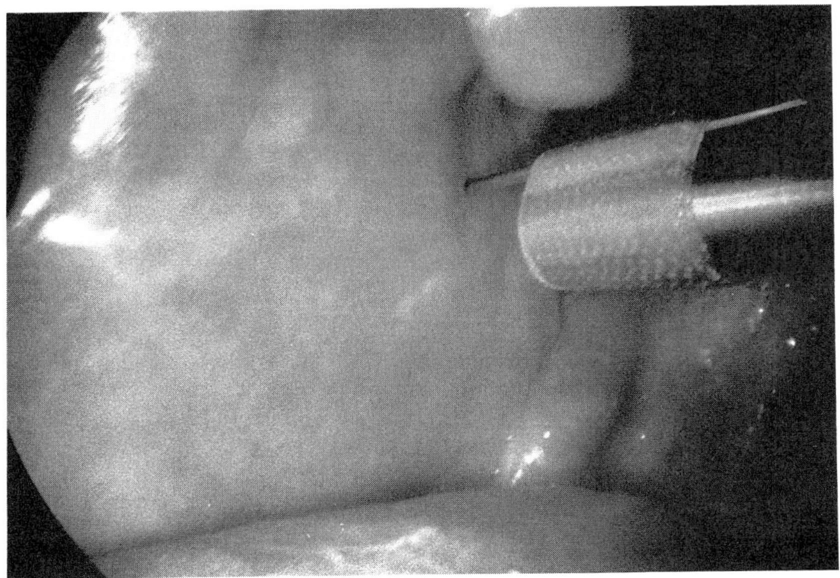

Figure 3b: Result at 4 days post-PDT. Distinct necrosis is present at the site of irradiation. This was observed in all cases, the exudate being slightly less pronounced with low irradiation doses (60 joules/cm^2).

Table IV
PDT of 25 Early Pharyngo-Esophageal Carcinomas: Results versus Staging

	Recurrence			
Site	*Carcinoma in situ*	*Microinvasive Carcinoma*	*Submucosal Carcinoma*	*Total*
Pharynx	0/3	3/7	—	3/10
Esophagus	0/2	1/7	2/6	3/15
Total	0/5	4/14	2/6	6/25

References

1. Dougherty TJ: Photodynamic therapy (PDT) of malignant tumors. Crit Rev Oncol Hematol 2:83, 1984.
2. Kessel D: Hematoporphyrin and HpD: Photophysics, photochemistry and phototherapy. Photochem Photobiol 34:851, 1984.
3. Berenbaum MC, Bonnett R, Scourides PA: In vivo biological activity of the components of haematoporphyrin derivate. Br J Cancer 45:571, 1982.
4. Hayata Y, Kato H, Konaka C, et al: Fiberoptic bronchoscopic photoradiation in experimentally induced canine lung cancer. Cancer 51:50, 1983.
5. Kinsey JH, Cortese DA, Moses HL, et al: Photodynamic effect of hematoporphyrin derivative as a function of optical spectrum and incident energy density. Cancer Res 41:5020, 1981.
6. Mack HP, Diehl WK, Peck GC, et al: Evaluation of the combined effects of hematoporphyrin and radiation. Cancer 10:529, 1957.
7. Moan J, Pettersen EO, Christensen T: The mechanism of photodynamic inactivation of human cells in vitro in the presence of haematoporphyrin. Br J Cancer 39:398, 1979.
8. Wile AG, Dahlman A, Burns RG, et al: Laser photoradiation therapy of cancer following hematoporphyrin sensitization. Laser Surg Med 2:163, 1982.
9. Zalar GL, Poh-Fitxpatrick M, Krohn DL, et al: Induction of drug photosensitization in man after parenteral exposure to hematoporphyrin. Arch Dermatol 113:1392, 1977.
10. Cortese DA, Kinsey JH: Endoscopic management of lung cancer with hematoporphyrin derivative phototherapy. Mayo Clin Proc 57:543, 1982.
11. Jocham D, Staehler G, Chaussy C, et al: Laserbehandlung von Blasentumoren nach photosensibilisierung mit Hamatoporphyrin- Derivat. Urologue A 20:340, 1981.
12. Figge FH, Weiland GS, Manganiello LO: Cancer detection and therapy. Proc Soc Exp Biol Med 68:640, 1948.
13. Lipson RL, Baldes EJ: The photodynamic properties of a particular hematoporphyrin derivate. Arch Dermatol 82:508, 1960.
14. Lipson RL, Baldes EJ, Olsen AM: The use of a derivative of hematoporphyrin in tumor detection. J Natl Cancer Inst 26:1, 1961.
15. Lipson RL, Baldes EJ, Gray MJ: Hematoporphyrin derivative for detection and management of cancer. Cancer 20:2255, 1967.
16. Doughtery TJ: Activated dyes as antitumor agents. J Natl Cancer Inst 52:1333, 1974.
17. Diamond I, Granelli SG, McDonagh AF, et al: Photodynamic therapy of malignant tumors. Lancet 2:1175, 1972.
18. Kelly JF, Snell ME, Berenbaum MC: Photodynamic destruction of human bladder carcinoma. Br J Cancer 31:237, 1975.
19. Monnier P, Savary M, Anani P: Endoscopic morphology of "early" esophageal carcinoma. In: Esophageal Disorders. DeMeester TR, Skinner DB (eds), New York, Raven Press, 1985, p 333.
20. Mandard AM, Tourneux J, Gignoux M, et al: In situ carcinoma of the esophagus: Macroscopic study with particular reference to the Lugol test. Endoscopy 12:51, 1980.

21. Monnier P, Savary M, Pasche R, et al: Intraepithelial carcinoma of the esophagus: Endoscopic morphology. Endoscopy 13:85, 1981.
22. Pasche P: Le staging endoscopique du cancer precoce pour la voie digestive superieure. ORL 12, Bern, Hans Huber Verlag, 1988, p 131.
23. Kato H, Kawagushi M, Konaka C, et al: Evolution of photodynamic therapy in gastric cancer. Lasers Med Sci 1:67, 1986.
24. Konaka C, Kato H, Hayata Y: Lung cancer treated by photodynamic therapy alone. Lasers Med Sci 2:17, 1987.
25. Gluckman JL, Weissler MC: Role of photodynamic therapy in the management of early cancers of the upper aerodigestive tract. Lasers Med Sci 1:217, 1986.

43

Management of Esophageal Carcinoma with Respiratory Tract Fistula

Alberto Peracchia, Andrea Segalin, Romeo Bardini, Alberto Ruol, Carlo Castoro, Carlo Tremolada

Introduction

The development of a fistula between the esophagus and the respiratory tract (RTF) is one of the most severe complications of esophageal carcinoma.[1] Its incidence ranges between 5% and 10% of all patients with esophageal carcinoma.[2,3] In these patients, the continued aspiration of food, saliva, and refluxed gastric contents results in coughing and rapid development of pulmonary infections, with a major influence on the quality and the length of survival.

The management of malignant RTF is not yet determined. Attempts at curative resection have been reported with a prohibitively high operative mortality rate and poor long-term results,[4] so that few surgeons would advocate such an approach today. In these patients, the main goal of treatment is represented by palliation, which should relieve dysphagia and protect the respiratory tract from continued contamination with saliva and food.

In order to define the best palliative approach, we have reviewed our experience with malignant RTF in a series of 1,338 unselected patients with esophageal carcinoma observed between 1980 and 1987.

Ferguson MK, Little AG, Skinner DB: Diseases of the Esophagus, Vol. I: Malignant Diseases. Futura Publishing Company, Inc., Mount Kisco, NY, © 1990.

Patients and Methods

Between 1980 and 1987, 1338 unselected patients with esophageal carcinoma were admitted to the 1st Department of Surgery of the University of Padova. Patients with adenocarcinoma of the cardia were excluded from this study. A prospective computerized data collection was performed and data on age, sex, general condition, concomitant diseases, preoperative evaluation, site and stage of the tumor, type and intent of the treatment, and postoperative morbidity and mortality were specifically sought in each instance. Clinical and pathological staging was performed according to the most recent TNM guidelines.[5] Most patients were followed-up in the clinics and a complete follow-up to December 1988 was available in almost all cases.

A malignant respiratory tract fistula was observed in 57 patients (4.2%). The mean age was 58.2 years (range 26–84); 47 were male and 10 were female. The tumor was located in the cervical, upper thoracic, and middle thoracic esophagus in 9, 19, and 29 patients, respectively. The RTF was evident at initial presentaton of the esophageal carcinoma in 45 cases (78.9%), and developed after chemotherapy in four, after radiotherapy in three, after endoscopic Nd:YAG laser therapy in three, and after pulsion intubation in two cases. The trachea was involved in 28 patients (49.2%), the left main bronchus in 26 (45.6%), and the right bronchus in three (5.2%). The diagnosis of a malignant RTF was made by means of esophagogram with water-soluble contrast and/or endoscopy. An esophagogram was performed in 49 patients and showed an RTF in 47 cases (95.9%). Esophagoscopy in 40 patients showed an RTF in 24 cases (60.0%). Bronchoscopy in 45 patients showed tracheobronchial invasion or impingement in all, and fistulization in 18 (40.0%). Distant metastases were detected in nine patients (15.7%).

A bypass procedure was performed in 12 patients, 26 patients underwent intubation, six patients received a feeding gastrostomy, and four a nasogastric tube. Finally, in nine cases only medical supportive treatment was performed (Table I).

The quality of palliation was evaluated according to the patient's ability to swallow and to the control of respiratory aspiration, and was scored as follows: good – general diet with occasional dysphagia and good control of respiratory symptoms; fair – only able to swallow semi-liquids with occasonal respiratory symptoms; poor – severe and/or total dysphagia and no improvement in respiratory symptoms.[1,3]

Table I
Treatments of Esophageal RTF

Treatment	*Patients*	*Mortality*	*Mean (days) Hospitalization*	*Palliation* Good	Fair	Poor	*Median (mo.) Survival*
Bypass	12	1 (8.3%)	20.6	11	—	—	6
Intubation	26	2 (7.6%)	7.1	—	17	7	2
Gastrostomy	6	2 (33.3%)	8.3	—	—	4	1
Nothing/NGT	13	5 (38.4%)	3.7	—	—	8	1

NGT = nasogastric tube

Results

Bypass Procedures

The mean age of the 12 patients who underwent a bypass procedure was 52.5 years. Distant metastases were detected in only one patient. A retrosternal esophagogastrostomy was the procedure of choice in all cases. In eight patients, the whole stomach was transposed to the neck and the distal esophagus was decompressed by means of a Roux-en-Y esophagojejunostomy as originally proposed by Kirschner.[6] In four patients, an isoperistaltic gastric tube formed from the greater curvature, according to the Postlethwait technique, was used.[7] There were five anastomotic leaks (41.6%), two in the patients who were treated with the Kirschner procedure and three in the patients in whom the Postlethwait technique was used.

Three anastomotic leaks were successfully treated with antibiotics and hypercaloric parenteral nutrition. The other two cases required one and three reoperations, respectively. One patient underwent splenectomy for bleeding 3 days after the bypass procedure. The hospital mortality was 8.3%, consisting of a single patient in whom redo surgery failed to fix the leak, and who died in the hospital 70 days after the first procedure. The hospitalization time ranged from 14 to 62 days, with an average of 20.6 and a median of 15 days. All of the 11 operative survivors were discharged on a general diet and without respiratory symptoms. The mean survival of the patients who died during the follow-up was 7.3 months, and three patients are still alive at 2, 7, and 18 months after surgery. The quality of the palliation was evaluated in seven patients between 2 and 17 months after surgery and was excellent or good in all. Overall, four patients lived more than 10 months.

Intubation

The mean age of the 26 patients who underwent intubation was 58.4 years. Distant metastases were detected in five patients. Twenty-three patients underwent pulsion intubation with local pharyngeal anesthesia and intravenous premedication. The tumor was dilated by means of the Savary or American Endoscopy dilators and the tube was positioned by means of the Savary or Nottingham devices. Three other patients underwent traction intubation; in two cases the surgical approach was deemed necessary due to a previous unsuccessful attempt at pulsion intubation. After intubation, an esophagogram was always performed to assess the correct positioning of the tube and the exclusion of the fistula. In five and three patients, respectively, the tube dislocated or failed to control the respiratory symptoms. In two patients, the tube was endoscopically replaced, while it was removed and a feeding gastrostomy or a nasogastric tube were placed in one and three cases, respectively. One additional patient had an aspiration pneumonia which was successfully managed with medical treatment. Two patients died 17 and 7 days after intubation, one because of neoplastic cachexia and the other because of a massive bleeding from an aorto-esophageal fistulization. The mean and the median hospitalization time was 7.1 and 3 days, respectively. Seventeen patients were discharged on a liquid diet, experiencing only occasional respiratory symptoms. The mean survival was 2.8 months, and only four patients lived more than 6 months.

Feeding Gastrostomy

In six patients with a carcinoma of the cervical esophagus, a feeding gastrostomy was performed. In these patients, esophageal intubation was not possible. All these cases were in terminal or pre-terminal condition. Two patients died in the hospital from neoplastic cachexia and respiratory complications. The mean survival of the four patients, who were discharged on an average of 7 days after the procedure, was 1 month. No patient experienced a good or fair palliation.

Nasogastric Tube versus Nothing

In four patients, it was only possible to place a nasogastric tube and in nine more cases only medical supportive treatment was provided. These patients were in extremely poor general condition, and in three instances the tumor was located in the cervical esophagus. Five patients died in the hospital of pneumonia, generalized disease, and neoplastic cachexia; all the others died shortly after hospital discharge after 1 month on average. No palliation was achieved in these patients.

Discussion

The development of a malignant RTF has a major influence on the survival of patients with esophageal carcinoma. Moreover, the quality of the remaining life is strongly impaired by this devastating complication. The selection of appropriate palliative therapy is difficult since it involves both the choice of the best therapeutic procedure and the assessment of the patient's ability to withstand that procedure. The choices are few and the general condition of the patient and the preference of the surgeon should determine the procedure to be performed.

From a theoretical point of view, the best palliation can be achieved only by means of the exclusion of the esophagus with the RTF, and restoring upper digestive tract continuity with an esophageal bypass. Either the stomach or colon can be placed in the substernal position with the anastomosis performed in the neck. Interposition of the colon, necessitating several anastomoses, entails extremely high morbidity and mortality rates in patients with advanced malignant disease.[8] In our opinion, a patient with RTF in whom the stomach is not available should not be considered a candidate for a bypass procedure.

Several techniques using the stomach have been reported. Among these, the procedures using the whole stomach were used in the last years with higher success rates.[9–11] In our experience, a higher incidence of cervical anastomotic leaks was found in patients in whom we used an isoperistaltic gastric tube created from the greater curvature, according to Postlethwait's technique. On the contrary, the Kirschner operation was a safer procedure, which was mainly due to the effect that the vascular supply of the whole stomach was better than that of a small tube from the greater curvature. For this reason, we are performing only this operation when an esophageal bypass is needed.

To avoid the risk of a distal esophageal disruption which is reported to occur in patients in whom the distal esophagus is closed,[12] we have always drained the distal esophagus by means of an esophagojejunostomy, as originally described by Kirschner.[6] In disagreement with Roeher,[13] no complications were related to the distal esophageal anastomosis. We believe that performing a stapled end-to-side esophagojejeunostomy takes only a few minutes and has no influence on the morbidity or mortality of the procedure.

The bypass procedure still remains a major operation with the highest operative mortality rates of all palliative procedures performed for esophageal carcinoma, ranging from 24.0% to 41.5%.[11] On the other hand, the quality of palliation of survivors is good and the survival is similar to that achieved in patients undergoing palliative resections.[14,15] In our series, a gastric bypass was performed only in selected favorable-risk patients, with overall morbidity and mortality rates of 50% (6/12) and 8.3% (1/12), respectively. All operative survivors could eat a normal diet until death. Careful selection of these patients is mandatory in planning a bypass procedure in order to keep operative morbidity and mortality rates within acceptable levels. The main requisites are a relatively good general condition, no clinical signs of respiratory infection, and no distant metastases.

Intubation generally provides fair or poor palliation for this devastating complication, since the fistula is frequently not totally occluded and only a soft or liquid diet is allowed. On the other hand, using the pulsion technique, this procedure can be performed in high-risk patients, under local anesthesia with a very short hospitalization or on an outpatient basis.

In our series, the overall morbidity and mortality rates were 30.7% (8/26) and 7.6% (2/26), respectively. These results were satisfactory since major surgery was contraindicated in almost all of these patients. On the other hand, only 17 patients (70.8%) were discharged on a soft diet and with a fair control of the respiratory symptoms. Pulsion intubation is a simple method to restore a partial ability to swallow and to control respiratory symptoms in patients who are not candidates for a bypass procedure. The introduction of new cuffed tubes, specifically created for being used in presence of RTF, could perhaps improve the results of intubation.[16]

Feeding gastrostomy or jejunostomy were used in patients with a tumor of the cervical esophagus and an RTF involving the trachea. In all of these cases, the location of the tumor did not allow either the exclusion of the cervical esophagus by means of a cervical esophagostomy or intubation. As previously reported,[1] these procedures allow nutritional replenishment but they do not improve the quality of life of the patient. In fact, most of these patients died in the immediate postoperative period of pulmonary complications. Similarly, some terminal or pre-terminal patients with small fistulas can be managed for the short period of their remaining lives by using a nasogastric tube, but in none of these patients can a real palliation be achieved.

Conclusions

A malignant fistula between the esophagus and the tracheobronchial tree is relatively frequent and has a major influence on the survival of patients with esophageal cancer. If the fistula is effectively controlled, most of the patients can expect the same survival of those undergoing palliative resection. All of the therapeutic possibilities should be considered and tailored to the individual patient to offer the best quality of life with the lowest morbidity and mortality rates. A bypass procedure offers the most effective palliation in selected good-risk patients. Whenever a major operative procedure is contraindicated by poor general condition, concomitant diseases, and/or respiratory infection, pulsion intubation should be considered.

References

1. Little AG, Ferguson MK, DeMeester TR, et al: Esophageal carcinoma with respiratory tract fistula. Cancer 53:1322, 1984.
2. Martini N, Goodner JT, D'Angio GJ, et al: Tracheoesophageal fistula due to cancer. J Thorac Cardiovasc Surg 59:319, 1970.
3. Duranceau A, Jamieson GG: Malignant tracheoesophageal fistula. Ann Thorac Surg 37:346, 1984.
4. Ong GB, Kwong KH: Management of malignant esophagobronchial fistula. Surgery 67:293, 1970.
5. TNM Classification of malignant tumours. 4th edition UICC. Springer-Verlag, Berlin, 1987.
6. Kirschner MB: Ein neues verfahren der oesophagoplastik. Arch Klin Chir 114:606, 1920.
7. Postlethwait RW: Technique for isoperistaltic gastric tube for esophageal bypass. Ann Surg 187:673, 1979.

8. Orel J, Vidmar S, Hrabar B: Intrathoracic gastriic and jejunal bypass for palliation of nonresectable carcinoma of the esophagus and gastroesophageal junction. In: Diseases of the Esophagus, Siewert JR, Holscher H (eds), Springer-Verlag, Berlin, 1988, pp 758–761.
9. Sugimachi K, Hiroaki U, Hidenobu K, et al: Problems in esophageal bypass for unresectable carcinoma of the thoracic esophagus. J Thorac Cardiovasc Surg 84:62, 1982.
10. Akiyama H, Hiyama M: A simple esophageal bypass operation by the high gastric division. Surgery 75:674, 1974.
11. Wong, J. Lam KH, Wei WI, et al: Results of the Kirschner operation. World J Surg 5:547, 1981.
12. Orringer MB: Substernal gastric bypass of the excluded esophagus: Results of an ill-advised operation. Surgery 96:467, 1984.
13. Roeher HD, Horeyseck G: The Kirschner bypass operations: A palliation for complicated esophageal carcinoma. World J Surg 5:543, 1981.
14. Segalin A, Little AG, Ruol A, et al: Surgical and endoscopic palliation of esophageal carcinoma. Ann Thorac Surg 48:267, 1989.
15. Peracchia A, Bardini R, Ruol A, Segalin A, Castoro C: Palliative surgery for inoperable esophageal carcinoma. Lectures and Symposia of the 14th International Cancer Congress of the UICC, Oncological Surgery, Vol. 7, Lapis K, Eckhardt S (Eds), Akademiai Kaido, Budapest, 1987, pp 35–40.
16. Irving JD, Simson JNL: A new cuffed oesophageal prosthesis for the management of malignant oesophago-respiratory fistula. Ann R Coll Surg Engl 70:13, 1988.

Index